Frontiers in Anti-Infective Agents

(Volume 5)

Edited by

Parvesh Singh
School of Chemistry and Physics
University of Kwa-Zulu Natal (UKZN)
Westville campus, Durban
South Africa

Vipan Kumar
Department of Chemistry
Guru Nanak Dev University
Amritsar
India

&

Rajshekhar Karpoormath
Department of Pharmaceutical Chemistry
University of Kwa-Zulu Natal (UKZN)
Westville Campus, Durban
South Africa

Frontiers in Anti-Infective Agents

Volume # 5

Editors: Parvesh Singh, Vipan Kumar & Rajshekhar Karpoormath

ISSN (Online): 2705-1080

ISSN (Print): 2705-1072

ISBN (Online): 978-981-4998-39-0

ISBN (Print): 978-981-4998-40-6

ISBN (Paperback): 978-981-4998-41-3

©2021, Bentham Books imprint.

Published by Bentham Science Publishers Pte. Ltd. Singapore. All Rights Reserved.

BENTHAM SCIENCE PUBLISHERS LTD.
End User License Agreement (for non-institutional, personal use)

This is an agreement between you and Bentham Science Publishers Ltd. Please read this License Agreement carefully before using the ebook/echapter/ejournal (**"Work"**). Your use of the Work constitutes your agreement to the terms and conditions set forth in this License Agreement. If you do not agree to these terms and conditions then you should not use the Work.

Bentham Science Publishers agrees to grant you a non-exclusive, non-transferable limited license to use the Work subject to and in accordance with the following terms and conditions. This License Agreement is for non-library, personal use only. For a library / institutional / multi user license in respect of the Work, please contact: permission@benthamscience.net.

Usage Rules:

1. All rights reserved: The Work is the subject of copyright and Bentham Science Publishers either owns the Work (and the copyright in it) or is licensed to distribute the Work. You shall not copy, reproduce, modify, remove, delete, augment, add to, publish, transmit, sell, resell, create derivative works from, or in any way exploit the Work or make the Work available for others to do any of the same, in any form or by any means, in whole or in part, in each case without the prior written permission of Bentham Science Publishers, unless stated otherwise in this License Agreement.
2. You may download a copy of the Work on one occasion to one personal computer (including tablet, laptop, desktop, or other such devices). You may make one back-up copy of the Work to avoid losing it.
3. The unauthorised use or distribution of copyrighted or other proprietary content is illegal and could subject you to liability for substantial money damages. You will be liable for any damage resulting from your misuse of the Work or any violation of this License Agreement, including any infringement by you of copyrights or proprietary rights.

Disclaimer:

Bentham Science Publishers does not guarantee that the information in the Work is error-free, or warrant that it will meet your requirements or that access to the Work will be uninterrupted or error-free. The Work is provided "as is" without warranty of any kind, either express or implied or statutory, including, without limitation, implied warranties of merchantability and fitness for a particular purpose. The entire risk as to the results and performance of the Work is assumed by you. No responsibility is assumed by Bentham Science Publishers, its staff, editors and/or authors for any injury and/or damage to persons or property as a matter of products liability, negligence or otherwise, or from any use or operation of any methods, products instruction, advertisements or ideas contained in the Work.

Limitation of Liability:

In no event will Bentham Science Publishers, its staff, editors and/or authors, be liable for any damages, including, without limitation, special, incidental and/or consequential damages and/or damages for lost data and/or profits arising out of (whether directly or indirectly) the use or inability to use the Work. The entire liability of Bentham Science Publishers shall be limited to the amount actually paid by you for the Work.

General:

1. Any dispute or claim arising out of or in connection with this License Agreement or the Work (including non-contractual disputes or claims) will be governed by and construed in accordance with the laws of Singapore. Each party agrees that the courts of the state of Singapore shall have exclusive jurisdiction to settle any dispute or claim arising out of or in connection with this License Agreement or the Work (including non-contractual disputes or claims).
2. Your rights under this License Agreement will automatically terminate without notice and without the

need for a court order if at any point you breach any terms of this License Agreement. In no event will any delay or failure by Bentham Science Publishers in enforcing your compliance with this License Agreement constitute a waiver of any of its rights.
3. You acknowledge that you have read this License Agreement, and agree to be bound by its terms and conditions. To the extent that any other terms and conditions presented on any website of Bentham Science Publishers conflict with, or are inconsistent with, the terms and conditions set out in this License Agreement, you acknowledge that the terms and conditions set out in this License Agreement shall prevail.

Bentham Science Publishers Pte. Ltd.
80 Robinson Road #02-00
Singapore 068898
Singapore
Email: subscriptions@benthamscience.net

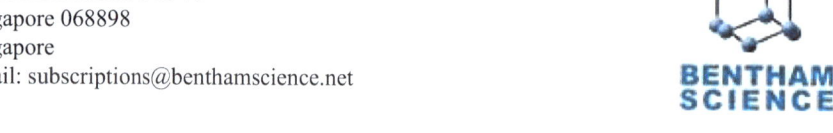

CONTENTS

PREFACE	i
LIST OF CONTRIBUTORS	iii
CHAPTER 1 ANTI-INFECTIVE AGENTS IN OCULAR TREATMENT AND NEW APPROACHES	1
Meltem Ezgi Durgun, Sevgi Güngör and *Yıldız Özsoy*	
INTRODUCTION	1
ANATOMY, PHYSIOLOGY, AND PHARMACOKINETIC OF EYE	3
OCULAR İNFECTİONS	4
Keratitis	4
Conjunctivitis	4
Endophthalmitis	5
Uveitis	6
Scleritis	7
ANTI-INFECTIVE AGENTS USED IN OCULAR TREATMENT	8
OCULAR DRUG DELIVERY SYSTEMS	9
Microparticles and Nanoparticles	9
Solid Lipid Microparticles and Nanoparticles	11
Microemulsions and Nanoemulsions	12
Nanosuspensions	13
Micelles	14
Liposomes	15
Niosomes	17
Spanlastics	17
Bilosomes	18
Cubosomes	18
Dendrimers	19
Hydrogels	19
Ocular Inserts, Implants, Lenses And Other Devices	20
CONCLUSION AND FUTURE PERSPECTIVES	24
CONSENT FOR PUBLICATION	25
CONFLICT OF INTEREST	26
ACKNOWLEDGEMENTS	26
REFERENCES	26
CHAPTER 2 PROPITIOUS DEVELOPMENT OF VACCINES FOR SARS-COV	42
Palaniswamy Rani, Balasubramanian Ayshwariya, Ramesh Harisharan and *Bhavananthi Ilackkeya*	
INTRODUCTION	42
SARS VIRUS	44
SARS Virus Family and Genome	44
SARS Virus Structure	44
Pathogenesis	45
Immune Response	47
Clinical symptoms, Diagnosis and Treatment	48
VACCINE DEVELOPMENT	49
Pipeline	49
Reverse Vaccinology Approach in SARS-COV-2 Vaccine Design	55
Vaccine Platform	56
Oral Vaccines	56

Live Attenuated Vaccines	57
Inactivated Vaccines	58
Protein Subunit Vaccine	59
Viral Vector Vaccines	61
mRNA Vaccine	63
DNA Vaccines	64
Animal Models	65
CHALLENGES IN VACCINE DEVELOPMENT	66
CONCLUSION	67
CONSENT FOR PUBLICATION	68
CONFLICT OF INTEREST	68
ACKNOWLEDGEMENTS	68
REFERENCES	68

CHAPTER 3 POTASSIUM PERMANGANATE, THE VIKUT® FORMULA, AN INNOVATION USING NON-ANTIBIOTIC ANTIMICROBIAL AGENTS TO TREAT BOTH CHRONIC AND NON-CHRONIC WOUNDS: A CLINICAL APPROACH WITH SCIENTIFIC EVIDENCE 76

Agustín Lara-Esqueda, Iván Delgado-Enciso, Agustín D. Lara-Basulto and *Margarita Balayan*

INTRODUCTION	77
THE ADVENT OF THE ANTIBIOTIC RESISTANCE	78
Antibiotics: What are They, and How do They Work?	78
CLASSIFICATION BASED ON THE MOLECULAR STRUCTURE	78
β-lactams	79
Macrolides	79
Tetracycline	80
Quinolones	80
Aminoglycosides	80
Sulfonamides	81
Glycopeptides (GPA's)	81
Polymyxins	81
Oxazolidinones	81
CLASSIFICATION BASED ON ITS MECHANISM OF ACTION	81
Inhibition of cell wall synthesis	81
Disruption of the structure or function of the cell membrane	82
Inhibition of nucleic acid structure or function	82
Inhibition of protein synthesis	82
Blocking key metabolic pathways	82
The bacteria strike back: mechanisms of resistance to antibiotics	82
Enzyme inhibition	82
Modification of molecular targets	83
Efflux pumps	83
Porin modification	83
LOOKING FOR ANSWERS: THE CAUSES OF ANTIBIOTIC RESISTANCE	83
INTRINSIC RESISTANCE IN NATURE	83
EXCESSIVE AND INAPPROPRIATE USE	84
EXTENSIVE USE IN THE AGRICULTURAL SECTOR	84
UNAVAILABILITY OF NEW ANTIBIOTICS	84
REGULATORY BARRIERS	84
POSSIBLE SOLUTIONS: HOW CAN WE DEAL WITH ANTIBIOTIC RESISTANCE?	85

PREVENTION OF TRANSMISSION OF BACTERIAL INFECTIONS	85
TRACKING METHODOLOGIES	85
IMPROVING THE USES OF EXISTING ANTIBIOTICS	85
Antibiotic Stewardship Programs	85
IMPROVEMENT OF PRESCRIPTION PRACTICES AND THERAPEUTIC TIME LENGTH	85
PROMOTION OF THE DEVELOPMENT OF NEW ANTIBIOTICS AND DIAGNOSTIC TESTS	86
Improvement of Diagnostic Tools	86
INCREASE THE VARIETIES OF ANTIMICROBIAL TREATMENTS	86
Conclusion: Persist or Perish	86
UNDERSTANDING THE WOUND HEALING PROCESS AND ITS RELATION TO THE CHRONICITY OF WOUNDS	86
Wounds and their Normal Healing Process	86
Proliferation	87
Remodeling	88
Chronic Injuries: When Things Go the Wrong Way	88
Types of Chronic Wounds	88
Chronic Wound Profile: What Went Wrong?	88
The Presence of ROS and Other Metabolic By-Products	89
An Increased Presence of Slough and Necrotic Tissue	90
The Occupation of Microorganism: Unwanted Visitors	90
The Biofilm: The Invaders' Fortress	90
The Treatment of Chronic Wounds: Untying a Gordian Knot	92
Patient and Wound Assessment	92
Topical Wound Therapy	92
New Therapies	92
Conclusion: Thinking Out of the Box	93
THE APPLICATION OF NON-ANTIBIOTIC ANTIMICROBIAL AGENTS FOR THE TREATMENT OF WOUNDS: THE EMERGENCE OF VIKUT®	93
Non-antibiotic Antimicrobial Agents: A Possible Solution?	93
Emulsifiers	94
Oxidizers	94
Acids	94
Heavy Metals	95
The inception of Vikut®: a synergetic surprise.	95
Potassium Permanganate: an Unexpected ally	95
Ethanol: the perfect mixer	96
Salicylic and Benzoic Acids: An Old but good team	96
Comparison Between Topical Antiseptics and Topical Antibiotics	97
The Synergies within the Vikut® Formula	98
Turning the Alcohol into Acetic Acid	98
Hypothesis I: Transforming the Oxidizer in Oxygen	98
Hypothesis II: The ROS Thief	99
Conclusion: Toward Unknown Waters	99
CLINICAL EVIDENCE OF THE FORMULA BASED ON POTASSIUM PERMANGANATE FOR THE TREATMENT OF BOTH ACUTE AND CHRONIC WOUNDS	100
Comparative Analysis Between Vikut® and the Conventional Treatment	100
Patients' Selection	100
Statistical Analysis	101

  RESULTS 102
  DISCUSSION 103
    The Use of Vikut® 5% Potassium Permanganate-based Formula in Both Acute and Chronic Wounds: Several Clinical Cases 103
    Cases of Acute wounds 103
      Clinical Case 1: Neglected Post- caesarian Wound 103
      Clinical Case 2: Post-surgical Wound 104
    Cases of Chronic Wounds 105
      Clinical Case 3: Diabetic Foot Ulcer on the Big Toe 105
      Clinical Case 4: Diabetic Ulcer in the Leg 107
      Clinical Case 5: Osteomyelitis-caused Injury 108
  CONCLUSION: GATHERING THE INFORMATION 110
  ECONOMIC AND FUNCTIONAL COMPARATIVE ANALYSIS BETWEEN THE FORMULA BASED ON POTASSIUM PERMANGANATE AND OTHER TOPICAL TREATMENTS 110
    Which is the goal? 111
  RESULTS OBTAINED REGARDING VIKUT® 111
  CONCLUSION: LOOKING AT THE FOREST 113
  CONSENT FOR PUBLICATION 113
  CONFLICT OF INTEREST 113
  ACKNOWLEDGEMENTS 113
  REFERENCES 113

CHAPTER 4 APPROACHES TO ANTI INFECTIVE THERAPIES 120
Sonia Sethi
  INTRODUCTION 120
    History of Antibiotics and their Resistance Mechanism 121
    Antibiotics Resistance Mechanisms 123
    Impact of Antibiotic Resistance 124
    Factors Contributing to the Emergence of Antibiotic Resistance 124
    Antibiotic Resistance in Human Medicine 125
    Use of Antibiotics in Food-producing Animals and Agriculture 125
    Resistance Spread and The Environment 125
    Prevention of Antibiotic Resistance 125
  APPROACHES FOR ANTIINFECTIVE THERAPIES 126
    Role of Reactive Oxygen and Nitrogen Species 126
    Mechanism of ROI and RNI against various microbes 127
    Host Innate Immunity Defense Systems 128
      Immune Modulators Expression and Secretion 129
      Avoiding Immune Detection 131
      Existing and Potential Innate Immune Targets for The Development of Anti-infectives 132
  ANTIMICROBIAL PEPTIDES AS ANTI-INFECTIVES 132
    Mode of Action 133
    Therapeutic Potential 135
  BACTERIOPHAGES AS ANTI-INFECTIVE AGENTS 136
    Phage Endolysins as Therapeutics 137
    Phage therapy as a Therapeutic Approach to Mycobacterial Infections 138
  THERAPY BASED ON ANTIBODY 138
  PROBIOTICS AS BIOTHERAPEUTIC AGENTS 140
  NANOTECHNOLOGY-BASED ANTI-INFECTIVES TO FIGHT MICROBIAL INTRUSIONS 142

  Nanomaterials for the Infections Control 143
  Carbon Nanotubes 143
  Nanocomposites 145
  Mechanism of Nanoparticles Against Bacteria 146
  Antiviral Mechanism of Nanoparticles 148
 CONCLUSION 148
 CONSENT FOR PUBLICATION 149
 CONFLICT OF INTEREST 149
 ACKNOWLEDGEMENTS 149
 LIST OF ABBREVIATIONS 149
 REFERENCES 151

CHAPTER 5 ANTI-INFECTIVE AGENTS AGAINST SEVERE ACUTE RESPIRATORY SYNDROME CORONAVIRUS 2 (SARS COV-2) 164
Ramadevi Mohan and *Subhashree Venugopal*
 INTRODUCTION 164
  Structure of SARS- CoV-2 165
  Structural Proteins 166
  S (Spike) Glycoprotein 166
  M (Membrane) Glycoprotein 166
  E (Envelope) Glycoprotein 167
  N (Nucleocapsid) Protein 167
  Clinical Outcomes 167
 TRANSMISSION OF INFECTION 168
  Intermediate Host Transmission 168
  Human-to-human Transmission 168
  Entry of COVID-19 and Interaction with a Host Cell Receptor 169
  Replication Process of SARS-CoV- 2 169
 TREATMENT 170
  Repurposing of Drugs for COVID-19 Treatment 171
  Role of Artificial Intelligence (AI) in Drug Repositioning 171
  Polymerase Inhibitors 172
  Remdesivir (GS-5734) 173
  Favipiravir (T-705) 174
  Sofosbuvir/Velpatasvir (EPCLUSA) 174
  β-D-N4-hydroxycytidine (NHC) 174
  Ribavirin 175
  Galidesivir (BCX4430) 175
  Gemcitabine Hydrochloride 176
 PROTEASES INHIBITORS 176
  SARS-CoV-2 Main Protease Inhibitors 176
  Serine Protease Inhibitors 178
  Malaria Drugs in COVID-19 178
  Lipid Lowering Statins 181
  Rheumatoid Arthritis Drugs 181
  Tocilizumab (TCZ) 181
  Sarilumab 182
  Baricitinib 182
  Corticosteroids 183
  Miscellaneous Drugs 183
 CONCLUDING REMARKS 183

CONSENT FOR PUBLICATION	184
CONFLICT OF INTEREST	184
ACKNOWLEDGEMENTS	184
REFERENCES	184

CHAPTER 6 BILAYER TABLET - APPROACH FOR THE TREATMENT OF SEXUALLY TRANSMITTED DISEASES WITH FIXED DOSE COMBINATION   197
Swati S. Gaikwad and *Mansi L. Patil*

INTRODUCTION	197
Benefits of Antimicrobial Combination	198
BI-LAYER TABLET TECHNOLOGY	198
ADVANTAGES OF BILAYER TABLET	198
GENERAL PROPERTIES OF BI-LAYER TABLETS	199
NEED	199
OBJECTIVE	199
PLAN OF WORK	199
MATERIAL AND METHODS	200
Drug Profile	200
Cefixime Trihydrate	200
Ofloxacin	201
POLYMER/ EXCIPIENTS PROFILE	202
Hydroxy Propyl Methylcellulose	202
Microcrystalline Cellulose	202
Crosscarmellose Sodium	202
Sodium Starch Glycolate	203
Crospovidone	203
Lactose, Monohydrate	203
EXPERIMENTAL METHODS	204
Confirmation of Drugs	204
Fourier Transformed Infrared Spectroscopy (FT-IR)	204
Spectrophotometric Analysis of Drug	204
Preformulation Studies	204
Drug-excipients Compatibility Study	204
Method of Preparation of Blend or Granules	204
Preparation of Powder Blend for Immediate Release Layer	204
Preparation of Granules for Sustained Release (SR) Layer	205
Evaluation study of Physical Properties of Blend/granules	205
Formulation of Cefixime Trihydrate Immediate Release Tablets	205
Evaluation Study of Cefixime Trihydrate Tablets	206
Formulation of Ofloxacin SR Tablets	206
Evaluation Study of Sustained Release Tablets	206
Bilayer Tablets Preparation	207
Evaluation Study of Bilayer Tablets	207
In-vitro Drug Release Study of Bilayer Tablets	207
Stability Studies and Storage Condition	209
RESULTS AND DISCUSSION	209
Confirmation of Drug	209
Fourier Transform Infrared Spectroscopy (FT-IR) Study	209
Preformulation Studies	209
Drug-excipient Compatibility Study	209

Evaluation of Precompression Parameters for Cefixime Trihydrate Immediate Release Tablets 212
   Physical Properties of Blend of Cefixime Trihydrate Tablets 212
Evaluation of Post Compression Parameters of Cefixime Trihydrate (IR) Tablets 212
In-vitro Drug Release Studies of Cefixime Trihydrate (IR) Tablets 213
Precompression evaluation parameters for ofloxacin SR tablets 213
Evaluation of Post Compression Parameters of Ofloxacin (SR) Tablets 214
In-vitro Drug Release Studies of Ofloxacin (SR) Tablets 214
Release Kinetics Study 215
Mechanism of Drug Release 215
Bilayer Tablets 215
   Evaluation of Bilayer Tablets 215
   In-vitro Drug Dissolution Test of Bilayer Tablet 215
   Dissolution Test 216
   Stability Study 217

SUMMARY AND CONCLUSION 217
CONSENT FOR PUBLICATION 218
CONFLICT OF INTEREST 218
ACKNOWLEDGEMENTS 218
REFERENCES 218

SUBJECT INDEX 220

PREFACE

Bacteria, viruses, fungi, protozoa, or parasites are the causative agents for various infectious diseases and are responsible for morbidity and mortality at large scale worldwide. Although remarkable accomplishments have been achieved in recent years in developing new anti-infectives, the widespread emergence of drug resistance has been the main obstacle and continues to provide a strong stimulus to develop new strategies in drug design and discovery. For instance, despite the exuberant therapeutic success of antibiotics, acute infections are still responsible for 25% of deaths worldwide, killing around 17 million people per year. Apart from de novo drug discovery, the re-positioning, and re-engineering of existing drugs or drug-like molecules with known pharmacokinetics and established target profiles have now become ideal starting points for identifying new chemical entities as new anti-infectives. The quantum of research in this field has shown a tremendous increase in recent years and thus keeping oneself abr/east of recent developments is rather challenging.

The book series **"Frontiers in Anti-infective Agents"** is aimed to update the scientific community on recent accomplishments and provide critical commentaries on the most exciting developments in the field of anti-infectives. The present volume 5 of the series has six comprehensive reviews, contributed by leading practitioners in these fields. These reviews broadly cover the clinical use of Vikut® for chronic and non-chronic wounds, drug delivery systems for ocular drug targeting, aspects of vaccination against SARS-CoV virus categories, nanotechnological interventions for the diagnosis and treatment of infectious diseases, repurposing and re-engineering of various drugs for targeting SARS-CoV-2 and a bilayer tablet approach for the treatment of sexually transmitted diseases.

The 1st chapter by Durgun *et al*. explicates ocular drug targeting as one of the most challenging research areas because of the presence of natural barriers of the eye. It discusses in detail the various drug delivery systems approved by USFDA for the treatment of ocular infections wherein the bioavailability is enhanced using micro and nano-carriers. The 2nd chapter by Rani *et al*. includes the various aspects of vaccination, its importance in the current scenario, and methods of implementation specifically targeting SARS-CoV virus categories.

The 3rd chapter by Lara-Esqueda *et al*. describes the healing properties of each of the components of Vikut® and the results of its use in the clinical case obtained by healthcare professionals in the treatment of both chronic and non-chronic wounds. Sonia Sethi discussed the nanotechnological interventions for the diagnosis and treatment of infectious diseases, particularly resistant to conventional antibiotics, in the 4th chapter. In particular, the use of nanomaterials with intrinsic anti-infective properties as carriers for targeted and site-specific delivery of potential drugs is discussed in detail.

Mohan and Venugopal, in the 5th chapter, highlight the successful repurposing and re-engineering of various drugs for assessing their activities on SARS-CoV-2 and are in various phases of clinical trials. A particular emphasis was given on protease inhibitors, polymerase inhibitors, antimalarial drugs, rheumatoid drugs, and lipid-lowering statins with promising SARS-CoV-2 activities. The 6th chapter by Gaikwad and Patil delineats a bilayer tablet approach for the treatment of sexually transmitted diseases. The combination of Cefixime and ofloxacin was employed to prepare the bilayered tablets to maintain the peak plasma level of the drug.

We are indeed grateful to all the authors of the above-cited articles for their excellent contributions and hope that these contributions will help readers in gaining a better understanding of this field. We would also like to express our gratitude to the entire team of Bentham Science Publishers, particularly Ms. Fariya Zulfiqar (Manager Publications), and Mr. Mahmood Alam (Editorial Director), for the timely production of the 5th volume.

Parvesh Singh
School of Chemistry and Physics
University of Kwa-Zulu Natal (UKZN)
Westville campus, Durban
South Africa

Vipan Kumar
Department of Chemistry
Guru Nanak Dev University
Amritsar
India

&

Rajshekhar Karpoormath
Department of Pharmaceutical Chemistry
University of Kwa-Zulu Natal (UKZN)
Westville Campus, Durban
South Africa

List of Contributors

Agustín D. Lara-Basulto	Department of Psychology and Human Communication Therapy, University of Durango, Durango, CO 81301, United States
Agustín Lara-Esqueda	Department of Psychology and Human Communication Therapy, University of Durango, Durango, CO 81301, United States
Balasubramanian Ayshwariya	Department of Biotechnology, PSG College of Technology, Coimbatore, Tamil Nadu 641004, India
Bhavananthi Ilackkeya	Department of Biotechnology, PSG College of Technology, Coimbatore, Tamil Nadu 641004, India
Iván Delgado-Enciso	Department of Psychology and Human Communication Therapy, University of Durango, Durango, CO 81301, United States
Mansi L. Patil	Department of Pharmaceutical Sciences, R. T. M. Nagpur University, Nagpur 440033, Maharashtra, India
Margarita Balayan	Department of Psychology and Human Communication Therapy, University of Durango, Durango, CO 81301, United States
Meltem Ezgi Durgun	Department of Pharmaceutical Technology, Faculty of Pharmacy, Istanbul University, Istanbul, Turkey
Palaniswamy Rani	Department of Biotechnology, PSG College of Technology, Coimbatore, Tamil Nadu 641004, India
Ramesh Harisharan	Department of Biotechnology, PSG College of Technology, Coimbatore, Tamil Nadu 641004, India
Ramadevi Mohan	Department of Integrative Biology, VIT University, Vellore-632014, Tamil Nadu, India
Sevgi Güngör	Department of Pharmaceutical Technology, Faculty of Pharmacy, Istanbul University, Istanbul, Turkey
Sonia Sethi	Dr. B. Lal Institute of Biotechnology Malviya Industrial Area, Malviya Nagar, Jaipur, India
Subhashree Venugopal	Department of Integrative Biology, VIT University, Vellore-632014, Tamil Nadu, India
Swati S. Gaikwad	Nagpur College of Pharmacy, Wanadongri, Hingna Road, Nagpur, India
Yıldız Özsoy	Department of Pharmaceutical Technology, Faculty of Pharmacy, Istanbul University, Istanbul, Turkey

CHAPTER 1

Anti-Infective Agents in Ocular Treatment and New Approaches

Meltem Ezgi Durgun[1,*], **Sevgi Güngör**[1] and **Yıldız Özsoy**[1]

[1] *Department of Pharmaceutical Technology, Faculty of Pharmacy, Istanbul University, Istanbul, Turkey*

Abstract: Ocular drug targeting is one of the most interesting and challenging research topics due to the presence of natural barriers of the eye that attract pharmaceutical technologists. It is important to treat ocular infections, which are frequently encountered and affect people of all ages, in order to protect the integrity of the eye. For this reason, anti-infective agents used in the treatment of ocular infections are frequently the subject of ocular drug delivery system studies. The ocular bioavailability of anti-infective agents is also increased, thanks to micro and nano-carriers, where the dose strength of drugs and frequency of administration can be reduced. On the other hand, the fact that there are products approved by the USFDA among these delivery systems which have completed clinical phase studies shows that these drug delivery systems are promising in the ocular field.

Keywords: Anti-infective agents, Ocular drugs, Ocular drug delivery systems, Nanotechnology, Ocular anatomy, Ocular physiology, Pharmacokinetic.

INTRODUCTION

The eye, the organ of vision, is located in the orbita and is protected by the orbital bones. It is one of the most complex organs in the human body due to its anatomy and physiology and consists of three different layers as fibrous, vascular, and neural structures. Since the eye is in contact with the external environment, it contains natural protective mechanisms. The protective mechanisms known as ocular barriers are tear film, cornea, conjunctiva, sclera, blood-aqueous humor, and blood-retina barrier. They are mainly tasked with minimizing the toxic effects of external agents such as liquids and dissolved molecules on the eyes. However, these protective mechanisms also reduce ocular bioavailability of drugs. Different drug delivery strategies have been developed in order to eliminate the effect of

---

[*] **Corresponding author Meltem Ezgi Durgun:** Department of Pharmaceutical Technology, Faculty of Pharmacy, Istanbul University, Istanbul, Turkey; E-mails:m.ezgidurgun@gmail.com

Parvesh Singh, Vipan Kumar & Rajshekhar Karpoormath (Eds.)
All rights reserved-© 2021 Bentham Science Publishers

ocular barriers, which are more effective in topically applied drugs, and thus increase ocular bioavailability. However, most of Ocular drugs are differentiated into conventional dosage forms and drug delivery systems. 90% of commercial products are conventional dosages and are applied topically to the eye. In response to these drugs with low ocular bioavailability, the development of new drug delivery systems is one of the most interesting and challenging areas for scientists. These systems can cross the ocular barriers, accumulate in the target area, show a longer retention time, and do not cause systemic toxicity. Micro and nanoparticles, microemulsions, nanosuspensions, solid lipid nanoparticles, liposomes, cubosomes, dendrimers, niosomes, hydro-gelling systems, ocular lens/inserts/implants, and micelles have been developed as ocular drug delivery systems.

Depending on the anatomical and physiological structure of the eye, any ocular disease or disorder can easily trigger a secondary disease/disorder. In particular, ocular infections can quickly involve other tissues. Also, alterations in tissue because of infection cause activation of opportunistic pathogens and aggravation of infection. To maintain the structural integrity of the eye, it is imperative to treat ocular infection quickly, accurately, and effectively. Otherwise, serious complications such as visual loss or spreading of infection to different organs can be seen. The primary group of commercial ocular products is intended to treat ocular infections. Artificial tears and lens solutions are used for the treatment of dry eye disease. However, both dry eye disease and lenses that are not used or stored properly cause ocular infection. For this reason, we can evaluate artificial tears and lens solutions as prophylactic products against ocular infection.

The development of new dosage forms for the treatment of ocular infections is one of the main topics in pharmaceutical science. The subject of these studies may be anti-infective agents that have been used for a long time in the treatment of ocular diseases, and those the effectiveness of which has been proven by *in vivo* experiments. Also, newly developed anti-infective agents that have not yet been studied in the ocular field may be a subject. All studies have the aim of increasing the ocular bioavailability of anti-infective agents with a suitable drug delivery system.

In this chapter, anti-infective agents used in the treatment of ocular infections, commercial products, and new approaches to anti-infective therapies will be examined. Also, the anatomy and physiology of the eye will be discussed with the aspects that affect the ocular bioavailability of drugs and should be considered in the development of new ocular drugs. This chapter will be informative for people working on drug delivery systems for ocular targeted drugs and anti-infective agents. It will also provide insight for clinicians who follow promising new approaches among treatment options and participate in clinical trials.

ANATOMY, PHYSIOLOGY, AND PHARMACOKINETIC OF EYE

The eye, the organ of vision, is located in the orbita and is protected by the orbital bones. The lens divides the eye into two as anterior and posterior segments. The eyeball consists of three layers, from the outside to the inside, the tunica fibrosa bulbi, the tunica vasculosa bulbi, and the tunica interna bulbi [1]. Inside the eyeball limited by these three layers, the corpus vitreum, lens, and aqueous humor are located. Tunicae Fibrosa Bulbi (Corneal-Scleral Layer) is the fibrous layer of the eyeball. Tunica vasculosa bulbi is the vascular layer, and tunica interna bulbi is the innermost neural layer [2]. The anatomy and segments of the eye are shown in Fig. (**1**).

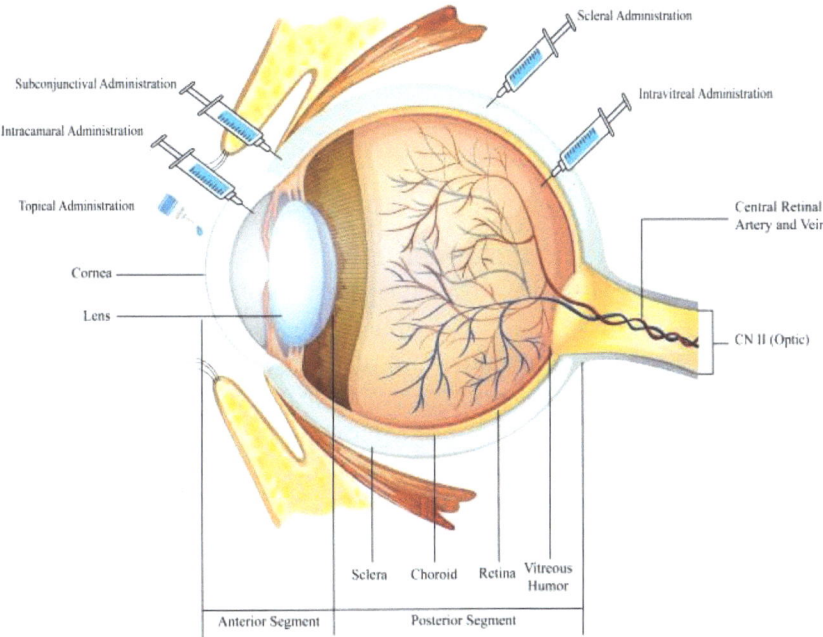

Fig. (1). Anatomy of the eye and ocular drug administration routes.

The eye contains natural barriers that limit the passage of liquids or dissolved substances into the anterior and posterior segments of the eye, depending on its anatomy and physiology. These barriers also affect the ocular absorption and the bioavailability of drugs. These barriers are in an anatomical order; tear film, cornea, conjunctiva, sclera, blood-aqueous humor or iris-ciliary body, lens, and blood-retinal barriers. While tear film acts as the first barrier for the drugs applied, it dilutes the drugs due to continuous production of tear fluid and nasolacrimal drainage. The cornea has a lipophilic and hydrophilic character at the same time due to tight junctions and collagen fibers in its structure. For this reason, the corneal epithelium acts as a barrier for hydrophilic drugs, while the stroma prevents the passage of lipophilic drugs to internal tissues. The sclera also acts as a barrier to lipophilic drugs with the collagen fibers it contains [3 - 6]. Besides, the pores of the cornea and sclera affect the passage of drugs to internal tissues. Drugs with particle size smaller than 100 nm and particle sizes in the range of 20-80 nm, respectively, can pass through the cornea and sclera [7, 8].

Drugs are administrated to the eye with different methods in order to increase bioavailability in the presence of ocular barriers. In addition to topical application, subconjunctival, scleral, and intravitreal injection are other ocular drug administration routes. However, the difficulty of applying these methods and possible complications limit their use.

OCULAR İNFECTİONS

Keratitis

Keratitis is one of the most common causes of visual impairment among adults. It is a rapidly progressing disease. Corneal opacification due to keratitis is the fourth underlying cause of blindness [9]. Contact lenses, ocular surgery, physical or chemical injury, diabetes, immunosuppressive diseases, topical steroids and agricultural activities in developing societies may be the predisposing factors of keratitis formation. The type of microorganism that causes keratitis depends on the geographical location and climate of the region where the person lives. Keratitis is divided into three main groups as infectious, interstitial, and non-infectious, as shown in Table **1** [10 - 15].

Conjunctivitis

Conjunctivitis is an infection of the conjunctiva due to bacteria, viruses, irritant substances, or allergens. It is a common ocular disease that affects people of all ages and socio-economic segments. The fact that 70% of acute conjunctivitis cases present to primary care centers or emergency services instead of an ophthalmologist is one of the data showing the prevalence of the disease [20 - 23].

Fungi species do not play a role in the development of conjunctivitis. However, conjunctival involvement can also be seen in allergic conjunctivitis or in cases of fungal keratitis and/or scleritis [24 - 26]. Depending on the pathogen type, topical drugs are preferred in the treatment.

Table 1. Classification of keratitis.

Type	Subtype	Treatment Agents	References
Infectious keratitis	Bacterial	Topical antibiotics, tetracycline group antibiotics, and corticosteroids	[11,12]
	Viral	Trifluridine, acyclovir, and ganciclovir	[11,12]
	Fungal	5% natamycin, 0.3-0.5% amphotericin B (AMB), 1% voriconazole, oral, intravenous (i.v.) or intrastromal VRC and intracameral AMB	[12]
	Acanthamoeba	Combined treatment with 0.1% propamidine and 1% neomycin, 0.02% concentration of polyhexamethylene biguanide (PHMB) and topical neomycin, miconazole, prednisolone and metronidazole, oral ketoconazole	[11,12,16,17]
Interstitial keratitis	-	Since it is a multidisciplinary disease, a multidisciplinary approach is essential in its treatment: corticosteroids such as prednisolone, methotrexate, cyclophosphamide, azotropine, infliximab, rituximab, cyclosiporin a, anti TNF-α, tocilizumab, etanercept, and adalimumab are included	[18]
Non-Infectious keratitis	Exposure keratitis	Medical therapy: steroids Physical intervention: Bandaging to eliminate eyelid looseness, application of amniotic membrane	[19]
	Neuroparalytic keratitis	Topical steroids or nonsteroidal anti-inflammatory drugs (NSAIDs) to relieve eye infection	[15]

Endophthalmitis

It is an infection of the intraocular cavities, the aqueous humor, and the vitreous humor that fills these cavities. It is basically divided into two groups as infective and non-infective. The infection seen in infective endophthalmitis is usually of bacteria or fungus origin. The development of viral or parasitic infections is not a common condition [27].

Infectious endophthalmitis is divided into exogenous and endogenous endophthalmitis. Exogenous endophthalmitis is a type of endophthalmitis that occurs after eye surgery or trauma. Possible contamination in sterile equipments and solutions used during intravitreal injection and surgical procedure, the risk of contamination from the personnel of the surgery, and the flora of the eyelid or conjunctiva may be factors in the development of infection [27 - 30]. Endogenous

Endophthalmitis accounts for 5-15% of total endophthalmitis cases. The infectious agent is bacteria or fungal. It occurs when a possible infectious agent in any tissue reaches the eye. Gram positive bacteria such as S. aureus, streptococci and Gram negative bacteria such as Pseudomonas and E. coli [28]. Infectious endophthalmitis is treated with antibiotics or anti-fungal agents, depending on the type of pathogen. These drugs are the same as the active ingredient used in the treatment of infectious keratitis and are applied topically, systemically, or intravitreally [28].

Non-infectious endophthalmitis is an uncommon type of endophthalmitis seen with infection caused by an allergen substance independent of any microorganism infection. Corticosteroids are used in their treatment [31, 32].

Uveitis

Uveitis is the infection of the uvea, or vascular layer of the eye due to various reasons. Although it is defined as ocular infection, it is actually a multidisciplinary disease since it may develop due to another underlying disease. Determining the agent by performing a detailed examination in an individual diagnosed with uveitis can enable the diagnosis of another disease [33 - 35]. It is thought that more than 2 million people in the world are affected with uveitis and 10% of blindness worldwide is due to uveitis. The incidence in the age range of 16-65, defined as the working population, is higher than in other age groups [35 - 39].

The International Uveitis Working Group (IUSG) classifies uveitis clinically into infectious, non-infectious, and masked uveitis [40]. In some sources, endophthalmitis is considered uveitis [35, 41].

Infectious uveitis is a type of uveitis that develops due to bacterial, viral, protozoal, fungal, helminthic, or intestinal worms. Its incidence is 50% more common in less developed and / or tropical countries than in developed countries. It is seen in the USA and European countries with a rate of 13-21%. While varicella-zoster, herpes simplex, or toxoplasma are the main factors in the USA and European countries, mycobacterium leprae, Mycobacterium tuberculosis, toxoplasma, and onchocerciasis causing river blindness are the main factors in tropical and/or underdeveloped countries [35 ,42]. Infectious uveitis is generally seen in the posterior segment. Therefore, the main drug administration method in treatment is intravitreal injection. It is extremely important to determine the pathogen type to choose the correct active ingredient. Ganciclovir and foscarnet as anti-virals, vancomycin, gentamicin, ceftazidime, moxifloxacin, and amikacin as anti-bacterials, clindamycin, and Trimethoprim/sulfamethoxazole as an antiprotozoal, AMB and VRC as anti-fungal are preferred [35].

Non-infectious uveitis is associated with systemic disease [40]. In the absence of systemic disease, uveitis may develop due to trauma, an ocular surgical procedure, idiopathic diseases, and the use of drugs such as cidofovir or rifabutin. Diseases such as sarcoidosis, juvenile idiopathic arthritis, and Behçet's disease are given as examples of uveitis due to systemic diseases [35]. Treatment in non-infectious uveitis is generally performed with corticosteroids or alternative agents that will suppress the immune system [35].

Masked uveitis is a type of uveitis that develops due to cancer. It is divided into neoplastic or non-neoplastic [40].

Scleritis

Scleritis is a type of ocular infection that is centered in the sclera and can often involve adjacent tissues such as the episclera, cornea, and uvea. It is a rare ocular disease with severe pain and blinding potential [43 - 45].

Considering the etiology, the incidence of the systemic disease has been reported to be 39-50% in individuals with scleritis [46 - 48]. Posterior scleritis is more likely to be associated with anterior scleritis in an individual with underlying systemic disease [46]. Infection, autoimmune diseases, surgical interventions, intraocular tumors such as melanomas, conjunctival tumors, lymphoma, trauma, congenital erythropoietic porphyria after allogeneic bone marrow transplantation, rare systemic diseases such as graft- *versus* -host disease can cause scleritis [43, 49,50].

Infection is a rare cause of scleritis (5-10%). However, it is a common belief that infected scleritis begins with an autoimmune basis and appears with a progressively worsening condition and has worse results than autoimmune scleritis. Although the reason for this is not known exactly, it is thought to be caused by the late diagnosis or the aggressiveness of the pathogens causing the infection. Bacteria, protozoa, fungus, coinfections are the most common causes of scleritis due to infection. Many pathogenic organisms have been shown to be among the possible causes of scleritis in cases seen over the years [43,44]. Fungal scleritis generally gives worse results than bacterial or viral scleritis [51]. Studies showed that despite the treatment, rapid cataract, serous retinal or choroidal detachments, or endophthalmitis were observed in many patients [43].

Surgery (pterygium, cataract, glaucoma, vitroretinal or conjunctival tumor surgery) [45], immunosuppressants [52,53], traumas, Mitomycin C, and radiation use [54 - 59] are among the most common infectious scleritis factors.

Watson and Hayreh classified the scleritis by anatomy. This classification system is considered to be the most common predisposing factors of infectious scleritis. Table **2** includes the agents used in this classification and treatment [45].

Table 2. Classification of scleritis.

Type	Subtype	Treatment Agents	References
Episcleritis	Diffused	Artificial tears, topical corticosteroids, and topical nonsteroidal anti-inflammatory drugs (NSAIDs)	[49,60,61]
	Nodular		
Anterior scleritis	Diffused	Topical corticosteroids, oral NSAIDs (COX inhibitors), oral corticosteroids, immunosuppressive agents, and subconjunctival corticosteroid injection	[24,47,62 - 64]
	Nodular		
	Necrotized • With infection • Without infection • Scleromalasia perforans		
Posterior scleritis	Diffused	oral NSAIDs (COX inhibitors), oral corticosteroids and immunosuppressive agents	[24,62,65]
	Nodular		
	Necrotized		

ANTI-INFECTIVE AGENTS USED IN OCULAR TREATMENT

The eye is separated from other organs due to its unique anatomy and physiology. It has a small size and volume but has rich vascular and neural networks. On the other hand, tear, aqueous humor, and vitreous humor turnover are rapid. Due to this unique anatomy and physiology, it is common for an infection that begins in any ocular tissue to spread to other ocular tissues. Also, as ocular immunity is suppressed by infection, the eye becomes suitable for the activation of other opportunistic pathogens. Therefore, the treatment of ocular infections should be done quickly with a suitable agent. Anti-bacterial, anti-viral, anti-fungal, and anti-parasitic drugs are used in the treatment of ocular infections. The anti-infective agent should be selected according to the type of pathogens that caused the infection. For this reason, it is very important to be able to isolate the strain that is the cause of infection. Anti-infective agents used in ocular infection, approved by the USFDA, are listed in Table **3**.

Most of the commercial products used in the treatment of any disease are in a conventional dosage form. 90% of the products in the treatment of ocular diseases are also included in this group. Conventional dosage forms applied to the eyes are solutions, suspensions, ointments, and gels (4-6). These dosage forms, also known as traditional medicines, generally target the anterior segment of the eye and do not show much effect on a possible disease in the posterior segment. On the other hand, the ocular bioavailability of these drugs is low due to the ocular barriers. Because of their low bioavailability, the dose frequency during the day is high, and this reduces patient compliance. Also, the fact that gels and ointments cause blurry vision is another factor that reduces patient compliance. To address these issues, drug delivery systems targeting ocular tissues have been developed.

OCULAR DRUG DELIVERY SYSTEMS

Microparticles and Nanoparticles

Microparticles and nanoparticles are colloidal drug delivery systems with particle sizes between 1-10 μm and 10-1000 nm, respectively [66, 67]. They are often preferred for ocular drug targeting. Prolonged drug release and slow ocular drainage due to particle size are important advantages compared to conventional dosage forms. Because the particle size of microparticles is larger than nanoparticles, their ocular tolerability is less than nanoparticles [68 - 70].

Cortesi *et al* prepared acyclovir loaded microparticles using different Eudragit types. It was found that the prepared microparticles had an extended release for 8 hours, and their anti-viral activity was similar to that of acyclovir solution [71]. Gavini *et al*. produced ciprofloxacin loaded microparticles using chondroitin 6-sulfate or lambda-carrageenan. Also, they examined the mucoadhesion properties by adding carbomer (Carbopol 934P®) to the microparticles. They reported that the microparticles were suitable for ocular application in terms of particle size, and high mucoadhesion was seen in all formulations, although it was higher in those with carbomer added [72].

Liu *et al* prepared cyclosporin A loaded poly-lactic acid (PLA) nanoparticles and compared them with Restasis®, which is used to treat dry eye disease. It has been observed that nanoparticles have a longer retention time with ocular tissues than Restasis® thanks to their mucoadhesion feature and significantly reduces the dose of cyclosporine A to be used (50- to 100-fold). Although Restasis® is normally used twice a day, it was determined that nanoparticles were applied once a week to eliminate infection. In addition, it has been reported that goblet cells regenerate within one month in the treatment applied with nanoparticles, and this regeneration is not seen in the treatment with Restasis® [73]. Poly(lactic-c--glycolic acid) (PLGA) is a copolymer commonly used in the preparation of ocular delivery systems [74]. Gupta *et al*. produced levofloxacin loaded PLGA nanoparticles and compared with a commercial product. It has been determined that the nanoparticles remain in the pre-corneal area for 24 hours and their efficiency is better than the commercial product in *in vivo* rabbit model [75]. In another ocular study with PLGA, acyclovir loaded nanoparticles were produced using PLGA combined with TPGS. Alkholief *et al*. reported that AUC_{0-24h}, $t_{1/2}$ (h), and MRT_{0-24h} values of nanoparticles were 2.78-fold, 1.71-fold, and 2.2-fold higher, respectively, compared to acyclovir solution [76]. Clarithromycin is another anti-infective agent studied with PLGA. In anti-fungal activity studies, the minimum inhibitory concentration (MIC) of nanoparticles on S.aureus was 8-fold lower than clarithromycin solution. Although this study was not conducted with direct ocular drug targeting, Mohammadi *et al*. underlined that the nanoparticles were suitable for ocular application due to their particle size (in the range of 180-280 nm) [77].

Table 3. Anti-infective agents approved by the USFDA.

Active Ingredient	Dosage Form
Azithromycin	Solution
Bacitracin/ Zinc/ Hydrocortisone Acetate/ Neomycin Sulfate/ Polymyxin B Sulfate	Ointment
Bacitracin/ Zinc/ Neomycin Sulfate/ Polymyxcin B Sulfate	Ointment
Bacitracin/ Zinc/ Polymyxin B Sulfate	Ointment
Bepotastine Besilate	Solution
Besifloxacin Hydrochloride	Suspensions
Ciprofloxacin Hydrochloride	Ointment
Cyclosporine	Solution / Emulsion
Cysteamine Hydrochloride	Solution
Dexamethasone/ Neomycin Sulfate / Polymyxin B Sulfate	Ointment/ Suspension
Dexamethasone/ Tobramycin	Ointment/ Suspension
Erythromycin	*Ointment*
Gancyclovir	Gel
Gatifloxacin	Solution
Gentamicin Sulfate	Solution/ Ointment
Gentamicin Sulfate/ Prednisolone Acetate	Solution/ Ointment/ Suspension
Gramicidin/ Neomycin Sulfate/ Polymyxin B Sulfate	Solution
Hydrocortisone/ Gramicidin/ Neomycin Sulfate/ Polymyxin B Sulfate	Suspension
Ketorolac Tromethamine	Solution
Levofloxacin	Solution
Loteprednol Etabonate/ Tobramycin	Suspension
Moxifloxacin Hydrochloroide	Solution
Natamycin	Suspension
Ofloxacin	Solution

(Table 3) cont.....

Active Ingredient	Dosage Form
Polymyxin B Sulfate/ Trimethoprim Sulfate	Solution
Povidone - Iodine	Solution
Prednisolone Sodium/ Sulfacetamide Sodium	Solution
Sulfacetamide Sodium	Solution/ Ointment
Tobramycin	Solution/ Ointment
Trifluridine	Solution
Tropicamide	Solution

Solid Lipid Microparticles and Nanoparticles

Despite the advantages of micro and nanoparticles, their use is limited because of the long-term potential toxicity of the polymers used in their preparation. Solid lipid microparticles (SLM) and solid lipid nanoparticles (SLN) are drug delivery systems developed in the 1990s as an alternative to the emulsion, polymeric nanoparticles, and liposomes. Their lipid part formed by the liquid lipid (oil) has been substituted by a solid lipid. While SLNs have smaller diameters than 1 µm, SLMs have a larger particle size [78, 79].

SLM or SLN are often preferred for ocular targeting of anti-bacterial drugs. Wolska *et al.* prepared SLMs of cyclosporine A using Compritol 888 ATO and Tween 80, and emulsions of cyclosporine A using soybean oil or castor oil for comparison. In the studies, the concentration of cyclosporin A in the precorneal tissues in the SLM groups was found to be higher than the therapeutic value and emulsion groups [80]. Gökçe *et al.* also developed SLN drug delivery systems containing cyclosporine A. It has been shown that the cumulative corneal permeation value of cyclosporin A of these formulations was higher 2-fold than the cyclosporin A solution, and the formulations were not cytotoxic and did not cause irritation in cell culture studies [81]. In studies conducted with another antibiotic ofloxacin, it was observed that SLNs had extended release for 8 hours, and *in vivo* corneal permeation of SLNs in rabbit eyes after 24 hours were 2.5-fold higher than commercial eye drops (Oflox®) [82]. In the study done by Pignatello *et al.* with ciprofloxacin, it was reported that SLNs have anti-bacterial effects on different strains, even nine months after their production [83].

Tobramycin is an antibiotic with commercial ocular drops, suspension, and ointment [84]. Chetoni *et al.* applied the tobramycin SLNs they developed both topically to the eye and intravenously to two separate groups. In these *in vivo* rabbit studies, it has been observed that tobramycin SLNs accumulate in the retina, regardless of the route of administration. It was also reported that SLNs show more bactericidal activity against Pseudomonas aeruginosa compared to tobramycin solution [85].

Baig *et al* developed SLNs of levofloxacin using the Box-Behnken experimental design. In comparative studies with levofloxacin commercial eye drops, levofloxacin SLNs have been reported to provide extended release for 12 hours. It has also been observed that SLNs, whose anti-fungal activity is similar to eye drops, were not toxic with the hen's egg-chorioallantoic membrane test (HET-CAM test) [86]. Khames *et al.* also made a different SLN study using the Box-Behnken experimental design. They produced natamycin SLNs with different lipid types and chose the most appropriate formulation using the Box-Behnken experimental design. It was shown that the final natamycin SLN had extended release over 10 hours, and the anti-fungal activity of SLNs was 2.5-fold higher than the natamycin suspension [87].

Valacyclovir is an anti-viral drug. *ex vivo* corneal permeation and ocular bioavailability of valacyclovir SLNs were found to be 7-fold and 2-fold higher, respectively, compared to valacyclovir solution. Also, HETCAM analysis was demonstrated that the developed SLNs were non-toxic [88].

Although tuberculosis is a disease that generally affects the lungs, orbital and external eye infections were detected in 15% of 6.3 million tuberculosis cases in 2016 [89]. Isoniazid is used in the treatment of tuberculosis caused by Mycobacterium tuberculosis. Singh *et al.* prepared SLNs of isoniazid considering this situation. Compared to isoniazid solution, SLNs with extended release for 48 hours increased *ex vivo* corneal permeability and ocular bioavailability of isoniazid 1.6-fold and 4.2-fold, respectively. The MIC value was also five-fold lower than isoniazid solution [90].

Microemulsions and Nanoemulsions

Micro and nanoemulsions are systems that are created by means of an aqueous phase, an oily phase, one or more surfactants. Despite the different definitions in the literature, microemulsions generally define systems with a droplet size of less than 100 nm and nanoemulsions with a droplet size higher than 100 nm. However, there is still a use of the definition of nanoemulsion for systems smaller than 100 nm. Microemulsions are thermodynamically more stable than nanoemulsions [91].

Seyfoddin *et al* reported that the acyclovir nanoemulsions increased the anti-viral activity of acyclovir 3.5-fold after 24 hours. It was observed that nanoemulsions increase the bioavailability of acyclovir by 4.5-fold in comparative *in vivo* rabbit studies performed with commercial acyclovir ophthalmic ointment [92].

Bharti *et al* showed that the moxifloxacin microemulsions remained stable for three months. Microemulsions were found to be more effective than commercial moxifloxacin eye drops in *in vivo* rabbit studies [93].

Kumar *et al* examined the voriconazole microemulsions in terms of toxicity and ocular permeability. It was found that the microemulsions developed are suitable for ocular use, and *ex vivo* corneal permeation is higher than voriconazole suspension. Also, *in vivo* studies showed that microemulsions had less nasolacrimal drainage than suspension [94].

Nanosuspensions

Nanosuspensions are colloidal systems formed by suspending poorly soluble or insoluble drugs in a suitable dispersion medium. Their stability is provided by surface-active agents. They do not show the potential irritant properties of microemulsions, as their size is smaller than 1 μm [69, 95, 96].

Mugdil *et al* compared their moxifloxacin nanosuspensions with commercial eye drops. It has been observed that the nanosuspension structure increases the corneal permeability of moxifloxacin *in vitro* by almost 2-fold compared to commercial eye drops. Also, the anti-bacterial activity of nanosuspensions was also found to be high [97]. Ambhore *et al.* prepared nanosuspensions of sparfloxacin using hydroxypropylmethylcellulose (HPMC) or chitosan. It has been observed that chitosan nanosuspension had sustained drug released for 9 hours, while HPMC nanosuspensions had 6 hours. The effectiveness of nanosuspensions, which were well tolerated by ocular tissues, were proven by *in vivo* rabbit studies [98]. When the cyclosporine A nanosuspension developed by Kim *et al.* was compared with the commercial eye product in terms of toxicity, both products were found to be irritating in the Draize test, while in the Schirmer tear test, the nanosuspension was found to be safer than the commercial product [99].

Maged *et al* produced a series of nanosuspensions of econazole nitrate using different surfactants. It was observed that the nanosuspension containing hydroxypropyl-β-cyclodextrin and Tween 80 was stable for one year at room temperature. This selected formulation was suspended in chitosan HCl to improve bioavailability by increasing mucoadhesion. In *in vivo* studies, the AUC values of econazole nanosuspension and nanosuspension added to chitosan HCL were 2.5-fold and 5-fold higher, respectively, than econazole suspension [100]. Voriconazole was used in another nanosuspension study with anti-fungal agents. It was observed that the nanosuspension increased the anti-fungal effect of voriconazole and produced more inhibition in less concentration on the Candida albicans strain. Also, nanosuspensions showed better ocular permeability than commercial voriconazole injection in both *in vitro* and *in vivo* studies [101].

Micelles

Micelles are another nanocarrier frequently used in ocular drug targeting. Micelles are self-emulsifying systems containing amphiphilic copolymer or surfactant. The hydrophobic core and hydrophilic shell of micelles provide an advantage for targeting hydrophobic drugs to hydrophilic environments. Therefore, the lipophilic property of micelles made them pass through the corneal epithelium more easily [102].

Micelles are easy to manufacture and scale-up. For this reason, micellar carrier systems are very likely to turn into commercial products. Cequa® is one of the most recent examples of this. Phase III studies of cyclosporine A loaded micellar eye drops developed by Mandal *et al* have also been successfully completed. USFDA approved Cequa® in the treatment of dry eye disease [103 - 105]. Apart from Cequa®, cyclosporine A emulsions are also used in the treatment of dry eye disease [84]. For this reason, many micellar carrier system studies have been conducted with cyclosporine A for the treatment of dry eye disease. It has been reported that the corneal permeation of the lyophilized cyclosporine A micelles developed by Yu *et al*. was better than the cyclosporine A emulsion and the micelle structure reduces the elimination of cyclosporine A [106]. Luschmann *et al*. examined the effectiveness of cyclosporine A loaded micelles in an *in situ* porcine model. It has been reported that micellar structure increases cyclosporine A uptake 3.5-fold and 3-fold, respectively, compared to cyclosporin A in olive oil and Restasis® (cyclosporine nanoemulsion) [107]. The micelles developed by Li *et al*. increased the corneal penetration of cyclosporine A *in vitro* and *in vivo* mice model [108].

Kanoujia *et al* developed a micellar ocular delivery system with another anti-bacterial drug, gatifloxacin. They have shown that micelles increase corneal permeation of gatifloxacin compared to commercial eye drops and gatifloxacin solution [109]. In a study conducted with Neomycin B, Kanamycin B, and DNA aptamers, it has been shown that micelles increase corneal permeation and inhibit bacterial growth. Willem de Vries *et al*. reported that micelles could be applied to the human eye [110].

Micelles are also suitable carrier systems for anti-fungal drugs. Triazole group anti-fungal agents, which are used as the first choice in the treatment of fungal infections [111], may be the subject of ocular targeted micellar drug delivery systems. Sertaconazole nitrate loaded micelles developed by Younes *et al* increased corneal permeation and corneal uptake of sertaconazole 2-fold compared to sertaconazole suspension [112]. Posaconazole, which has a similar chemical structure to itraconazole and has the most penetrating spectrum of triazole agents, is used off-label in cases of severe keratitis and sclerokeratitis [10, 113, 114]. Durgun *et al* reported that optimized posaconazole loaded micelles that had extended drug release in simulated tear fluid for 8 hours and increased the total amount of drug released 30-fold to 110-fold compared to posaconazole suspension [115]. Terbinafine is an anti-fungal agent not included in the triazole group. Terbinafine hydrochloride loaded micelles developed by Zhou *et al* increased corneal permeation compared to oily terbinafine hydrochloride. However, it has been reported that the micelle structure did not change the ocular bioavailability of terbinafine [116].

Aciclovir, ganciclovir, famciclovir, valaciclovir, and trifluorothymidine are drugs used in the treatment of viral ocular infections [117]. Varela-Garcia *et al* reported that acyclovir loaded micelles and acyclovir solution were similar to corneal permeation coefficients, but micelles significantly shortened the permeation lag time through the cornea. In *ex vivo* studies, it was observed that the total amount of acyclovir in the cornea and sclera tissues was 6-fold and 4-fold higher in micelles, respectively, compared to acyclovir solution. It has also been reported that the scleral permeation of micelles is 10-fold higher than the corneal permeation [118]. Biotin12Hydroxystearicacid-Acyclovir (B-12HS-ACV) is a prodrug of acyclovir. Vadlapudi *et al.* reported that B-12HS-ACV loaded TPGS micelles had extended release and were compatible with human corneal epithelial cells [119]. Cidofovir and its cyclic analogs (cCDF), unlike other anti-viral drugs, are used in the treatment of viral retinitis in AIDS patients [120, 121]. Mandal *et al.* produced Biotin12Hydroxystearicacid-cCDF (B-12HS-cCDF) is also a prodrug loaded micelles. In studies conducted with human retinal pigment epithelial, human corneal epithelial, and human conjunctival epithelial cells, they found that B-12HS-cCDF micelles are compatible with human ocular tissues and their intracellular uptake is higher than free cCDF [122].

Liposomes

Liposomes are drug delivery systems in which a hydrophilic center is surrounded by one or more phospholipid layers. It is an effective dosage form for both hydrophilic and lipophilic drugs because it contains hydrophilic and lipophilic structures together [68,96]. They are an effective dosage form in the ocular field because of their high ocular penetration and low ocular elimination.

Abdelbary produced a total of 19 different liposomes of ciprofloxacin hydrochloride by using different lipids, and a total of 9 different chitosan-coated liposomes of 3 different formulations selected from these 19 liposomes. İn vivo studies have shown that certain liposomal and chitosan-coated liposomal formulations had a long retention time in the eye compared to the ciprofloxacin commercial eye drops (Ciprocin®) [123]. Fusidic acid is a commercially available anti-bacterial agent used in the treatment of ocular infections [117]. The efficacy of fusidic acid liposomes developed by Nicolasi *et al.* was investigated *in vitro* on different gram-positive and gram-negative strains. It has been reported that liposomes have lower MIC values than free fusidic acid and also showed therapeutic efficacy on strains where free fusidic acid did not show anti-bacterial activity [124].

Fresta *et al* showed that liposomal structure increased acyclovir concentration in rabbit aqueous humor by 40-fold compared to free acyclovir in their study with acyclovir in 1999 [125]. In another study, Chetoni *et al.* compared the acyclovir liposomes with acyclovir ointment and its aqueous solution. It was observed that the AUC value of liposomes increased 12-fold and 7-fold, respectively, compared to ointment and an aqueous solution having the same amount of acyclovir as the liposome. The AUC value of Zovirax ointment, which contains almost 10-fold more acyclovir than liposomes, was only 2-fold higher than liposomes. With this study, it was shown that liposomes reduce ocular elimination, achieving higher ocular bioavailability with lower doses [126]. Ferreira *et al* developed moxifloxacin liposomes and reported that liposomes reached their maximum concentration 2 hours after intracameral administration and that the therapeutic moxifloxacin concentration in ocular tissues was maintained for 24 hours [127]. In another study, Ren *et al* found that the corneal permeability of azithromycin ion-pair liposomes, which they developed for use in the treatment of dry eye disease, was 2-fold higher than the azithromycin solution. In *in vivo* rat pharmacodynamic studies compared with commercial hyaluronic acid sodium eye drops, they showed that liposomes were better than commercial products in reducing the main symptoms of the disease [128].

Distamycin A is an antibiotic that acts on the Herpes simplex virus and Varicella zoster virus by a mechanism different from acyclovir and its analogues [129]. Chetoni *et al.* developed distamycin A liposomes. They reported that the amount of distamycin A in the tear fluids of rabbits after application of liposomes was found in therapeutic concentrations, and the liposome structure also reduced the toxicity of distamycin A [130].

Different ocular drug delivery systems of voriconazole, an anti-fungal agent in the triazole group, are being studied frequently. De Sa *et al* developed voriconazole liposomes with cholesterol, soybean phosphatidylcholine, and 1,2-dioleoyl-3-trimethylammonium-propane. When they applied the liposomes to the *ex vivo* porcine cornea, they reported that the amount of voriconazole permeated to the cornea at the end of 30 minutes was above the therapeutic concentration based on the the MIC value [131].

Niosomes

Niosomes are the dosage form developed because of the chemical stability problems of liposomes. It has a double-layer structure composed of non-ionic surfactants and has a size of 10-1000 nm. Because of its amphiphilic character, both lipophilic and hydrophilic drugs can be loaded in it. It is structurally non-toxic and has high biocompatibility [69, 95].

Khalil *et al* examined the effectiveness of lomefloxacin niosomes *in vivo* (rabbit). The anti-bacterial efficacy and the AUC value in the first 12 hours of niosomes was higher than commercial lomefloxacin eye drops (Orchacin®). There was a significant improvement in therapeutic response has been noted after eight days of treatment [132].

The natamycin-loaded niosomes developed by El-Nabarawi *et al* had extended release over 24 hours. In comparative studies with ketoconazole and natamycin commercial ocular suspensions (Natacyn®), it was reported that liposomes showed similar anti-fungal activity with commercial products, whereas free natamycin failed. *in vivo* rabbit studies, liposomes had better results on corneal infiltration and hypopyon level compared to ketoconazole and natamycin commercial ocular suspensions [133]. Clotrimazole is another anti-fungal agent. Basha *et al* compared clotrimazole niosomes to clotrimazole suspension in *in vivo* rabbit model. It was reported that niosomes had a 3-fold higher AUC value than the suspension without any ocular toxicity [134].

Spanlastics

Spanlastics are drug delivery systems that were first developed by Kakkar and Kaur by giving elasticity to the vesicles of conventional niosomes with surfactants [135]. These aimed to increase the corneal permeation with the increase of the elasticity of niosomes. Kakkar and Kaur developed the spanlastics and conventional niosome of ketoconazole. In studies with *ex vivo* porcine cornea, it was found that the corneal permeation of spanlastics was 1.3-fold and 1.8-fold higher than conventional niosome and ketoconazole suspension, respectively. In *in vivo* studies, spanlastics was detected in ocular tissues without any deformation after the application of 2 hours. Spanlastics, which may have a safety risk due to their high surfactant content, were found to be compatible with ocular tissues in cytotoxic studies. ElMeshad *et al.*, found that spanlastics increased the *ex vivo* permeation of itraconazole from conventional niosomes by 1.34-fold in their studies with itraconazole spanlastics and conventional niosomes. Also, it was observed that the structure of spanlastics significantly increased the inhibition zone of itraconazole in *in vitro* anti-fungal activity studies [136].

Bilosomes

Since a drug delivery system with bioadhesive property penetrates the target tissues better, it is expected to increase the bioavailability of the drug. Bile salts are widely used in the pharmaceutical industry as a natural penetration enhancing agent. Bilosomes are carrier systems formed by the amphiphilic bilayer of niosomes containing bile salt [137]. In fact, although they were developed with the aim of increasing oral bioavailability, different tissue-targeted bilosomes have been developed over time [138, 139]. Bilosomes have also been used in ocular drug targeting in recent years.

Yousry *et al* developed ocular targeted terconazole bilosomes. It was observed that the structure of the bilisome significantly reduced the cytotoxic effect of the suspension and solution of terconazole. IC50 dose of bilosomes was found 11-fold higher than suspension and solution in *in vitro* cell culture studies. İn vivo studies have also supported these results. After that, researchers prepared the integrated nanovesicular / self-nano emulsifying system (INV/SNES) of these bilosomes. It was found that INV/SNES is more effective than the terconazole suspension in treating ocular fungal infections in *in vivo* efficacy studies [140]. Another study with terconazole was done by Abdelbary *et al*. Developing the conventional niosomes and bilosomes of terconazole, they also developed the ultradeformable bilosomes (UBs) carrier system, which increases corneal permeation by providing extra flexibility to the vesicles of the bilosomes. After examinations, it was found that *ex vivo* corneal permeation of UBs was 1.5-fold, 2-fold, and 3-fold more than conventional bilozomes, niosomes, and drug suspension, respectively. Also, it has been observed that UBs are compatible with ocular tissues *in vivo* studies [141].

Cubosomes

Nanoparticles produced with liquid crystals are called cubosomes [96]. Antifungal drugs come to the fore in studies of ocular cubosomes. Fluconazole cubosomes have been evaluated *ex vivo* and *in vivo* . *ex vivo* corneal permeability of cubosomal fluconazole was found to be 2-fold higher than the fluconazole solution. Also, in *in vivo* studies, cubosomes reduced corneal opacity 2-fold more than fluconazole solution [142]. Younes *et al* reported that corneal permeation of sertaconazole nitrate cubosomes was better than sertaconazole suspension in both *ex vivo* and *in vivo* studies [143]. In studies conducted with natamycin, it was observed that cubosomal structure increased *ex vivo* corneal permeation compared to the suspension dosage form [144].

Dendrimers

Dendrimers contain a nucleus at their center and functional groups attached to this nucleus. These structures resemble trees. For this reason, they got their name from the word "dendro," which means tree in Greek. These functional groups can be single or they can repeat themselves by being connected to each other. If functional groups are connected to each other and branched, other generations occur, and the repetition of these groups is called the "number of generations." The generation number is expressed with "G." If there is only one functional group directly connected to the nucleus, these dendrimers are called G-0, *i.e* .the zeroth generation. If the number of branches of a functional group that is directly connected to the center is 2, for example, that dendrimer is called the 2nd generation or G-2 [69,95,145].

Polyguanidylated translocators dendrimers (DPTs) are formed triolyl branches and surface guanidine groups [146]. Durairaj *et al*.produced gatifloxacin dendrimers using DPTs. Dendrimers were found to have anti-bacterial activity 3-fold faster than free gatifloxacin. In cell uptake studies, it was observed that dendrimers showed permeability to human corneal epithelial cells within 5 minutes and to bovine sclera-choroid-retina pigment epithelium within 6 hours [147].

Ciprofloxacin-triazine dendrimers, developed by Vembu *et al.*, were found to be 5-fold more effective than the ciprofloxacin standard in the anti-bacterial activity test performed on different strains [148]. Although ocular permeation and penetration studies of these dendrimers have not been performed, it was predicted that dendrimers would increase the ocular bioavailability of ciprofloxacin.

Hydrogels

Hydrogels are drug delivery systems that are produced by polymers forming three-dimensional networks in water and increase ocular bioavailability by extending the drug retention time in the conjunctival cul-de-sac [69,145]. Hydrogels are differentiated into two groups as pre-gelled systems and *In-situ* systems [149]. Pre-gelled systems are simple viscous solutions applied to the eyes [150]. *In-situ* gels are drug delivery systems that are becoming gel form after being applied as a solution depending on the pH, temperature, and ion balance of the range of application. Hydrogels are safe, simple, and repeatable products, especially for anterior eye diseases [151]. HyloTM (Candorvision, Montreal, QC, Canada), Aqualarm® (Bausch + Lomb, Bridgewater, NJ, USA), Vismed® (Horus Pharma, Saint-Laurent-du-Var, France), and Geltim® (LP, Thea, Clermont-Ferrand, France) are examples of commercial ocular hydrogel products [150].

Hydrogels can be prepared either directly from a free drug with gelling agents or with any ocular drug delivery system. There are many hydrogel studies in the literature for ocular drug targeting. Some of these studies are summarized in Table 4 below. Proniosomes in compact liquid crystal gel form, which can be easily obtained from niosomes by means of hydration [152], are also included in this group.

Ocular Inserts, Implants, Lenses And Other Devices

Although ocular implants and inserts are described as the same dosage form in many sources, they differ mainly in the way they are applied to the eye. Ocular inserts are the dosage form placed right between the eyelid and the sclera on the conjunctival ridge. Implants are systems that are surgically placed in the eye [167]. Ocusert containing pilocarpine for use in the treatment of ocular hypertension is the first known successful ocular insert [168].

Ocular lenses are thin, transparent, curved and round systems according to the shape of the eyeball, placed directly on the eye surface. They increase the contact time of the drug with the ocular tissue. It is one of the applicable methods for the treatment of anterior ocular diseases. Oxygen permeability is one of the most important challenging steps in its production. The risk of contamination is their major disadvantage, and they can cause any ocular infection to develop in the event of possible contamination [150,169].

Table 4. Hydrogelling ocular drug delivery system studies.

Loaded Drug	Hydrogel Based Nanocarrier	Polymers/ Surfactants/ Lipids	Comments	References
Ciprofloxacin	Nanostuctered lipid carriers	Tween 80/ Poloxamer 188/ Glycerin/ Precirol ATO 5/ Oleic acid/ Gellan gum	• Increased transcorneal and permeability compared to ciprofloxacin nanolipid carriers and commercial eye drop.	[153]
Curcumin	Micelles	Pluronic P123/ TPGS/ Gellan gum	• Increased cumulative corneal penetration (*ex vivo* rabbit cornea).	[154]

(Table 4) cont.....

Fluconazole	Niosomes	Span® 60/ Span® 80/ Castor oil/ Olive oil/ Soya oil/ Tween® 80/ PEG 400	• Increased bioavailability of fluconazole 2-fold compared to fluconazole microemulsion in *in vivo* rabbit models.	[155]
	Liposomes	Hyaluronic acid/ Lipoid S100/ Cholesterol Tween 80/ Transcutol HP/ Caproyl 90	• Increased corneal permeability of fluconazole 2.99-fold and 4.18-fold compared to fluconazole liposome and suspension, respectively. • Retention in therapeutic dose for fluconazole in ocular tissues for 24 hours in *in vivo* (rabbit) studies.	[156]
Itraconazole	Micelles	Pluronic F127/ Pluronic F68/ Carbopol 934P	• Increased *ex vivo* corneal permeation 5-fold compared to itraconazole eye drops (Itral®) and pure drug suspension • Increased *in vitro* mucoadhesive strength 40-fold higher than the ocular shear stress. • Increased *in vitro* anti-fungal activity compared to itraconazole eye drops (Itral®).	[157]
		Synperonic® F108/ Synperonic® P84/ β-cyclodextrin	• Increase ocular permeation and anti-fungal activity of itraconazole compared to itraconazole suspension in *ex vivo* and *in vivo* rabbit models.	[158]
Ketoconazole	Proniosomes	Span 20/ Span 60/ Span 65/ Span80/ Tween 80/ Brij 35/ Brij 72/ Brij 92/ Pluronic F68/ Pluronic L121/ L---phosphatidylcholine from egg Yolk/ Cholesterol	• Increased bioavailability of ketoconazol 20-fold compared to ketoconazole suspension in *in vivo* rabbit models.	[159]
Levofloxacin	Nanoparticles	PLGA/ Poly vinyl alcohol (PVA)	• Increased corneal permeability with nanoparticle *In-situ* gels compared to nanoparticle or free levofloxacin *In-situ* gel in *in vivo* rabbit models.	[160]

(Table 4) cont.....

Lomefloxacin	Proniosomes	Brij 35*/ Span 20*/ Span 40*/ Span 60*/ Tween 80*/ Brij 98*/ Brij 72*/ Tween 40*/ Tween 60*/ Cholesterol	• Increased anti-bacterial activity compared to commercial lomefloxacin eye drops (Orchacin*) in *in vivo* rabbit models.	[152]
	Niosomes	Span 20*/ Span 60*/ Span* 80/ Poluronic* F127/ Poluronic* F68/ HPMC	• Increased corneal penetration compared to lomefloxacin solution. • Increased lomefloxacin concentration 2-fold to 5-fold in ocular tissues compared to commercial lomefloxacin eye drops (Orchacin*) in *in vivo* (rabbit) studies. • Increased antimicrobial efficacy of lomefloxacin 35-fold compared to free lomefloxacin.	[161]
Natamycin	Bilosomes	Sodium taurocholate/ Span 60*/ Cholesterol/ Gellan Gum/ Xanthum gum	• Increased corneal penetration in *in vivo* rabbit models 9-fold and 1.5-fold compared to commercial natamycin ocular suspension (Natacyn*) and natamycin bilosomes, respectively.	[162]
	Transfersomes	Phospholipon* 90H/ TPGS/ Span 60*/ Gellan Gum	• Increased transcorneal permeability and ocular disposition compared to natamycin suspension (Natacyn*) in *in vivo* rabbit models.	[163]
Ofloxacin	Micelles	Poluronic* F127/ Poluronic* F68	• Increased *in vitro* and *in vivo* (rabbit) retention time of hydrogels based on micelles	[164]
Tobramycin	Microparticles	Chitosan/ Poloxamer 407	• Increased *in vitro* ocular permeability of tobramycin 2-fold compared to commercial eye drop (Toba*).	[165]
Vancomycin	Niosomes	Tween 40/ Span 60/ Cholesterol/ Carbopol 934P/ HPMC	• Increased anti-bacterial efficacy of vancomycin 180-fold and 2.5-fold compared to the untreated animals (rabbit) and the animals (rabbit) treated with the vancomycin free drug solution, respectively.	[166]

Pawar *et al.* produced moxifloxacin inserts using different types of Eudragit. It was found that inserts, which were observed to maintain their stability for 2 years, release the drug from 7 hours to 9 hours, and *ex vivo* ocular permeation was high [170]. Samanta *et al*.reported that the developed inserts released the ciprofloxacin at the therapeutic dose for two days in *in vivo* rabbit studies [171]. Polat *et al.* produced besifloxacin loaded nanofibers using cyclodextrin. They used Ussing Chamber in *ex vivo* transport experiments, which is specially designed to measure epithelial membrane properties by the Danish zoologist and physiologist Hans Henriksen Ussing [172]. *ex vivo* transport of besifloxacin loaded nanofibrous ocular inserts was similar to the commercial product (Besivance®) in rabbit cornea. They also showed the anti-bacterial activity of nanofibrous in *in vivo* rabbit models [173].

Bozdağ Pehlivan *et al.* prepared implants of cyclosporine A nanoparticles produced with PLGA or PCL using molding and electrospinning methods. They showed that the release of cyclosporine A from the implants was extended between 30 and 60 days. They also concluded that the implants were compatible with ocular tissues due to relatively high cell viability (77.4% -99.0%). The effectiveness of the implants was proven by *in vivo* studies (mice) [174]. Another implant study with PLGA was done by Fernandes-Cunha *et al.* Clindamycin implants have been shown to be non-toxic in cell culture and *in vivo* studies both rabbit and rat [175].

Ciolino *et al.* loaded econazole in contact lenses. It has been observed that the contact lenses were effective on the Candida albicans strain. They also found that the amount of econazole-PLGA film loaded on contact lenses affects the effectiveness of fungicidal activity [176]. Danion *et al.* reported that contact lenses decorated with levofloxacin liposomes had an anti-bacterial activity for 24 hours [177].

Microneedles are drug delivery systems manufactured as solid, hollow, or soluble needles ranging from 50-1000 μm in an area of 0.5-1.5 cm^2 [178]. Microneedles, a suitable carrier system for large molecules, hormones, and proteins, have been used transdermally in cosmetics and vaccine fields for years [179]. Examples of approved products for microneedles are Dermaroller®, BD Soluvia™ (BD Company), and MicronJet 600™ (NanoPass Technologies Ltd) [180]. Microneedles are made into patch form using various materials such as metals, ceramics, silicon, and polymers [178]. These patches are not only used transdermally but are also preferred for drug targeting to different tissues [179, 181].

The first study of microneedles in the ocular drug delivery was done by Jiang *et al*. They coated 500-750 μm length microneedles using protein, DNA, sodium fluorescein, or pilocarpine [182]. They examined these microneedles both in the human sclera they isolated from the cadaver and in *in vivo* rabbit experiments. It was reported that the drug was rapidly dissolved from the needles in the scleral tissue within 30 seconds after insertion. For sodium fluorescein microneedles, the fluorescence concentration in the anterior segment of rabbits was 60 times higher than that of topical application in studies with sodium fluorescein. The rapid and widespread narrowing was observed in the rabbit pupil with pilocarpine microneedles.

Bhatnagar *et al*. tested besifloxacin microneedles on human cornea isolated from cadaver. They found that the application of microneedles for 5 min significantly improved the besifloxacin deposition and permeation through the cornea compared with free besifloxacin solution [183]. Roy *et al*. compared amphotericin B microneedle ocular patch with amphotericin B liposomes and free amphotericin B. Ocular patches were found to increase the *ex vivo* corneal permeation of amphotericin B. Also, the anti-fungal activity of ocular patches was determined by *ex vivo* and *in vivo* (rabbit) experiments [184].

CONCLUSION AND FUTURE PERSPECTIVES

Ocular infections may occur due to contamination with bacterial, viral, fungal, or parasitic strains, as well as when an underlying systemic disorder activates opportunistic pathogens. These infections that are not treated quickly with the suitable agent can cause loss of visual function. For this reason, it is very important to isolate the pathogen species causing the infection and to select the appropriate anti-infective agent.

0% of commercial ocular products currently available are in a conventional dosage form. For this reason, their ocular bioavailability is very low. Also, different methods used in the administration of ocular drugs can cause complications and decrease patient compliance. On the other hand, new drug delivery systems developed to reduce the dose and frequency of drugs have a potential to increase ocular bioavailability and patient compliance, also enable drugs to be targeted to the organ or tissue. The development of ocular drug delivery systems is one of the most challenging topic in pharmaceutical technology due to the limitations of natural barriers created by the anatomy and physiology of the eye.

Anti-infective agents are frequently the subject of ocular drug delivery systems. The efficiency of many micro and nanocarriers developed in this field has been demonstrated by *in vitro* and *in vivo* studies. The fact that there are products approved by the USFDA, EMA or other regulatory authority among these delivery systems by completing phase studies that show that drug delivery systems are promising in the ocular field. Some examples of approved drug delivery systems are given in Table 5. In addition to Table 5, clinical studies of cyclosporine products named PADciclo™ (a carbomer hydrogel), CyclASol® (semi-fluorinated alkanes solution) and ApidSOL® (micelles) are ongoing [185].

Table 5. List of novel ocular products approved by different regulatory authorities.

Active Ingredient	Trade Name	Dosage Form	Approved Authority	References
Cyclosporine	Cequa®	Micellar eye drop	USFDA	[104]
	Papilock mini®		PMDA	[185]
	TJ Cyporin®		MFDS	[185]
	Restasis®	Nanoemulsions	USFDA	[84]
	Ikervis®		EMA	[185]
	Vekacia®			[186]
	Clacier™		MFDS	[187]
	Cyporin N®			[188]
Fluocinolone acetonide	Retisert®	Intravitreal implant	USFDA, EMA	[84,189]
	Iluvien®			[84,190]
Ganciclovir	Vitrasert®	Implant		[84,191]

Thanks to the drug delivery systems, a drug known to have ocular toxicity can be compatible with ocular tissues. However, the ocular safety of the polymers or surfactants used in the preparation of drug delivery systems should also be considered. Some of the polymers and surfactants are biocompatible, and their ocular safety has been proven over the years. However, the ocular toxicity of some polymers and surfactants that may be created by long-term use is still unclear. Moreover, the long-term effects of high doses of lipids or surfactants used in carrier systems produced with natural lipids are not known.

Based on the aforementioned background, together with the necessity of closely monitoring their ocular safety, drug delivery systems appear to be important in ocular drug targeting of anti-infective agents and increasing bioavailability.

CONSENT FOR PUBLICATION

Not Applicable.

CONFLICT OF INTEREST

The author declares no conflict of interest, financial or otherwise.

ACKNOWLEDGEMENTS

Declared none.

REFERENCES

[1] Kels BD, Grzybowski A, Grant-Kels JM. Human ocular anatomy. Clin Dermatol 2015; 33(2): 140-6. https://linkinghub.elsevier.com/retrieve/pii/S0738081X1400234X [Internet].
[http://dx.doi.org/10.1016/j.clindermatol.2014.10.006] [PMID: 25704934]

[2] Beuerman RW, Pedroza L. Ultrastructure of the human cornea. Microsc Res Tech 1996; 33(4): 320-35. https://onlinelibrary.wiley.com/doi/10.1002/(SICI)1097-0029(19960301)33:4%3C320::AI--JEMT3%3E3.0.CO;2-T [Internet].
[http://dx.doi.org/10.1002/(SICI)1097-0029(19960301)33:4<320::AID-JEMT3>3.0.CO;2-T] [PMID: 8652889]

[3] Durairaj C. Ocular Pharmacokinetics.Pharmacologic Therapy of Ocular Disease. Cham: Springer 2016; pp. 31-55.http://link.springer.com/10.1007/164_2016_32 Internet
[http://dx.doi.org/10.1007/164_2016_32]

[4] Urtti A. Challenges and obstacles of ocular pharmacokinetics and drug delivery. Adv Drug Deliv Rev 2006; 58(11): 1131-5. https://linkinghub.elsevier.com/retrieve/pii/S0169409X06001578 [Internet].
[http://dx.doi.org/10.1016/j.addr.2006.07.027] [PMID: 17097758]

[5] Nettey H, Darko Y, Bamiro OA, Addo RT. Ocular Barriers.Ocular Drug Delivery: Advances, Challenges and Applications. Cham: Springer International Publishing 2016; pp. 27-36.http://link.springer.com/10.1007/978-3-319-47691-9_3 Internet
[http://dx.doi.org/10.1007/978-3-319-47691-9_3]

[6] Winter KN, Anderson DM, Braun RJ, Sharma NSR, Thrimawithana T, Young S, *et al.* A model for wetting and evaporation of a post-blink precorneal tear film. Drug Deliv Lett 2009; 37(3): 40-4.
[PMID: 19861501]

[7] Pepic I, Lovric J, Filipovic-Grcic J. Polymeric Micelles in Ocular Drug Delivery: Rationale, Strategies and Challenges. Chem Biochem Eng Q 2012; 26(4): 365.

[8] Cholkar K, Gunda S, Earla R, Pal D, Mitra AK. Nanomicellar Topical Aqueous Drop Formulation of Rapamycin for Back-of-the-Eye Delivery. AAPS PharmSciTech 2015; 16(3): 610-22.http://link.springer.com/10.1208/s12249-014-0244-2 [Internet].
[http://dx.doi.org/10.1208/s12249-014-0244-2] [PMID: 25425389]

[9] Pascolini D, Mariotti SP. Global estimates of visual impairment: 2010. Br J Ophthalmol 2012; 96(5): 614-8.http://bjo.bmj.com/lookup/doi/10.1136/bjophthalmol-2011-300539 [Internet].
[http://dx.doi.org/10.1136/bjophthalmol-2011-300539] [PMID: 22133988]

[10] Sponsel WE, Graybill JR, Nevarez HL, Dang D. Ocular and systemic posaconazole(SCH-56592) treatment of invasive Fusarium solani keratitis and endophthalmitis. Br J Ophthalmol 2002; 86(7): 829-30.http://bjo.bmj.com/cgi/doi/10.1136/bjo.86.7.829-a [Internet].
[http://dx.doi.org/10.1136/bjo.86.7.829-a] [PMID: 12084760]

[11] Watson S, Cabrera-Aguas M, Khoo P. Common eye infections. Aust Prescr 2018; 41(3): 67-72.
[http://dx.doi.org/10.18773/austprescr.2018.016] [PMID: 29922000]

[12] Austin A, Lietman T, Rose-Nussbaumer J. Update on the Management of Infectious Keratitis. Ophthalmology 2017; 124(11): 1678-89. https://linkinghub.elsevier.com/retrieve/pii/S0161642 016325295 [Internet].

[http://dx.doi.org/10.1016/j.ophtha.2017.05.012] [PMID: 28942073]

[13] Petrovic A, Hashemi K, Blaser F, Wild W, Kymionis G. Characteristics of Linear Interstitial Keratitis by *in vivo* Confocal Microscopy and Anterior Segment Optical Coherence Tomography. Cornea 2018; 37(6): 785-8.http://journals.lww.com/00003226-201806000-00020 [Internet].
[http://dx.doi.org/10.1097/ICO.0000000000001552] [PMID: 29543661]

[14] Vantieghem G, Maudgal PC. Neuroparalytic keratopathy as the first sign of a cerebral meningioma. Bull Soc Belge Ophtalmol 2007; (303): 81-6.http://www.ncbi.nlm.nih.gov/pubmed/17894293 [Internet].
[PMID: 17894293]

[15] Sacchetti M, Lambiase A, Lambiase A. Diagnosis and management of neurotrophic keratitis. Clin Ophthalmol 2014; 8(Mar): 571-9. http://www.dovepress.com/diagnosis-and- management-o--neurotrophic-keratitis-peer-reviewed-article-OPTH [Internet].
[PMID: 24672223]

[16] Lorenzo-Morales J, Khan NA, Walochnik J. An update on Acanthamoeba keratitis: diagnosis, pathogenesis and treatment. Parasite 2015; 22: 10. http://www.parasite-journal.org/10.1051/parasite/2015010 [Internet].
[http://dx.doi.org/10.1051/parasite/2015010] [PMID: 25687209]

[17] Bairagi SH. Acanthamoeba Keratitis: Diagnosis and Treatment. J Rare Disord Diagnosis Ther [Internet] 2018; 03(04) http://raredisorders.imedpub.com/acanthamoeba-keratitis -diagnosis- and-treatment.php?aid=19803

[18] D'Aguanno V, Ralli M, de Vincentiis M, Greco A. Optimal management of Cogan's syndrome: a multidisciplinary approach. J Multidiscip Healthc 2017; 11: 1-11. https://www.dovepress.com/optimal-management-of-cogans-syndrome-a-multidisciplinary-approach -peer-reviewed-article-JMDH [Internet].
[http://dx.doi.org/10.2147/JMDH.S150940] [PMID: 29317827]

[19] Rajaii F, Prescott C. Management of Exposure Keratopathy. Eyenet 2014; pp. 37-8.

[20] Visscher KL, Hutnik CML, Thomas M. Evidence-based treatment of acute infective conjunctivitis: Breaking the cycle of antibiotic prescribing. Can Fam Physician 2009; 55(11): 1071-5.http://www.ncbi.nlm.nih.gov/pubmed/19910590 [Internet].
[PMID: 19910590]

[21] Kaufman HE. Adenovirus advances: new diagnostic and therapeutic options. Curr Opin Ophthalmol 2011; 22(4): 290-3.http://journals.lww.com/00055735-201107000-00015 [Internet].
[http://dx.doi.org/10.1097/ICU.0b013e3283477cb5] [PMID: 21537185]

[22] Rietveld RP, ter Riet G, Bindels PJ, Schellevis FG, van Weert HC. Do general practitioners adhere to the guideline on infectious conjunctivitis? Results of the Second Dutch National Survey of General Practice. BMC Fam Pract 2007; 8(1): 54. https://bmcfampract.biomedcentral.com/articles/10.1186/1471-2296-8-54 [Internet].
[http://dx.doi.org/10.1186/1471-2296-8-54] [PMID: 17868475]

[23] Sheikh A, Hurwitz B. Antibiotics versus placebo for acute bacterial conjunctivitis.Cochrane Database of Systematic Reviews. Chichester, UK: John Wiley & Sons, Ltd 2006.http://doi.wiley.com/10.1002/14651858.CD001211.pub2 Internet
[http://dx.doi.org/10.1002/14651858.CD001211.pub2]

[24] Daniel Diaz J, Sobol EK, Gritz DC. Treatment and management of scleral disorders. Surv Ophthalmol 2016; 61(6): 702-17. https://linkinghub.elsevier.com/retrieve/pii/S0039625715300825 [Internet].
[http://dx.doi.org/10.1016/j.survophthal.2016.06.002] [PMID: 27318032]

[25] Sridhar MS, Gopinathan U, Rao GN. Fungal keratitis associated with vernal keratoconjunctivitis. Cornea 2003; 22(1): 80-1.http://journals.lww.com/00003226-200301000-00020 [Internet].
[http://dx.doi.org/10.1097/00003226-200301000-00020] [PMID: 12502957]

[26] Reddy JC, Murthy SI, Reddy AK, Garg P. Risk factors and clinical outcomes of bacterial and fungal scleritis at a tertiary eye care hospital. Middle East Afr J Ophthalmol 2015; 22(2): 203-11. http://www.meajo.org/text.asp?2015/22/2/203/150634 [Internet].
[http://dx.doi.org/10.4103/0974-9233.150634] [PMID: 25949079]

[27] Barry P, Cordovés L, Gardner S. ESCRS Guidelines for Prevention and Treatment of Endophthalmitis Following Cataract Surgery: Data, Dilemmas and Conclusions 2013. https://www.escrs.org/downloads/Endophthalmitis -Guidelines.pdf

[28] Yenerel NM, Dinc UA, Gorgun E. A case of sterile endophthalmitis after repeated intravitreal bevacizumab injection. J Ocul Pharmacol Ther 2008; 24(3): 362-3. http://www.liebertpub.com/doi/10.1089/jop.2007.0126 [Internet].
[http://dx.doi.org/10.1089/jop.2007.0126] [PMID: 18476807]

[29] Durand ML. Endophthalmitis. Clin Microbiol Infect 2013; 19(3): 227-34. https://linkinghub.elsevier.com/retrieve/pii/S1198743X14601282 [Internet].
[http://dx.doi.org/10.1111/1469-0691.12118] [PMID: 23438028]

[30] Artunay O, Yuzbasioglu E, Rasier R, Sengül A, Bahcecioglu H. Incidence and management of acute endophthalmitis after intravitreal bevacizumab (Avastin) injection. Eye (Lond) 2009; 23(12): 2187-93.http://www.nature.com/articles/eye20097 [Internet].
[http://dx.doi.org/10.1038/eye.2009.7] [PMID: 19218994]

[31] Sharma SM, Jackson D. Uveitis and spondyloarthropathies. Best Pract Res Clin Rheumatol 2017; 31(6): 846-62. [Internet].
[http://dx.doi.org/10.1016/j.berh.2018.08.002] [PMID: 30509444]

[32] Sonmez K, Ozturk F. Complications of intravitreal triamcinolone acetonide for macular edema and predictive factors for intraocular pressure elevation. Int J Ophthalmol 2012; 5(6): 719-25.
[PMID: 23275907]

[33] Durrani OM, Meads CA, Murray PI. Uveitis: a potentially blinding disease. Ophthalmologica 2004; 218(4): 223-36. https://www.karger.com/Article/FullText/78612 [Internet].
[http://dx.doi.org/10.1159/000078612] [PMID: 15258410]

[34] Krishna U, Ajanaku D, Denniston AK, Gkika T. Uveitis: a sight-threatening disease which can impact all systems. Postgrad Med J 2017; 93(1106): 766-73. http://pmj.bmj.com/lookup/doi/10.1136/postgradmedj-2017-134891 [Internet].
[http://dx.doi.org/10.1136/postgradmedj-2017-134891] [PMID: 28942431]

[35] Guly CM, Forrester JV. Investigation and management of uveitis. BMJ 2010; 341(oct13 3): c4976-6. http://www.bmj.com/cgi/doi/10.1136/bmj.c4976
[http://dx.doi.org/10.1136/bmj.c4976]

[36] Deschenes J, Murray PI, Rao NA, Nussenblatt RB. International Uveitis Study Group (IUSG) Clinical Classification of Uveitis. Ocul Immunol Inflamm 2008; 16(1-2): 1-2. http://www.tandfonline.com/doi/full/10.1080/09273940801899822

[37] Hwang D-K, Chou Y-J, Pu C-Y, Chou P. Epidemiology of uveitis among the Chinese population in Taiwan: a population-based study. Ophthalmology 2012; 119(11): 2371-6. https://linkinghub.elsevier.com/retrieve/pii/S0161642012004526 [Internet].
[http://dx.doi.org/10.1016/j.ophtha.2012.05.026] [PMID: 22809756]

[38] Gritz DC, Wong IG. Incidence and prevalence of uveitis in Northern California; the Northern California Epidemiology of Uveitis Study. Ophthalmology 2004; 111(3): 491-500. https://linkinghub.elsevier.com/retrieve/pii/S0161642003014891 [Internet].
[http://dx.doi.org/10.1016/j.ophtha.2003.06.014] [PMID: 15019324]

[39] Foster CS, Kothari S, Anesi SD, et al. The Ocular Immunology and Uveitis Foundation preferred practice patterns of uveitis management. Surv Ophthalmol 2016; 61(1): 1-17. https://linkinghub.elsevier.com/retrieve/pii/S0039625715001137 [Internet].

[http://dx.doi.org/10.1016/j.survophthal.2015.07.001] [PMID: 26164736]

[40] Moothy RS, Read RW, Birnbaum AD, Levy-Clarke GA, Rao PK, Thorne JA. Uveitis Practising ophthalmologist curriculum 2014-2016 american Academy of ophthalmology 2014. https://www.aao.org/assets/8f1bff17-b02c-4750-b05c.../uveitis-2014-pdf

[41] London NJS, Rathinam SR, Cunningham ET Jr. The epidemiology of uveitis in developing countries. Int Ophthalmol Clin 2010; 50(2): 1-17.http://journals.lww.com/00004397-201005020-00003 [Internet].
[http://dx.doi.org/10.1097/IIO.0b013e3181d2cc6b] [PMID: 20375859]

[42] Miserocchi E, Fogliato G, Modorati G, Bandello F. Review on the worldwide epidemiology of uveitis. Eur J Ophthalmol 2013; 23(5): 705-17.http://journals.sagepub.com/doi/10.5301/ejo.5000278 [Internet].
[http://dx.doi.org/10.5301/ejo.5000278] [PMID: 23661536]

[43] Jabs DA, Mudun A, Dunn JPP, Marsh MJ. Episcleritis and scleritis: clinical features and treatment results. Am J Ophthalmol 2000; 130(4): 469-76. https://linkinghub.elsevier.com/retrieve/pii/S0002939400007108 [Internet].
[http://dx.doi.org/10.1016/S0002-9394(00)00710-8] [PMID: 11024419]

[44] Watson PG, Hayreh SS. Scleritis and episcleritis. Br J Ophthalmol 1976; 60(3): 163-91.http://bjo.bmj.com/cgi/doi/10.1136/bjo.60.3.163 [Internet].
[http://dx.doi.org/10.1136/bjo.60.3.163] [PMID: 1268179]

[45] Okhravi N, Odufuwa B, McCluskey P, Lightman S. Scleritis. Surv Ophthalmol 2005; 50(4): 351-63. https://linkinghub.elsevier.com/retrieve/pii/S0039625705000391 [Internet].
[http://dx.doi.org/10.1016/j.survophthal.2005.04.001] [PMID: 15967190]

[46] McCluskey PJ, Watson PG, Lightman S, Haybittle J, Restori M, Branley M. Posterior scleritis: clinical features, systemic associations, and outcome in a large series of patients. Ophthalmology 1999; 106(12): 2380-6.http://www.ncbi.nlm.nih.gov/pubmed/10599675 [Internet].
[http://dx.doi.org/10.1016/S0161-6420(99)90543-2] [PMID: 10599675]

[47] Watson PG, Young RD. Scleral structure, organisation and disease. A review. Exp Eye Res 2004; 78(3): 609-23. https://linkinghub.elsevier.com/retrieve/pii/S0014483503002124 [Internet].
[http://dx.doi.org/10.1016/S0014-4835(03)00212-4] [PMID: 15106941]

[48] Sainz de la Maza M, Jabbur NS, Foster CS. Severity of scleritis and episcleritis. Ophthalmology 1994; 101(2): 389-96.http://www.ncbi.nlm.nih.gov/pubmed/8115160 [Internet].
[http://dx.doi.org/10.1016/S0161-6420(94)31325-X] [PMID: 8115160]

[49] Veenashree MP, Sangwan VS, Vemuganti GK, Parthasaradhi A. Acute scleritis as a manifestation of congenital erythropoietic porphyria. Cornea 2002; 21(5): 530-1.http://journals.lww.com/00003226-200207000-00018 [Internet].
[http://dx.doi.org/10.1097/00003226-200207000-00018] [PMID: 12072732]

[50] Kim RY, Anderlini P, Naderi AA, Rivera P, Ahmadi MAA, Esmaeli B. Scleritis as the initial clinical manifestation of graft- *versus* -host disease after allogenic bone marrow transplantation. Am J Ophthalmol 2002; 133(6): 843-5. https://linkinghub.elsevier.com/retrieve/pii/S0002939402014253 [Internet].
[http://dx.doi.org/10.1016/S0002-9394(02)01425-3] [PMID: 12036687]

[51] DeCroos FC, Garg P, Reddy AK, *et al.* Hyderabad Endophthalmitis Research Group. Optimizing diagnosis and management of nocardia keratitis, scleritis, and endophthalmitis: 11-year microbial and clinical overview. Ophthalmology 2011; 118(6): 1193-200. https://linkinghub.elsevier.com/retrieve/pii/S0161642010011589 [Internet].
[http://dx.doi.org/10.1016/j.ophtha.2010.10.037] [PMID: 21276615]

[52] Hwang Y-S, Chen Y-F, Lai C-C, Chen HS-L, Hsiao C-H. Infectious scleritis after use of immunomodulators. Arch Ophthalmol (Chicago, Ill 1960) 1960; 120(8): 1093-4. http://www.ncbi.nlm.nih.gov/pubmed/12149068

[53] Moreno Honrado M, del Campo Z, Buil JA. A case of necrotizing scleritis resulting from Pseudomonas aeruginosa. Cornea 2009; 28(9): 1065-6.http://journals.lww.com/00003226-200910000-00021 [Internet].
[http://dx.doi.org/10.1097/ICO.0b013e3181971213] [PMID: 19724201]

[54] Helm CJ, Holland GN, Webster RG Jr, Maloney RK, Mondino BJ. Combination intravenous ceftazidime and aminoglycosides in the treatment of pseudomonal scleritis. Ophthalmology 1997; 104(5): 838-43. https://linkinghub.elsevier.com/retrieve/pii/S0161642097302255 [Internet].
[http://dx.doi.org/10.1016/S0161-6420(97)30225-5] [PMID: 9160031]

[55] Moriarty AP, Crawford GJ, McAllister IL, Constable IJ. Bilateral streptococcal corneoscleritis complicating beta irradiation induced scleral necrosis. Br J Ophthalmol 1993; 77(4): 251-2.http://bjo.bmj.com/cgi/doi/10.1136/bjo.77.4.251 [Internet].
[http://dx.doi.org/10.1136/bjo.77.4.251] [PMID: 8494865]

[56] Paula JS. Sim??o MLH, Rocha EM, Rom??o E, Velasco Cruz AA. Atypical Pneumococcal Scleritis After Pterygium Excision. Cornea 2006; 25(1): 115-7.http://journals.lww.com/00003226-200601000-00021 [Internet].
[http://dx.doi.org/10.1097/01.ico.0000164784.18290.45] [PMID: 16331053]

[57] Moriarty AP, Crawford GJ, McAllister IL, Constable IJ, Mc Allister IL, Constable IJ. Fungal corneoscleritis complicating beta-irradiation-induced scleral necrosis following pterygium excision. Eye (Lond) 1993; 7(Pt 4): 525-8.http://www.nature.com/articles/eye1993114 [Internet].
[http://dx.doi.org/10.1038/eye.1993.114] [PMID: 8253231]

[58] Moriarty AP, Crawford GJ, McAllister IL, Constable IJ. Severe corneoscleral infection. A complication of beta irradiation scleral necrosis following pterygium excision. Arch Ophthalmol 1993; 111(7): 947-51. http://archopht.jamanetwork.com/article.aspx?doi=10.1001/archopht.1993.01090070065021 [Internet].
[http://dx.doi.org/10.1001/archopht.1993.01090070065021] [PMID: 8328937]

[59] MacKenzie FD, Hirst LW, Kynaston B, Bain C. Recurrence rate and complications after beta irradiation for pterygia. Ophthalmology 1991; 98(12): 1776-80. https://linkinghub.elsevier.com/retrieve/pii/S0161642091320517 [Internet].
[http://dx.doi.org/10.1016/S0161-6420(91)32051-7] [PMID: 1775309]

[60] Kolomeyer AM, Ragam A, Shah K, Do BK, Shah VP, Chu DS. Cyclo-oxygenase inhibitors in the treatment of chronic non-infectious, non-necrotizing scleritis and episcleritis. Ocul Immunol Inflamm 2012; 20(4): 293-9.http://www.tandfonline.com/doi/full/10.3109/09273948.2012.689075 [Internet].
[http://dx.doi.org/10.3109/09273948.2012.689075] [PMID: 22642498]

[61] Williams CPRR, Browning AC, Sleep TJ, Webber SK, McGill JI. A randomised, double-blind trial of topical ketorolac vs artificial tears for the treatment of episcleritis. Eye (Lond) 2005; 19(7): 739-42.http://www.nature.com/articles/6701632 [Internet].
[http://dx.doi.org/10.1038/sj.eye.6701632] [PMID: 15359265]

[62] Wakefield D, Di Girolamo N, Thurau S, Wildner G, McCluskey P. Scleritis: Immunopathogenesis and molecular basis for therapy. Prog Retin Eye Res 2013; 35: 44-62. https://linkinghub.elsevier.com/retrieve/pii/S1350946213000189 [Internet].
[http://dx.doi.org/10.1016/j.preteyeres.2013.02.004] [PMID: 23454614]

[63] Albini TA, Rao NA, Smith RE. The diagnosis and management of anterior scleritis. Int Ophthalmol Clin 2005; 45(2): 191-204.
[http://dx.doi.org/10.1097/01.iio.0000155900.64809.b2] [PMID: 15791166]

[64] Erkanli L, Akova YA, Guney-Tefekli E, Tugal-Tutkun I. Clinical features, prognosis, and treatment results of patients with scleritis from 2 tertiary eye care centers in Turkey. Cornea 2010; 29(1): 26-33.http://journals.lww.com/00003226-201001000-00006 [Internet].
[http://dx.doi.org/10.1097/ICO.0b013e3181ac9fad] [PMID: 19907295]

[65] McCluskey PJ, Wakefield D, Penny R. Scleritis and the spectrum of external inflammatory eye

disease. Aust N Z J Ophthalmol 1985; 13(2): 159-64.
[http://dx.doi.org/10.1111/j.1442-9071.1985.tb00416.x] [PMID: 4052263]

[66] Zimmer A, Kreuter J. Microspheres and nanoparticles used in ocular delivery systems. Adv Drug Deliv Rev 1995; 16(1): 61-73. https://linkinghub.elsevier.com/retrieve/pii/0169409X95000172 [Internet].
[http://dx.doi.org/10.1016/0169-409X(95)00017-2]

[67] Bu H-Z, Gukasyan HJ, Goulet L, Lou X-J, Xiang C, Koudriakova T. Ocular disposition, pharmacokinetics, efficacy and safety of nanoparticle-formulated ophthalmic drugs. Curr Drug Metab 2007; 8(2): 91-107. http://www.eurekaselect.com/openurl/content.php?genre=article&issn=1389-2002&volume=8&issue=2&spage=91 [Internet].
[http://dx.doi.org/10.2174/138920007779815977] [PMID: 17305490]

[68] Rupenthal ID, Alany RG. Ocular Drug Delivery.Pharmaceutical Manufacturing Handbook. 729-67.http://doi.wiley.com/10.1002/9780470259818.ch19 Internet

[69] Wadhwa S, Paliwal R, Paliwal SR, Vyas SP. Nanocarriers in ocular drug delivery: an update review. Curr Pharm Des 2009; 15(23): 2724-50.
[http://dx.doi.org/10.2174/138161209788923886] [PMID: 19689343]

[70] Gouda R, Baishya H, Qing Z. Application of Mathematical Models in Drug Release Kinetics of Carbidopa and Levodopa ER Tablets. J Dev Drugs 2017; 06(02) https://www.omicsonline.org/open-access/application-of-mathematical-models-in-drug-release-kinetics-of-carbidopaand--evodopa-er-tablets-2329-6631-1000171.php?aid=92315 [Internet].

[71] Cortesi R, Ajanji SC, Sivieri E, *et al.* Eudragit microparticles as a possible tool for ophthalmic administration of acyclovir. J Microencapsul 2007; 24(5): 445-56.http://www.tandfonline.com/doi/full/10.1080/02652040701374889 [Internet].
[http://dx.doi.org/10.1080/02652040701374889] [PMID: 17578734]

[72] Gavini E, Bonferoni MC, Rassu G, *et al.* Engineered microparticles based on drug-polymer coprecipitates for ocular-controlled delivery of Ciprofloxacin: influence of technological parameters. Drug Dev Ind Pharm 2016; 42(4): 554-62. https://www.tandfonline.com/doi/full/10.3109/03639045.2015.1100201 [Internet].
[http://dx.doi.org/10.3109/03639045.2015.1100201] [PMID: 26482534]

[73] Liu S, Dozois MD, Chang CN, *et al.* Prolonged Ocular Retention of Mucoadhesive Nanoparticle Eye Drop Formulation Enables Treatment of Eye Diseases Using Significantly Reduced Dosage. Mol Pharm 2016; 13(9): 2897-905. https://pubs.acs.org/doi/10.1021/acs.molpharmaceut.6b00445 [Internet].
[http://dx.doi.org/10.1021/acs.molpharmaceut.6b00445] [PMID: 27482595]

[74] Jain RA. The manufacturing techniques of various drug loaded biodegradable poly(lactide-c--glycolide) (PLGA) devices. Biomaterials 2000; 21(23): 2475-90. https://linkinghub.elsevier.com/retrieve/pii/S0142961200001150 [Internet].
[http://dx.doi.org/10.1016/S0142-9612(00)00115-0] [PMID: 11055295]

[75] Gupta H, Aqil M, Khar RK, Ali A, Bhatnagar A, Mittal G. Biodegradable levofloxacin nanoparticles for sustained ocular drug delivery. J Drug Target 2011; 19(6): 409-17.http://www.tandfonline.com/doi/full/10.3109/1061186X.2010.504268 [Internet].
[http://dx.doi.org/10.3109/1061186X.2010.504268] [PMID: 20678034]

[76] Alkholief M, Albasit H, Alhowyan A, *et al.* Employing a PLGA-TPGS based nanoparticle to improve the ocular delivery of Acyclovir. Saudi Pharm J 2019; 27(2): 293-302. https://linkinghub.elsevier.com/retrieve/pii/S1319016418305796 [Internet].
[http://dx.doi.org/10.1016/j.jsps.2018.11.011] [PMID: 30766442]

[77] Mohammadi G, Nokhodchi A, Barzegar-Jalali M, *et al.* Physicochemical and anti-bacterial performance characterization of clarithromycin nanoparticles as colloidal drug delivery system. Colloids Surf B Biointerfaces 2011; 88(1): 39-44.

https://linkinghub.elsevier.com/retrieve/pii/S0927776511003262 [Internet].
[http://dx.doi.org/10.1016/j.colsurfb.2011.05.050] [PMID: 21752610]

[78] Mukherjee S, Ray S, Thakur RS. Solid lipid nanoparticles: a modern formulation approach in drug delivery system. Indian J Pharm Sci 2009; 71(4): 349-58.http://www.ijpsonline.com/text.asp?2009/71/4/349/57282 [Internet].
[http://dx.doi.org/10.4103/0250-474X.57282] [PMID: 20502539]

[79] Üstündağ Okur N, Homan Gökçe E, Okur NÜ, Gökçe EH. Lipid Nanoparticles for Ocular Drug Delivery. Int J Ophthalmic Res 2015; 1(3): 77-82.
[http://dx.doi.org/10.17554/j.issn.2409-5680.2015.01.29]

[80] Wolska E, Sznitowska M, Chorążewicz J, et al. Ocular irritation and cyclosporine A distribution in the eye tissues after administration of Solid Lipid Microparticles in the rabbit model. Eur J Pharm Sci 2018; 121: 95-105. https://linkinghub.elsevier.com/retrieve/pii/S0928098718302343 [Internet].
[http://dx.doi.org/10.1016/j.ejps.2018.05.015] [PMID: 29777856]

[81] Gokce EH, Sandri G, Bonferoni MC, et al. Cyclosporine A loaded SLNs: evaluation of cellular uptake and corneal cytotoxicity. Int J Pharm 2008; 364(1): 76-86. https://linkinghub.elsevier.com/retrieve/pii/S0378517308005218 [Internet].
[http://dx.doi.org/10.1016/j.ijpharm.2008.07.028] [PMID: 18725276]

[82] Eid HM, Elkomy MH, El Menshawe SF, Salem HF. Development, Optimization, and *in vitro / in vivo* Characterization of Enhanced Lipid Nanoparticles for Ocular Delivery of Ofloxacin: the Influence of Pegylation and Chitosan Coating. AAPS PharmSciTech 2019; 20(5): 183.http://link.springer.com/10.1208/s12249-019-1371-6 [Internet].
[http://dx.doi.org/10.1208/s12249-019-1371-6] [PMID: 31054011]

[83] Pignatello R, Leonardi A, Fuochi V, Petronio Petronio G, Greco AS, Furneri PM. A Method for Efficient Loading of Ciprofloxacin Hydrochloride in Cationic Solid Lipid Nanoparticles: Formulation and Microbiological Evaluation. Nanomaterials (Basel) 2018; 8(5): 304.http://www.mdpi.com/2079-4991/8/5/304 [Internet].
[http://dx.doi.org/10.3390/nano8050304] [PMID: 29734771]

[84] Orange Book FDA. Orange Book: Approved Drug Products with Therapeutic Equivalence Evaluations https://www.accessdata.fda.gov/scripts/cder/ob/search_product.cfm

[85] Chetoni P, Burgalassi S, Monti D, et al. Solid lipid nanoparticles as promising tool for intraocular tobramycin delivery: Pharmacokinetic studies on rabbits. Eur J Pharm Biopharm 2016; 109: 214-23. https://linkinghub.elsevier.com/retrieve/pii/S0939641116307202 [Internet].
[http://dx.doi.org/10.1016/j.ejpb.2016.10.006] [PMID: 27789355]

[86] Baig MS, Ahad A, Aslam M, Imam SS, Aqil M, Ali A. Application of Box-Behnken design for preparation of levofloxacin-loaded stearic acid solid lipid nanoparticles for ocular delivery: Optimization, *in vitro* release, ocular tolerance, and antibacterial activity. Int J Biol Macromol 2016; 85: 258-70. https://linkinghub.elsevier.com/retrieve/pii/S0141813015302634 [Internet].
[http://dx.doi.org/10.1016/j.ijbiomac.2015.12.077] [PMID: 26740466]

[87] Khames A, Khaleel MA, El-Badawy MF, El-Nezhawy AOH. Natamycin solid lipid nanoparticles - sustained ocular delivery system of higher corneal penetration against deep fungal keratitis: preparation and optimization. Int J Nanomedicine 2019; 14: 2515-31. https://www.dovepress.com/natamycin-solid-lipid-nanopartic-es-sustained-ocular-delivery-system-o-peer-reviewed-article-IJN [Internet].
[http://dx.doi.org/10.2147/IJN.S190502] [PMID: 31040672]

[88] Kumar R, Sinha VR. Lipid Nanocarrier: an Efficient Approach Towards Ocular Delivery of Hydrophilic Drug (Valacyclovir). AAPS PharmSciTech 2017; 18(3): 884-94.http://link.springer.com/10.1208/s12249-016-0575-2 [Internet].
[http://dx.doi.org/10.1208/s12249-016-0575-2] [PMID: 27368921]

[89] WHO; World Health Organization. Global tuberculosis report 2017; 1-249.

https://www.who.int/tb/publications/global_report/gtbr2017_main_text.pdf?ua=1

[90] Singh M, Guzman-Aranguez A, Hussain A, Srinivas CS, Kaur IP. Solid lipid nanoparticles for ocular delivery of isoniazid: evaluation, proof of concept and *in vivo* safety & kinetics. Nanomedicine (Lond) 2019; 14(4): 465-91. https://www.futuremedicine.com/doi/10.2217/nnm-2018-0278 [Internet].
[http://dx.doi.org/10.2217/nnm-2018-0278] [PMID: 30694726]

[91] Gibaud S, Attivi D. Microemulsions for oral administration and their therapeutic applications. Expert Opin Drug Deliv 2012; 9(8): 937-51.http://www.tandfonline.com/doi/full/10.1517/17425247.2012.694865 [Internet].
[http://dx.doi.org/10.1517/17425247.2012.694865] [PMID: 22663249]

[92] Seyfoddin A, Sherwin T, Patel DV, *et al. ex vivo* and *in vivo* Evaluation of Chitosan Coated Nanostructured Lipid Carriers for Ocular Delivery of Acyclovir. Curr Drug Deliv 2016; 13(6): 923-34.
http://www.eurekaselect.com/openurl/content.php?genre=article&issn=1567-2018&volume=13&issue=6&spage=923 [Internet].
[http://dx.doi.org/10.2174/1567201813666151116142752] [PMID: 26568139]

[93] Bharti SK, Kesavan K. Phase-transition W/O Microemulsions for Ocular Delivery: Evaluation of Antibacterial Activity in the Treatment of Bacterial Keratitis. Ocul Immunol Inflamm 2017; 25(4): 463-74. https://www.tandfonline.com/doi/full/10.3109/09273948.2016.1139136 [Internet].
[http://dx.doi.org/10.3109/09273948.2016.1139136] [PMID: 26943481]

[94] Kumar R, Sinha VR. Evaluation of Ocular Irritation and Bioavailability of Voriconazole Loaded Microemulsion. Curr Drug Deliv 2017; 14(5): 718-24.http://www.eurekaselect.com/144855/article [Internet].
[http://dx.doi.org/10.2174/1567201813666160816105905] [PMID: 27538459]

[95] Gaudana R, Jwala J, Boddu SHS, Mitra AK. Recent perspectives in ocular drug delivery. Pharm Res 2009; 26(5): 1197-216.
[http://dx.doi.org/10.1007/s11095-008-9694-0] [PMID: 18758924]

[96] Bachu RD, Chowdhury P, Al-Saedi ZHF, Karla PK, Boddu SHS. Ocular Drug Delivery Barriers-Role of Nanocarriers in the Treatment of Anterior Segment Ocular Diseases. Pharmaceutics 2018; 10(1): 28.http://www.mdpi.com/1999-4923/10/1/28 [Internet].
[http://dx.doi.org/10.3390/pharmaceutics10010028] [PMID: 29495528]

[97] Mudgil M, Pawar PK. Preparation and *in vitro / ex vivo* Evaluation of Moxifloxacin-Loaded PLGA Nanosuspensions for Ophthalmic Application. Sci Pharm 2013; 81(2): 591-606.http://www.mdpi.com/2218-0532/81/2/591 [Internet].
[http://dx.doi.org/10.3797/scipharm.1204-16] [PMID: 23833723]

[98] Ambhore NP, Dandagi PM, Gadad AP. Formulation and comparative evaluation of HPMC and water soluble chitosan-based sparfloxacin nanosuspension for ophthalmic delivery. Drug Deliv Transl Res 2016; 6(1): 48-56.http://link.springer.com/10.1007/s13346-015-0262-y [Internet].
[http://dx.doi.org/10.1007/s13346-015-0262-y] [PMID: 26545605]

[99] Kim JH, Jang SW, Han SD, Hwang HD, Choi H-G. Development of a novel ophthalmic ciclosporin A-loaded nanosuspension using top-down media milling methods. Pharmazie 2011; 66(7): 491-5.http://www.ncbi.nlm.nih.gov/pubmed/21812323 [Internet].
[PMID: 21812323]

[100] Maged A, Mahmoud AA, Ghorab MM. Nano Spray Drying Technique as a Novel Approach To Formulate Stable Econazole Nitrate Nanosuspension Formulations for Ocular Use. Mol Pharm 2016; 13(9): 2951-65. https://pubs.acs.org/doi/10.1021/acs.molpharmaceut.6b00167 [Internet].
[http://dx.doi.org/10.1021/acs.molpharmaceut.6b00167] [PMID: 27010795]

[101] Qin T, Dai Z, Xu X, *et al.* Nanosuspension as an Efficient Carrier for Improved Ocular Permeation of Voriconazole. Curr Pharm Biotechnol 2020; 21 https://www.eurekaselect.com/185160/article [Internet].

[PMID: 32867650]

[102] Durgun ME, Güngör S, Özsoy Y. Micelles: Promising Ocular Drug Carriers for Anterior and Posterior Segment Diseases. J Ocul Pharmacol Ther 2019; 36(6) https://www.liebertpub.com/doi/10.1089/jop.2019.0109 jop.2019.0109

[103] Smyth-Medina R, Johnston J, Devries DK, et al. Effect of OTX-101, a Novel Nanomicellar Formulation of Cyclosporine A, on Conjunctival Staining in Patients with Keratoconjunctivitis Sicca: A Pooled Analysis of Phase 2b/3 and 3 Clinical Trials. J Ocul Pharmacol Ther 2019; 35(7): 388-94. https://www.liebertpub.com/doi/10.1089/jop.2018.0154 [Internet]. [http://dx.doi.org/10.1089/jop.2018.0154] [PMID: 31373837]

[104] Mandal A, Gote V, Pal D, Ogundele A, Mitra AK. Ocular Pharmacokinetics of a Topical Ophthalmic Nanomicellar Solution of Cyclosporine (Cequa®) for Dry Eye Disease. Pharm Res 2019; 36(2): 36.http://link.springer.com/10.1007/s11095-018-2556-5 [Internet]. [http://dx.doi.org/10.1007/s11095-018-2556-5] [PMID: 30617777]

[105] Malhotra R, Devries DK, Luchs J, et al. Effect of OTX-101, a Novel Nanomicellar Formulation of Cyclosporine A, on Corneal Staining in Patients With Keratoconjunctivitis Sicca: A Pooled Analysis of Phase 2b/3 and Phase 3 Studies. Cornea 2019; 38(10): 1259-65.http://journals.lww.com/00003226-201910000-00010 [Internet]. [http://dx.doi.org/10.1097/ICO.0000000000001989] [PMID: 31306284]

[106] Yu Y, Chen D, Li Y, Yang W, Tu J, Shen Y. Improving the topical ocular pharmacokinetics of lyophilized cyclosporine A-loaded micelles: formulation, *in vitro* and *in vivo* studies. Drug Deliv 2018; 25(1): 888-99. [Internet]. [http://dx.doi.org/10.1080/10717544.2018.1458923] [PMID: 29631468]

[107] Luschmann C, Tessmar J, Schoeberl S, Strauß O, Luschmann K, Goepferich A. Self-assembling colloidal system for the ocular administration of cyclosporine A. Cornea 2014; 33(1): 77-81.http://journals.lww.com/00003226-201401000-00016 [Internet]. [http://dx.doi.org/10.1097/ICO.0b013e3182a7f3bf] [PMID: 24162754]

[108] Li J, Li Z, Zhou T, et al. Positively charged micelles based on a triblock copolymer demonstrate enhanced corneal penetration. Int J Nanomedicine 2015; 10: 6027-37. [http://dx.doi.org/10.2147/IJN.S90347] [PMID: 26451109]

[109] Kanoujia J, Kushwaha PS, Saraf SA. Evaluation of gatifloxacin pluronic micelles and development of its formulation for ocular delivery. Drug Deliv Transl Res 2014; 4(4): 334-43. [http://dx.doi.org/10.1007/s13346-014-0194-y] [PMID: 25787066]

[110] Willem de Vries J, Schnichels S, Hurst J, et al. DNA nanoparticles for ophthalmic drug delivery. Biomaterials 2018; 157: 98-106. [http://dx.doi.org/10.1016/j.biomaterials.2017.11.046] [PMID: 29258013]

[111] Lakhani P, Patil A, Majumdar S. Challenges in the Polyene- and Azole-Based Pharmacotherapy of Ocular Fungal Infections. J Ocul Pharmacol Ther 2019; 35(1): 6-22. https://www.liebertpub.com/doi/10.1089/jop.2018.0089 [Internet]. [http://dx.doi.org/10.1089/jop.2018.0089] [PMID: 30481082]

[112] Younes NF, Abdel-Halim SA, Elassasy AI. Solutol HS15 based binary mixed micelles with penetration enhancers for augmented corneal delivery of sertaconazole nitrate: optimization, *in vitro*, *ex vivo* and *in vivo* characterization. Drug Deliv 2018; 25(1): 1706-17. [Internet]. [http://dx.doi.org/10.1080/10717544.2018.1497107] [PMID: 30442039]

[113] Amiel H, Chohan AB, Snibson GR, Vajpayee R. Atypical fungal sclerokeratitis. Cornea 2008; 27(3): 382-3. [http://dx.doi.org/10.1097/ICO.0b013e31815e9298] [PMID: 18362676]

[114] Andes D. Optimizing antifungal choice and administration. Curr Med Res Opin 2013; 29(sup4): 13-8. http://www.tandfonline.com/doi/full/10.1185/03007995.2012.761135 [http://dx.doi.org/10.1185/03007995.2012.761135]

[115] Durgun ME, Kahraman E, Güngör S, Özsoy Y. Optimization and Characterization of Aqueous Micellar Formulations for Ocular Delivery of an Antifungal Drug, Posaconazole. Curr Pharm Des 2020; 26(14): 1543-55. https://www.eurekaselect.com/180211/article [Internet].
[http://dx.doi.org/10.2174/1381612826666200313172207] [PMID: 32167423]

[116] Zhou T, Zhu L, Xia H, *et al.* Micelle carriers based on macrogol 15 hydroxystearate for ocular delivery of terbinafine hydrochloride: *in vitro* characterization and *in vivo* permeation. Eur J Pharm Sci 2017; 109(March): 288-96. [Internet].
[http://dx.doi.org/10.1016/j.ejps.2017.08.020] [PMID: 28823856]

[117] Smit D. Anti-infective ophthalmic preparations in general practice. S Afr Fam Pract 2012; 54(4): 302-7. https://www.tandfonline.com/doi/full/10.1080/20786204.2012.10874239 [Internet].
[http://dx.doi.org/10.1080/20786204.2012.10874239]

[118] Varela-Garcia A, Concheiro A, Alvarez-Lorenzo C. Soluplus micelles for acyclovir ocular delivery: Formulation and cornea and sclera permeability. Int J Pharm 2018; 552(1-2): 39-47. [Internet].
[http://dx.doi.org/10.1016/j.ijpharm.2018.09.053] [PMID: 30253214]

[119] Vadlapudi AD, Cholkar K, Vadlapatla RK, Mitra AK. Aqueous nanomicellar formulation for topical delivery of biotinylated lipid prodrug of acyclovir: formulation development and ocular biocompatibility. J Ocul Pharmacol Ther 2014; 30(1): 49-58.http://www.liebertpub.com/doi/10.1089/jop.2013.0157 [Internet].
[http://dx.doi.org/10.1089/jop.2013.0157] [PMID: 24192229]

[120] De Clercq E. Clinical potential of the acyclic nucleoside phosphonates cidofovir, adefovir, and tenofovir in treatment of DNA virus and retrovirus infections. Clin Microbiol Rev 2003; 16(4): 569-96. https://cmr.asm.org/content/16/4/569 [Internet].
[http://dx.doi.org/10.1128/CMR.16.4.569-596.2003] [PMID: 14557287]

[121] Stewart MW. Optimal management of cytomegalovirus retinitis in patients with AIDS. Clin Ophthalmol 2010; 4(Apr): 285-99. http://www.dovepress.com/optimal-management-of-cytomegalovirus-retinitis-in-patients-with-aids-peer-reviewed-article-OPTH [Internet].
[http://dx.doi.org/10.2147/OPTH.S6700] [PMID: 20463796]

[122] Mandal A, Cholkar K, Khurana V, *et al.* Topical Formulation of Self-Assembled Antiviral Prodrug Nanomicelles for Targeted Retinal Delivery. Mol Pharm 2017; 14(6): 2056-69. https://pubs.acs.org/doi/10.1021/acs.molpharmaceut.7b00128 [Internet].
[http://dx.doi.org/10.1021/acs.molpharmaceut.7b00128] [PMID: 28471177]

[123] Abdelbary G. Ocular ciprofloxacin hydrochloride mucoadhesive chitosan-coated liposomes. Pharm Dev Technol 2011; 16(1): 44-56.http://www.tandfonline.com/doi/full/10.3109/10837450903479988 [Internet].
[http://dx.doi.org/10.3109/10837450903479988] [PMID: 20025433]

[124] Nicolosi D, Cupri S, Genovese C, Tempera G, Mattina R, Pignatello R. Nanotechnology approaches for antibacterial drug delivery: Preparation and microbiological evaluation of fusogenic liposomes carrying fusidic acid. Int J Antimicrob Agents 2015; 45(6): 622-6. https://linkinghub.elsevier.com/retrieve/pii/S0924857915000801 [Internet].
[http://dx.doi.org/10.1016/j.ijantimicag.2015.01.016] [PMID: 25816979]

[125] Fresta M, Panico AM, Bucolo C, Giannavola C, Puglisi G. Characterization and in-vivo ocular absorption of liposome-encapsulated acyclovir. J Pharm Pharmacol 1999; 51(5): 565-76.http://doi.wiley.com/10.1211/0022357991772664 [Internet].
[http://dx.doi.org/10.1211/0022357991772664] [PMID: 10411216]

[126] Chetoni P, Rossi S, Burgalassi S, Monti D, Mariotti S, Saettone MF. Comparison of liposome-encapsulated acyclovir with acyclovir ointment: ocular pharmacokinetics in rabbits. J Ocul Pharmacol Ther 2004; 20(2): 169-77.http://www.liebertpub.com/doi/10.1089/108076804773710849 [Internet].
[http://dx.doi.org/10.1089/108076804773710849] [PMID: 15117573]

[127] Ferreira KSA, dos Santos BMA, Lucena N de P, Ferraz MS, Carvalho R de SF. Ocular delivery of

moxifloxacin-loaded lipos. 2018; 81(6) http://www.gnresearch.org/doi/10.5935/0004-2749.20180090

[128] Ren T, Lin X, Zhang Q, *et al.* Encapsulation of Azithromycin Ion Pair in Liposome for Enhancing Ocular Delivery and Therapeutic Efficacy on Dry Eye. Mol Pharm 2018; 15(11): 4862-71. https://pubs.acs.org/doi/10.1021/acs.molpharmaceut.8b00516 [Internet].
[http://dx.doi.org/10.1021/acs.molpharmaceut.8b00516] [PMID: 30251864]

[129] Casazza AM, Fioretti A, Ghione M, Soldati M, Verini MA. Distamycin A, a new antiviral antibiotic. Antimicrob Agents Chemother 1965; 5: 593-8.http://www.ncbi.nlm.nih.gov/pubmed/4286925 [Internet].
[PMID: 4286925]

[130] Chetoni P, Monti D, Tampucci S, *et al.* Liposomes as a potential ocular delivery system of distamycin A. Int J Pharm 2015; 492(1-2): 120-6. https://linkinghub.elsevier.com/retrieve/pii/S0378517315004743 [Internet].
[http://dx.doi.org/10.1016/j.ijpharm.2015.05.055] [PMID: 26183332]

[131] de Sá FAP, Taveira SF, Gelfuso GM, Lima EM, Gratieri T. Liposomal voriconazole (VOR) formulation for improved ocular delivery. Colloids Surf B Biointerfaces 2015; 133: 331-8. https://linkinghub.elsevier.com/retrieve/pii/S0927776515004099 [Internet].
[http://dx.doi.org/10.1016/j.colsurfb.2015.06.036] [PMID: 26123854]

[132] Khalil RM, Abdelbary GA, Basha M, Awad GEA, El-Hashemy HA. Enhancement of lomefloxacin Hcl ocular efficacy *via* niosomal encapsulation: *in vitro* characterization and *in vivo* evaluation. J Liposome Res 2017; 27(4): 312-23. https://www.tandfonline.com/doi/full/10.1080/08982104.2016.1191022 [Internet].
[http://dx.doi.org/10.1080/08982104.2016.1191022] [PMID: 27241274]

[133] El-Nabarawi MA, Abd El Rehem RT, Teaima M, *et al.* Natamycin niosomes as a promising ocular nanosized delivery system with ketorolac tromethamine for dual effects for treatment of candida rabbit keratitis; *in vitro / in vivo* and histopathological studies. Drug Dev Ind Pharm 2019; 45(6): 922-36. https://www.tandfonline.com/doi/full/10.1080/03639045.2019.1579827 [Internet].
[http://dx.doi.org/10.1080/03639045.2019.1579827] [PMID: 30744431]

[134] Basha M, Abd El-Alim SH, Shamma RN, Awad GEA. Design and optimization of surfactant-based nanovesicles for ocular delivery of Clotrimazole. J Liposome Res 2013; 23(3): 203-10.http://www.tandfonline.com/doi/full/10.3109/08982104.2013.788025 [Internet].
[http://dx.doi.org/10.3109/08982104.2013.788025] [PMID: 23607316]

[135] Kakkar S, Kaur IP. Spanlastics--a novel nanovesicular carrier system for ocular delivery. Int J Pharm 2011; 413(1-2): 202-10. https://linkinghub.elsevier.com/retrieve/pii/S0378517311003541 [Internet].
[http://dx.doi.org/10.1016/j.ijpharm.2011.04.027] [PMID: 21540093]

[136] ElMeshad AN, Mohsen AM. Enhanced corneal permeation and antimycotic activity of itraconazole against Candida albicans *via* a novel nanosystem vesicle. Drug Deliv 2016; 23(7): 2115-23. https://www.tandfonline.com/doi/full/10.3109/10717544.2014.942811 [Internet].
[http://dx.doi.org/10.3109/10717544.2014.942811] [PMID: 25080226]

[137] Aburahma MH. Bile salts-containing vesicles: promising pharmaceutical carriers for oral delivery of poorly water-soluble drugs and peptide/protein-based therapeutics or vaccines. Drug Deliv 2014; 1-21.http://www.tandfonline.com/doi/full/10.3109/10717544.2014.976892 [Internet].
[http://dx.doi.org/10.3109/10717544.2014.976892] [PMID: 25390191]

[138] Al-Mahallawi AM, Abdelbary AA, Aburahma MH. Investigating the potential of employing bilosomes as a novel vesicular carrier for transdermal delivery of tenoxicam. Int J Pharm 2015; 485(1-2): 329-40. https://linkinghub.elsevier.com/retrieve/pii/S0378517315002495 [Internet].
[http://dx.doi.org/10.1016/j.ijpharm.2015.03.033] [PMID: 25796122]

[139] Shukla A, Khatri K, Gupta PN, Goyal AK, Mehta A, Vyas SP. Oral immunization against hepatitis B using bile salt stabilized vesicles (bilosomes). J Pharm Pharm Sci 2008; 11(1): 59-66. https://journals.library.ualberta.ca/jpps/index.php/JPPS/article/view/778 [Internet].

[http://dx.doi.org/10.18433/J3K01M] [PMID: 18445364]

[140] Yousry C, Zikry PM, Salem HM, Basalious EB, El-Gazayerly ON. Integrated nanovesicular/self-nanoemulsifying system (INV/SNES) for enhanced dual ocular drug delivery: statistical optimization, *in vitro* and *in vivo* evaluation. Drug Deliv Transl Res 2020; 10(3): 801-14. http://link.springer.com/10.1007/s13346-020-00716-5 [Internet].
[http://dx.doi.org/10.1007/s13346-020-00716-5] [PMID: 31989414]

[141] Abdelbary AA, Abd-Elsalam WH, Al-Mahallawi AM. Fabrication of novel ultradeformable bilosomes for enhanced ocular delivery of terconazole: *in vitro* characterization, *ex vivo* permeation and *in vivo* safety assessment. Int J Pharm 2016; 513(1-2): 688-96. https://linkinghub.elsevier.com/retrieve/pii/S0378517316309401 [Internet].
[http://dx.doi.org/10.1016/j.ijpharm.2016.10.006] [PMID: 27717916]

[142] Nasr M, Teiama M, Ismail A, Ebada A, Saber S. *in vitro* and *in vivo* evaluation of cubosomal nanoparticles as an ocular delivery system for fluconazole in treatment of keratomycosis. Drug Deliv Transl Res 2020. http://link.springer.com/10.1007/s13346-020-00830-4
[http://dx.doi.org/10.1007/s13346-020-00830-4]

[143] Younes NF, Abdel-Halim SA, Elassasy AI. Corneal targeted Sertaconazole nitrate loaded cubosomes: Preparation, statistical optimization, *in vitro* characterization, *ex vivo* permeation and *in vivo* studies. Int J Pharm 2018; 553(1-2): 386-97. https://linkinghub.elsevier.com/retrieve/pii/S0378517318308007 [Internet].
[http://dx.doi.org/10.1016/j.ijpharm.2018.10.057] [PMID: 30393167]

[144] DHAKNE R, DEHGHAN MH, KAZI M. Ocular delivery of natamycin based on monoolein/span 80/poloxamer 407 nanocarriers for the effectual treatment of fungal keratitis. J Res Pharm 2020; 24(2): 251-63. http://jrespharm.com/abstract.php?id=781

[145] Bennett L. Topical versus Systemic Ocular Drug Delivery.Ocular Drug Delivery: Advances, Challenges and Applications. Cham: Springer International Publishing 2016; pp. 53-74. http://link.springer.com/10.1007/978-3-319-47691-9_5 Internet
[http://dx.doi.org/10.1007/978-3-319-47691-9_5]

[146] Durairaj C, Kompella U. Dendritic polyguanidilyated translocators for ocular drug delivery. Drug Deliv Technol 2009; 9(9): 36-43.

[147] Durairaj C, Kadam RS, Chandler JW, Hutcherson SL, Kompella UB. Nanosized Dendritic Polyguanidilyated Translocators for Enhanced Solubility, Permeability, and Delivery of Gatifloxacin. Investig Opthalmology Vis Sci 2010; 51(11): 5804. http://iovs.arvojournals.org/article.aspx?doi=10.1167/iovs.10-5388

[148] Vembu S, Pazhamalai S, Gopalakrishnan M. Potential antibacterial activity of triazine dendrimer: Synthesis and controllable drug release properties. Bioorg Med Chem 2015; 23(15): 4561-6. https://linkinghub.elsevier.com/retrieve/pii/S0968089615005039 [Internet].
[http://dx.doi.org/10.1016/j.bmc.2015.06.009] [PMID: 26113186]

[149] Kirchhof S, Goepferich AM, Brandl FP. Hydrogels in ophthalmic applications. Eur J Pharm Biopharm 2015; 95(Pt B): 227-38. https://linkinghub.elsevier.com/retrieve/pii/S0939641115002489 [Internet].
[http://dx.doi.org/10.1016/j.ejpb.2015.05.016] [PMID: 26032290]

[150] Dubald M, Bourgeois S, Andrieu V, Fessi H. Ophthalmic Drug Delivery Systems for Antibiotherapy-A Review. Pharmaceutics 2018; 10(1): 10. http://www.mdpi.com/1999-4923/10/1/10 [Internet].
[http://dx.doi.org/10.3390/pharmaceutics10010010] [PMID: 29342879]

[151] Rajoria G, Gupta A. *In-situ* Gelling System: A Novel Approach for Ocular Drug Delivery. Am. J PharmTech Res 2012; 2(4): 24-53.

[152] Khalil RM, Abdelbary GA, Basha M, Awad GEA, El-Hashemy HA. Design and evaluation of proniosomes as a carrier for ocular delivery of lomefloxacin HCl. J Liposome Res 2017; 27(2): 118-29. https://www.tandfonline.com/doi/full/10.3109/08982104.2016.1167737 [Internet].
[http://dx.doi.org/10.3109/08982104.2016.1167737] [PMID: 27079800]

[153] Youssef A, Dudhipala N, Majumdar S. Ciprofloxacin Loaded Nanostructured Lipid Carriers Incorporated into *In-situ* Gels to Improve Management of Bacterial Endophthalmitis. Pharmaceutics 2020; 12(6): 572. https://www.mdpi.com/1999-4923/12/6/572 [Internet].
[http://dx.doi.org/10.3390/pharmaceutics12060572] [PMID: 32575524]

[154] Duan Y, Cai X, Du H, Zhai G. Novel *in situ* gel systems based on P123/TPGS mixed micelles and gellan gum for ophthalmic delivery of curcumin. Colloids Surf B Biointerfaces 2015; 128: 322-30. [Internet].
[http://dx.doi.org/10.1016/j.colsurfb.2015.02.007] [PMID: 25707750]

[155] Soliman OAE, Mohamed EA, Khatera NAA. Enhanced ocular bioavailability of fluconazole from niosomal gels and microemulsions: formulation, optimization, and *in vitro-in vivo* evaluation. Pharm Dev Technol 2019; 24(1): 48-62. https://www.tandfonline.com/doi/full/10.1080/10837450.2017.1413658 [Internet].
[http://dx.doi.org/10.1080/10837450.2017.1413658] [PMID: 29210317]

[156] Moustafa MA, Elnaggar YSR, El-Refaie WM, Abdallah OY. Hyalugel-integrated liposomes as a novel ocular nanosized delivery system of fluconazole with promising prolonged effect. Int J Pharm 2017; 534(1-2): 14-24. https://linkinghub.elsevier.com/retrieve/pii/S0378517317309572 [Internet].
[http://dx.doi.org/10.1016/j.ijpharm.2017.10.007] [PMID: 28987453]

[157] Jaiswal M, Kumar M, Pathak K. Zero order delivery of itraconazole *via* polymeric micelles incorporated *in situ* ocular gel for the management of fungal keratitis. Colloids Surf B Biointerfaces 2015; 130: 23-30. [Internet].
[http://dx.doi.org/10.1016/j.colsurfb.2015.03.059] [PMID: 25889081]

[158] Sayed S, Elsayed I, Ismail MM. Optimization of β-cyclodextrin consolidated micellar dispersion for promoting the transcorneal permeation of a practically insoluble drug. Int J Pharm 2018; 549(1-2): 249-60. https://linkinghub.elsevier.com/retrieve/pii/S0378517318305544 [Internet].
[http://dx.doi.org/10.1016/j.ijpharm.2018.08.001] [PMID: 30077759]

[159] Abdelbary GA, Amin MM, Zakaria MY. Ocular ketoconazole-loaded proniosomal gels: formulation, *ex vivo* corneal permeation and *in vivo* studies. Drug Deliv 2017; 24(1): 309-19. https://www.tandfonline.com/doi/full/10.1080/10717544.2016.1247928 [Internet].
[http://dx.doi.org/10.1080/10717544.2016.1247928] [PMID: 28165809]

[160] Gupta H, Aqil M, Khar RK, Ali A, Bhatnagar A, Mittal G. Nanoparticles laden *in situ* gel of levofloxacin for enhanced ocular retention. Drug Deliv 2013; 20(7): 306-9.http://www.tandfonline.com/doi/full/10.3109/10717544.2013.838712 [Internet].
[http://dx.doi.org/10.3109/10717544.2013.838712] [PMID: 24044648]

[161] Abdelbary A, Salem HF, Khallaf RA, Ali AMA. Mucoadhesive niosomal *in situ* gel for ocular tissue targeting: *in vitro* and *in vivo* evaluation of lomefloxacin hydrochloride. Pharm Dev Technol 2017; 22(3): 409-17. https://www.tandfonline.com/doi/full/10.1080/10837450.2016.1219916 [Internet].
[http://dx.doi.org/10.1080/10837450.2016.1219916] [PMID: 27476543]

[162] Janga KY, Tatke A, Balguri SP, Lamichanne SP, Ibrahim MM, Maria DN, *et al.* Ion-sensitive *in situ* hydrogels of natamycin bilosomes for enhanced and prolonged ocular pharmacotherapy: *in vitro* permeability, cytotoxicity and *in vivo* evaluation. Artif Cells, Nanomedicine, Biotechnol 2018; 46(sup1): 1039-50. https://www.tandfonline.com/doi/full/10.1080/21691401.2018.1443117
[http://dx.doi.org/10.1080/21691401.2018.1443117]

[163] Janga KY, Tatke A, Dudhipala N, *et al.* Gellan Gum Based *Sol-to-Gel* Transforming System of Natamycin Transfersomes Improves Topical Ocular Delivery. J Pharmacol Exp Ther 2019; 370(3): 814-22.http://jpet.aspetjournals.org/lookup/doi/10.1124/jpet.119.256446 [Internet].
[http://dx.doi.org/10.1124/jpet.119.256446] [PMID: 30872389]

[164] Al Khateb K, Ozhmukhametova EK, Mussin MN, *et al. in situ* gelling systems based on Pluronic F127/Pluronic F68 formulations for ocular drug delivery. Int J Pharm 2016; 502(1-2): 70-9. [Internet].
[http://dx.doi.org/10.1016/j.ijpharm.2016.02.027] [PMID: 26899977]

[165] Khan S, Warade S, Singhavi DJ. Improvement in Ocular Bioavailability and Prolonged Delivery of Tobramycin Sulfate Following Topical Ophthalmic Administration of Drug-Loaded Mucoadhesive Microparticles Incorporated in Thermosensitive *in situ* Gel. J Ocul Pharmacol Ther 2018; 34(3): 287-97.http://www.liebertpub.com/doi/10.1089/jop.2017.0079 [Internet].
[http://dx.doi.org/10.1089/jop.2017.0079] [PMID: 29211593]

[166] Allam A, El-Mokhtar MA, Elsabahy M. Vancomycin-loaded niosomes integrated within pH-sensitive *In-situ* forming gel for treatment of ocular infections while minimizing drug irritation. J Pharm Pharmacol 2019; 71(8): 1209-21. https://onlinelibrary.wiley.com/doi/abs/10.1111/jphp.13106 [Internet].
[http://dx.doi.org/10.1111/jphp.13106] [PMID: 31124593]

[167] Jervis LP. A Summary of Recent Advances in Ocular Inserts and Implants. J Bioequivalence Bioavailab 2016; 09(01) https://www.omicsonline.org/open-access/a-summary-of-recent-advanes-in-ocular-inserts-and-implants-jbb-1000318.php?aid=83552 [Internet].

[168] Armaly MF, Rao KR. The effect of pilocarpine Ocusert with different release rates on ocular pressure. Invest Ophthalmol 1973; 12(7): 491-6.
[PMID: 4742991]

[169] Baranowski P, Karolewicz B, Gajda M, Pluta J. Ophthalmic drug dosage forms: characterisation and research methods. ScientificWorldJournal 2014; 2014: 861904.http://www.hindawi.com/journals/tswj/2014/861904/ [Internet].
[http://dx.doi.org/10.1155/2014/861904] [PMID: 24772038]

[170] Pawar PK, Katara R, Majumdar DK. Design and evaluation of moxifloxacin hydrochloride ocular inserts. Acta Pharm 2012; 62(1): 93-104. https://content.sciendo.com/doi/10.2478/v10007-012-0002-5 [Internet].
[http://dx.doi.org/10.2478/v10007-012-0002-5] [PMID: 22472452]

[171] Samanta A, Ghosal SK. Prolonged delivery of ciprofloxacin hydrochloride from hydrophilic ocular inserts. Acta Pol Pharm 61(5): 343-9. http://www.ncbi.nlm.nih.gov/pubmed/15747690

[172] Larsen EH, Hans H. Hans H. Ussing--scientific work: contemporary significance and perspectives. Biochim Biophys Acta 2002; 1566(1-2): 2-15. https://linkinghub.elsevier.com/retrieve/pii/S0005273602005928 [Internet].
[http://dx.doi.org/10.1016/S0005-2736(02)00592-8] [PMID: 12421533]

[173] Polat HK, Bozdağ Pehlivan S, Özkul C, *et al.* Development of besifloxacin HCl loaded nanofibrous ocular inserts for the treatment of bacterial keratitis: *in vitro* , *ex vivo* and *in vivo* evaluation. Int J Pharm 2020; 585: 119552. https://linkinghub.elsevier.com/retrieve/pii/S0378517320305366 [Internet].
[http://dx.doi.org/10.1016/j.ijpharm.2020.119552] [PMID: 32569814]

[174] Pehlivan SB, Yavuz B, Çalamak S, *et al.* Preparation and *in vitro* / *in vivo* evaluation of cyclosporin A-loaded nanodecorated ocular implants for subconjunctival application. J Pharm Sci 2015; 104(5): 1709-20.
[http://dx.doi.org/10.1002/jps.24385] [PMID: 25716582]

[175] Fernandes-Cunha GM, Fialho SL, da Silva GR, Silva-Cunha A, Zhao M, Behar-Cohen F. Ocular safety of Intravitreal Clindamycin Hydrochloride Released by PLGA Implants. Pharm Res 2017; 34(5): 1083-92.http://link.springer.com/10.1007/s11095-017-2118-2 [Internet].
[http://dx.doi.org/10.1007/s11095-017-2118-2] [PMID: 28224388]

[176] Ciolino JB, Hudson SP, Mobbs AN, Hoare TR, Iwata NG, Fink GR, *et al.* A Prototype Antifungal Contact Lens. Investig Opthalmology Vis Sci 2011; 52(9): 6286. http://iovs.arvojournals.org/article.aspx?doi=10.1167/iovs.10-6935
[http://dx.doi.org/10.1167/iovs.10-6935]

[177] Danion A, Arsenault I, Vermette P. Antibacterial activity of contact lenses bearing surface-immobilized layers of intact liposomes loaded with levofloxacin. J Pharm Sci 2007; 96(9): 2350-63. https://linkinghub.elsevier.com/retrieve/pii/S0022354916323346 [Internet].

[http://dx.doi.org/10.1002/jps.20871] [PMID: 17541976]

[178] Garg P, Venuganti VVK, Roy A, Roy G. Novel drug delivery methods for the treatment of keratitis: moving away from surgical intervention. Expert Opin Drug Deliv 2019; 16(12): 1381-91. https://www.tandfonline.com/doi/full/10.1080/17425247.2019.1690451 [Internet].
[http://dx.doi.org/10.1080/17425247.2019.1690451] [PMID: 31701781]

[179] Jamaledin R, Yiu CKY, Zare EN, et al. Advances in Antimicrobial Microneedle Patches for Combating Infections. Adv Mater 2020; 32(33): e2002129. https://onlinelibrary.wiley.com/doi/abs/10.1002/adma.202002129 [Internet].
[http://dx.doi.org/10.1002/adma.202002129] [PMID: 32602146]

[180] Bhatnagar S, Dave K, Venuganti VVK. Microneedles in the clinic. J Control Release 2017; 260: 164-82. https://linkinghub.elsevier.com/retrieve/pii/S016836591730603X [Internet].
[http://dx.doi.org/10.1016/j.jconrel.2017.05.029] [PMID: 28549948]

[181] Moffatt K, Wang Y, Raj Singh TR, Donnelly RF. Microneedles for enhanced transdermal and intraocular drug delivery. Curr Opin Pharmacol 2017; 36: 14-21. https://linkinghub.elsevier.com/retrieve/pii/S1471489217300826 [Internet].
[http://dx.doi.org/10.1016/j.coph.2017.07.007] [PMID: 28780407]

[182] Jiang J, Gill HS, Ghate D, McCarey BE, Patel SR, Edelhauser HF, et al. Coated Microneedles for Drug Delivery to the Eye. Investig Opthalmology Vis Sci 2007; 4(9): 4038. http://iovs.arvojournals.org/article.aspx?doi=10.1167/iovs.07-0066
[http://dx.doi.org/10.1167/iovs.07-0066]

[183] Bhatnagar S, Saju A, Cheerla KD, Gade SK, Garg P, Venuganti VVK. Corneal delivery of besifloxacin using rapidly dissolving polymeric microneedles. Drug Deliv Transl Res 2018; 8(3): 473-83.http://link.springer.com/10.1007/s13346-017-0470-8 [Internet].
[http://dx.doi.org/10.1007/s13346-017-0470-8] [PMID: 29288357]

[184] Roy G, Galigama RD, Thorat VS, et al. Amphotericin B containing microneedle ocular patch for effective treatment of fungal keratitis. Int J Pharm 2019; 572: 118808. https://linkinghub.elsevier.com/retrieve/pii/S0378517319308531 [Internet].
[http://dx.doi.org/10.1016/j.ijpharm.2019.118808] [PMID: 31678387]

[185] Lallemand F, Schmitt M, Bourges J-L, Gurny R, Benita S, Garrigue J-S. Cyclosporine A delivery to the eye: A comprehensive review of academic and industrial efforts. Eur J Pharm Biopharm 2017; 117: 14-28. https://linkinghub.elsevier.com/retrieve/pii/S0939641116309080 [Internet].
[http://dx.doi.org/10.1016/j.ejpb.2017.03.006] [PMID: 28315447]

[186] Vekacia EMA. Vekacia: Withdrawal of the marketing authorisation application https://www.ema.europa.eu/en/medicines/human/withdrawn-applications/vekacia

[187] Kim HS, Kim TI, Kim JH, et al. Evaluation of Clinical Efficacy and Safety of a Novel Cyclosporin A Nanoemulsion in the Treatment of Dry Eye Syndrome. J Ocul Pharmacol Ther 2017; 33(7): 530-8.http://www.liebertpub.com/doi/10.1089/jop.2016.0164 [Internet].
[http://dx.doi.org/10.1089/jop.2016.0164] [PMID: 28759302]

[188] Kang M-J, Kim Y-H, Chou M, et al. Evaluation of the Efficacy and Safety of A Novel 0.05% Cyclosporin A Topical Nanoemulsion in Primary Sjögren's Syndrome Dry Eye. Ocul Immunol Inflamm 2020; 28(3): 370-8. https://www.tandfonline.com/doi/full/10.1080/09273948.2019.1587470 [Internet].
[http://dx.doi.org/10.1080/09273948.2019.1587470] [PMID: 30986119]

[189] EMA. Retisert 590 microgram Intravitreal Implant https://www.ema.europa.eu/en/documents/withdrawal-report/withdrawal-assessment-report-retisert_en.pdf

[190] EMA. fluocinolone acetonide (intravitreal implant in applicator) https://www.ema.europa.eu/en/documents/psusa/fluocinolone-acetonide-intravitreal-implant-applicator-list-nationally-authorised-medicinal-products/00010224/201608_en.pdf

[191] EMA. Vitrasert Implant https://www.ema.europa.eu/en/medicines/human/EPAR/vitrasert-implant

CHAPTER 2

Propitious Development of Vaccines for SARS-CoV

Palaniswamy Rani[1,*], **Balasubramanian Ayshwariya**[1], **Ramesh Harisharan**[1] and **Bhavananthi Ilackkeya**[1]

[1] *Department of Biotechnology, PSG College of Technology, Coimbatore, Tamil Nadu 641004, India*

Abstract: Anti-infective agents are effective for controlling infectious diseases by killing or inhibiting infectious organisms. Anti-infective agent encompasses antibiotics, antifungal agents and antiviral agents, *etc*. In this category, vaccines are major contributors in recent years to preventing infectious diseases. The emergence of COVID-19 (COronaVIrus Disease 2019) pandemic has caused a resurgence of interest in finding new vaccines. The vaccines are generally classified into conventional vaccines and recombinant vaccines. In this context, the recent development of Vaccines for SARS-CoV (Severe Acute Respiratory Syndrome Coronavirus) has to be focussed. SARS-CoV is a human virus that comes under the order of *Nidovirales* and the family of *Coronaviridae*. This virus primarily causes respiratory diseases by targeting ACE-2 (angiotensin-converting enzyme 2) receptor. This virus is categorized into SARS-CoV-1 and SARS-CoV-2 (COVID-19). In this essence, the contents embrace the various aspects regarding the common vaccine development pipeline, importance of vaccination for prevention of infectious diseases, types of vaccine production methods that are implemented for SARS-CoV virus categories, potential targets for SARS-CoV vaccines, difficulties or feasibilities involved in vaccine production, phases accomplished in vaccine production and involvement of vaccines in addressing the global pandemic. In conclusion, this chapter confers the outline of vaccine progression marked up-to-date for SARS-CoV.

Keywords: ACE-2 receptor, Animal model, COVID-19 vaccine, Nucleocapsid Protein, RBD, Respiratory failure, SARS-CoV, Spike protein, Vaccine development.

INTRODUCTION

Even before the scientific community could offer a breakthrough in providing an evident cure for the outbreak of SARS coronavirus-1 (SARS-CoV-1), the world is

---

[*] **Corresponding author Palaniswamy Rani:** Department of Biotechnology, PSG College of Technology, Avinashi Rd, Peelamedu, Coimbatore, Tamil Nadu 641004, India; Tel: 9443 161 653; Fax: 91-0422-2573833; E-mail: rani.bio@psgtech.ac.in

Parvesh Singh, Vipan Kumar & Rajshekhar Karpoormath (Eds.)
All rights reserved-© 2021 Bentham Science Publishers

faced with yet another challenging outbreak of SARS variant, SARS-CoV-2, posing a serious threat in the global community. Severe acute respiratory syndrome (SARS) is a fatal, contagious respiratory disease with symptoms similar to Pneumonia. SARS is caused by the coronaviruses that have a zoonotic origin known for upper respiratory tract infections. SARS-CoV infections appeared in 2002 and no longer spread after 2004 with the distribution to 24 countries. The variant SARS-CoV-2 is now spreading all over the world with an even higher degree of transmission and recombination because of the higher viral load in the upper respiratory tract, but the lethality of SARS-CoV-2 is comparatively lower than that of SARS-CoV-1 [1]. This alarming rise in the transmission of SARS virus has pushed us to identify new strategies to combat the novel coronavirus. The existing antiviral drugs and treatments, although being implemented across the world are found to be not promising enough to control the infection and defend the immune system in humans on a long term basis. This limitation encourages the researchers to develop a long term defense mechanism in a human system to fight back against the virus, which can only be fulfilled by developing therapeutic and prophylactic vaccines.

The parameters that are important for the SARS vaccine design are: (i) a long term effective immune response eliciting T lymphocytes against the SARS viral antigens which is crucial for viral infection/replication; (ii) the candidate vaccine's efficacy (>60%) is important so that it does not cause any serious adverse effects and cross-reactivity thereby ensuring the safety and successful herd immunity; (iii) the ease of administering the vaccine (preferably oral or intranasal) and the amount of dosage required, have to be considered especially for the pregnant/ lactating women/ in patients with other medical conditions such as elderly population and immunosuppressed individuals; (iv) The proposed vaccine should be easily scalable and the durability should also be ensured for availability in underdeveloped nations; (v) cost of the vaccine should be reasonable [2].

Existing knowledge on the mechanism of SARS virus, along with the advancement of other genomic tools and technologies, which enabled the availability of the genome sequence and structure of SARS-CoV-2 in a very short time has paved the way for vaccine development strategies for SARS-CoV-2 [3]. This helped in the identification of potential molecular and immunogenic determinants as targets for vaccines. This chapter will provide a brief walk through about the genome and structure of the virus, pathogenesis and exclusively about the vaccine development for SARS-CoV and the challenges faced while developing vaccines and a better scope in the near future from the lessons learnt.

SARS VIRUS

SARS Virus Family and Genome

SARS-CoV is a species of coronavirus classified from the genera *Betacoronavirus* sub-classified under lineage B, *Sarbecovirus*. SARS-CoV under *Sarbecovirus* is different from other genera by the presence of one papain-like proteinase (PLpro) instead of two in the open reading frame ORF1 [4 - 6].

SARS-CoV is an envelope, positive sense, single strand RNA virus. The genome of SARS-CoV is 29,740 base pairs in length. ORF1a and ORF1b encompass 75% of the viral genome. They have overlapping open reading frames that provide proteins needed for replication and transcription. The remaining part of the genome codes for four structural proteins and other accessory genes are also present in the structural region of the viral genome. These viral RNA have a high degree of recombination and it forms new recombinant RNA when infected in the host [7 - 9].

SARS Virus Structure

SARS coronaviruses are spherical to pleomorphic viral particles having an average diameter in a range of 85 nm to 125 nm. The club-shaped spike projections on the surface of coronaviruses under electron microscope recreates the similar image of solar corona from which the name originates. The SARS viruses have 4 structural proteins, namely E (envelope), S (spike), M (membrane) and N (nucleocapsid) (Fig. **1**). The envelope of the virus consists of a lipid bilayer membrane embedded with Spike, Envelope and Membrane proteins. Envelope and Membrane proteins are crucial for maintaining structural integrity. The inner genome comprises nucleocapsid protein scaffolded around the viral RNA. The outer spike protein enables the virus attachment to the receptor and facilitates host pathogen interaction. It belongs to the family of Class 1 fusion proteins. Spike protein has 2 subunits, namely, S1 subunit (head of spike protein which has Receptor Binding Domain (RBD), that binds with ACE-2 receptor) and S2 subunit (acts as the stem which anchors spike head and RBD; plays a role in receptor fusion following protease activity). The RBD has a Receptor Binding Motif (RBM) which plays a main role in ACE-2 receptor and SARS-CoV-2 interaction [10].

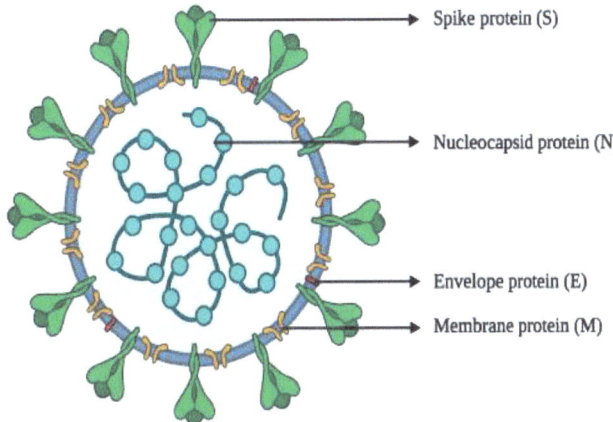

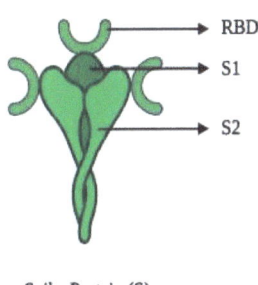

Spike Protein (S)

Fig. (1). Structure of SARS-CoV.

Pathogenesis

The binding and infection mechanisms are similar for SARS-CoV-1 and SARS-CoV-2. The SARS-CoV infection showed the peak of viral titers between 10-14 days of infection. SARS CoV-2 can generate 3.20 fold higher numbers of virulent particles than SARS-CoV-1. The binding of SARS-CoV-2 with ACE-2 receptor showed a higher affinity than SARS-CoV-1. SARS viruses are transmitted by respiratory epithelial droplets, which could spread from one person to another within 6 ft of distance by cough and sneeze, and indirectly transmitted *via* contaminated surfaces. Recent studies also suggested that the transmission could be airborne. Poor ventilation systems in hospitals are easily prone to the rapid spread of infection and airborne transmission [11]. Stool and semen samples from individuals showed viral RNA traces. The soaps and detergent have the ability to degrade the lipid coat of the virus; thereby, it can be used for personal disinfection [12 - 14].

The entry of the virus is mediated by the Spike protein (S) of SARS-CoV. The receptor binding domain (RBD) in spike protein binds with ACE-2 receptors in the host cells. SARS-CoV-1 and SARS-CoV-2 are similar in cell tropism and target the type 1 and 2 pneumocytes and alveolar macrophages (in lower and upper respiratory tract) which are rich in the ACE-2 receptors [15, 16]. This binding triggers the membrane and facilitates endocytosis. The released viral RNA gets translated into viral polymerase and enables the viral replication. The newly synthesized negative sense genomic RNA acts as a template for the formation of subgenomic positive sense RNA which is utilized for structural protein synthesis. The viral RNA and structural nucleocapsid proteins are replicated, transcribed and translated in the cytoplasm whereas the other structural proteins are transcribed and translated in Endoplasmic Reticulum (ER). The different structural proteins and RNA synthesized are assembled in the ER-Golgi intermediate compartment (ERGIC). Then the mature virions are released from the host cells and propagate the infection (Fig. **2**) [11].

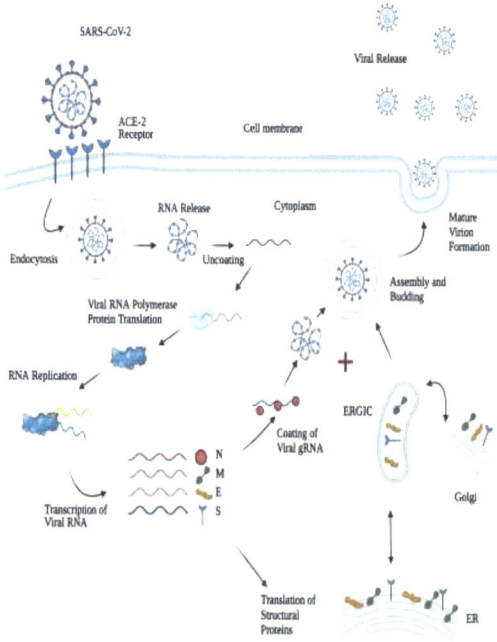

Fig. (2). Mechanism of infection by SARS-CoV (Structural proteins E- Envelope protein, N- Nucleocapsid protein, M- Membrane protein, S- Spike protein; Assembly of virions by translation and transportation by ERGIC - ER-Golgi intermediate compartment).

The prognosis of infection causes respiratory failure and death. In some cases, respiratory failure by brain stem damage is also observed. Autopsies of infected persons show detectable amounts of viral particles in the Central Nervous System (CNS). The virus may invade peripheral nerves which have low levels of ACE-2 receptors but the way of invading CNS remains unclear [17]. It can also cause acute myocardial injury and severe damage to the cardiovascular system because of the presence of ACE-2 receptors in the heart [18]. The evidence of thrombosis and venous thromboembolism is also observed in some infected patients. The mortality observed due to kidney failure was in about 30% of people who were newly affected with kidney related complications, without having prior kidney problems. Some autopsies also show Diffusive Alveolar Damage (DAD) [19].

Immune Response

The pathological effects in the lungs is due to the irregular innate immune response results in elevated levels of inflammatory cytokines and chemokines, such as: CXCL10 (IP-10), CCL2 (MCP-1), IL-6, IL-8, IL-12, IL-1 β, and IFN- γ. Host mechanism of sensing SARS-CoV remains unknown, but TLRs and RLRs may be involved in the innate immune sensing. SARS-CoV proteins modulate the innate immune responses, thereby antagonizing the IFN responses, which lead to the escape of viruses from host sensing mechanisms. Significantly, the type I IFNs are inhibited or delayed by the SARS-CoV infections. The usage of pegylated IFN-α as a prophylactic treatment has demonstrated a great reduction in the replication of SARS-CoV in lung infection. Regulation of IFN levels might play a significant role in the control of SARS [20, 21].

The T cells against Spike protein S and nucleocapsid N show evidence in long term memory and potent immune response. These responses also have an association with IgG and IgM levels. T lymphocytes, mainly CD4+ T cells, and CD8+ T cells were decreased in mild cases and also in severe cases, whereas CD4+/CD8+ ratio increased in the course of infection. A group of studies conducted on the direct *ex vivo* T cell assays using broad-based epitope pools and assays capable of detecting T cells of any cytokine polarization from the infected patients supports the evidence of a substantial increase in CD4+ T cell response against the SARS-CoV-2 [22]. In contrast, a study on mice that lack cellular immunity cleared the viral load in its body within 9 days of infection, thereby suggesting that cellular immunity may not be needed for viral clearance [23 - 25].

The total antibodies, IgG, IgM observed had median seroconversion time of 11-14 days after the onset of disease. 50 to 90% of people maintain the antibodies against SARS-CoV-1 up to three years after infection [23, 26], but the levels of IgG and IgM neutralizing antibodies in SARS-CoV-2 recovered patients start to decrease within 2–4 months after infection [27, 28]. Durability of SARS-CoV-2 vaccines cannot be assured at this time but can be compared with the elicited T cell immunity of genetically similar SARS-CoV-1, which confers immunity until 17 years post infection [29]. The neutralizing antibodies are developed in the body against different regions of Spike protein (S1 and S2) in SARS-CoV-1 and against the Nucleocapsid (N) and RBD in SARS-CoV-2 [30].

Clinical symptoms, Diagnosis and Treatment

The SARS-CoV-1 infection causes diseases in the lower respiratory tract that covers fever, peripheral T cell lymphocytopenia, decreased platelet count, prolonged coagulation profiles, gastrointestinal, urinary tract infection and mild elevation of serum hepatic enzyme levels [31]. COVID-19 has varied symptoms from patients to patients which include fever, nausea, cough, gastrointestinal problems such as diarrhea, loss of appetite, and loss of taste and smell. Some severe illness causes difficulty in breathing, fatigue, muscle and joint pains. Approximately, 40 to 45% of the COVID-19 infection cases are asymptomatic and undetectable [32]. The rate of intensive care and mortality depend upon the age of the patients [33, 34].

The standard method of diagnosis for SARS-CoV is Real time Reverse Transcriptase-Polymerase Chain Reaction (RT-PCR) for which the samples are obtained from the upper and lower respiratory tract. Most of the PCR assays target ORF1ab (open reading frame), RdRp (RNA dependent RNA polymerase gene), E (envelope protein coding gene), N (nucleocapsid protein gene) and S (Spike protein gene). The envelope gene is highly conserved among *Sarbecovirus* subgenus. Researchers proposed that the combinations of ELISA with real time RT-PCR have enhanced sensitivity and efficiency. CT scans are also used in serious cases of infection for "Ground Glass Opacities". In the case of non-availability of real time RT-PCR, newly advanced diagnostic kits like Lateral flow assays and CRISPR based detection strips are used. Most of the serological tests have low sensitivity; therefore real time RT-PCR is used as the confirmatory test [35 - 37].

Specific treatments for SARS-CoV infections are not yet recognized and even now there aren't any promising antiviral drugs available for the cure. General medicines like Paracetamol (acetaminophen), antiviral drugs (Ribavirin, Remdesivir), corticosteroids (Dexamethasone) are prescribed for early infections. Other than medications, people are provided with supportive care including fluid therapy, oxygen support (ECMO, ventilators) and treatments specific for affected vital organs [38, 39]. The convalescent plasma therapy is yet another promising solution to treat COVID-19 that has proved to be safe and effective without any serious threats [40, 41]. Even though the existing therapeutic drugs and treatment are available, the control of the disease has not been successful. This encourages the development of prophylactic approaches such as vaccines for the treatment and prevention.

VACCINE DEVELOPMENT

Pipeline

It is well known that the vaccines for SARS-CoV-1 are still in the progress (Table 1) even after its outbreak for the past 10-15 years, the expectation for effective production of vaccines against SARS-CoV-2 for COVID-19 is set high [42, 43]. Normally, the timeline for conducting clinical research is exhaustive. This pandemic situation requires a reduced timeline for vaccine production by also considering the essential strategies such as safety, efficacy and availability. Various established organizations like World Health Organization (WHO), the Coalition for Epidemic Preparedness Innovations (CEPI) and various other government and private sources are trying to collaborate by providing funds to innovative ideas for developing promising vaccines thereby reducing the timeline of 10+ years of vaccine development to 12-18 months in this current pandemic situation (Fig. 3). However, an appropriate timeline and strategy is required. Each of these vaccine platform strategies may have its own strengths and flaws [3]. In April 2020, the National Institutes of Health (NIH) announced the Accelerating COVID-19 Therapeutic Interventions and Vaccines (ACTIV) as a public private initiative to form an alliance with various pharmaceutical companies to develop a strong coordinated strategy for vaccine development at the earliest [2].

In July 2020, WHO has suggested Solidarity Clinical Trials as a globalized strategy which encourages randomized clinical trials enrolling worldwide participants for the vaccine development in a reduced time (20% of the conventional timeline). The development of vaccines should be based on prioritization of the research and strategies to fill the gaps between preclinical studies and manufacturing of final approved vaccines [44]. However, to produce vaccines on a reduced timeline, the vaccine manufacturers are adopting a strategy by employing the overlap of different phases of vaccine development without even bothering about the financial risk involved. This reduced timeline will overlap the phases of target vaccine candidate selection, preclinical studies (*in vivo* and in animal models) and shortened clinical stage thereby producing large capacity of vaccines when the results are observed with minimal (~70%) prescribed efficacy and safety [45].

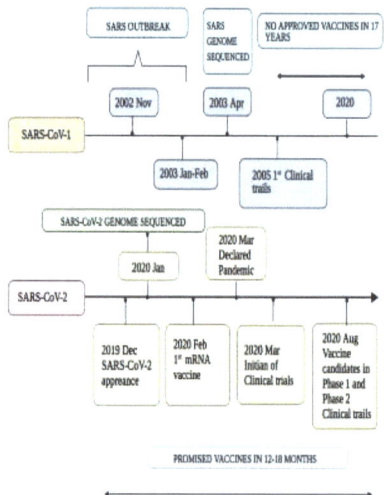

Fig. (3). Comparison of Timeline in Vaccine Development progress for SARS-CoV-1 and SARS-CoV-2 since its outbreak [2].

Table 1. State of Progress in SARS-CoV-1 Vaccine Development [93].

Vaccine Manufacturer	Vaccine Platform	Type of Candidate Vaccine	Current Stage of Development
Sinovac Biotech Ltd (/Beijing Kexing Bioproducts), Chinese Centre for Disease Control and Prevention; Chinese Academy of Medical Sciences	Inactivated Virus	ISCV	Phase I
CNB-CSIC; University of Iowa	Inactivated Virus	rSARSCoV-E	Pre-Clinical
University of North Carolina	Live Attenuated Virus	Live attenuated vaccine Nsp16 mutant lacking 2'-OMTase	Pre-Clinical
University of North Carolina	Live Attenuated Virus	Live attenuated SARS-CoV MA-ΔExoN	Pre-Clinical
University Health Network, Canada; Center for Disease Control and Prevention (CDC)	Replicating Viral Vector	Recombinant measles virus Spike protein	Pre-Clinical
Institut Pasteur	Replicating Viral Vector	MV-SARS recombinant measles virus vaccine expressing SARS CoV antigen	Pre-Clinical
International Vaccine Institute (IVI)	Non-Replicating Viral Vector	recombinant adenovirus expressing Trunctuated S protein (rADV-S)	Pre-Clinical
The Rockefeller University	Non-Replicating Viral Vector	MVA S alone, or MVA-S prime and Ad5-S boost	Pre-Clinical

(Table 1) cont.....

Vaccine Manufacturer	Vaccine Platform	Type of Candidate Vaccine	Current Stage of Development
Vaxine Pty Ltd, Australia	Protein Subunit	SARS recombinant spike protein plus delta inulin	Pre-Clinical
Baylor College Medicine; Sabin; New York Blood Center (NYBC); University of Texas Medical Branch (UTMB); Walter Reed Army Institute of Research (WRAIR); National Institute of Allergy and Infectious Diseases (NIAID)	Protein Subunit	receptor binding domain (RBD) of the SARS- CoV spike (S) protein	Pre-Clinical
Institute of ImmunoBiology, Shanghai Medical College of Fudan University, China	DNA	DNA prime–protein S437–459 and M1–2	Pre-Clinical
National Institute of Allergy and Infectious Diseases (NIAID)	DNA	DNAvaccine VRC-SRSDNA015- 00-VP ; Biojector used	Phase I
University of Texas Medical Branch (UTMB)	Virus-like Particle	Chimeric VLP (S protein SARS plus E, M and N proteins of mouse hepatitis virus)	Pre-Clinical
Novavax	Virus-like Particle	SARS VLPs S protein and influenza M1 protein	Pre-Clinical

As of 22nd December 2020, the World Health Organisation (WHO) has listed 61 vaccine candidates under clinical evaluation (Table **2**) and 172 vaccine candidates under pre-clinical evaluation for SARS-CoV-2 [46]. Newer options for vaccine design like chimeric viral vaccines and membrane vesicle-vaccines are coming up. Since the spike protein has been found to elicit an immune response, most of the vaccines have been targeting this protein at all molecular levels. The cryo-electron microscopy (cryo-EM) structure of SARS-CoV-2 S trimer has been shared recently, which seemed to accelerate the process of vaccine development [47].

Table 2. State of Progress in Clinical Development of Vaccines for SARS-CoV-2 [46].

Vaccine Manufacturer	Vaccine Platform	Type of Candidate Vaccine	No. of Doses	Timing of Doses	Route of Administration	Clinical Stage
Sinovac Research and Development Co., Ltd.	Inactivated virus	SARS-CoV-2 (Inactivated)	2	0, 14 days	IM	Phase 3
Wuhan Institute of Biological Products/ Sinopharm	Inactivated virus	Inactivated SARS-CoV-2 Vaccine (Vero cell)	2	0, 21 days	IM	Phase 3

(Table 2) cont.....

Vaccine Manufacturer	Vaccine Platform	Type of Candidate Vaccine	No. of Doses	Timing of Doses	Route of Administration	Clinical Stage
Beijing Institute of Biological Products/ Sinopharm	Inactivated virus	Inactivated SARS-CoV-2 Vaccine (Vero cell)	2	0, 21 days	IM	Phase 3
Institute of Medical Biology, Chinese Academy of Medical Sciences	Inactivated virus	SARS-CoV-2 Vaccine (Vero cell)	2	0,28 days	IM	Phase 1/2
Bharat Biotech International Limited	Inactivated virus	Whole-Virion Inactivated SARS-CoV-2 Vaccine (BBV152)	2	0, 14 days	IM	Phase 3
Research Institute for Biological Safety Problems, Rep of Kazakhstan	Inactivated virus	QazCovid-in- COVID-19 inactivated vaccine	2	0, 21 days	IM	Phase 1/2
Shenzhen Kangtai Biological Products Co., Ltd.	Inactivated virus	Inactivated SARS-CoV-2 vaccine (Vero cell)	1, 2 or 3	ND	IM	Phase 2
Valneva, National Institute for Health Research, United Kingdom	Inactivated virus	VLA2001	2	0, 21 days	IM	Phase 1/2
Codagenix/Serum Institute of India	Live attenuated virus	COVI-VAC	1/ 2	Day 0 or 0,28 days	IN	Phase 1
Institut Pasteur/Themis/ Univ. of Pittsburg CVR/Merck & co./Sharp &Dohme	Replicating Viral Vector	V591-001 Measles-vector based (TMV-o38)	1/ 2	0, 28 days	IM	Phase 1/2
Jiangsu Provincial Center for Disease Prevention and Control	Replicating Viral Vector	DelNS1-2019-nCo V-RBD-OPT1 (Intranasal flu-based-RBD)	1	Day 0	IN	Phase 2
Shenzhen Geno-Immune Medical Institute	Replicating Viral vector with APC	Covid-19/aAPC vaccine	3	0, 14, 28 days	SC	Phase 1
Aivita Biomedical, Inc.	Replicating Viral Vector with APC	Dendritic cell vaccine AV-COVID-19	1	Day 0	IM	Phase 1/ 2
Israel Institute for Biological Research	Replicating Viral Vector	rVSV-SARS-CoV-2-S Vaccine	1	Day 0	IM	Phase 1
Cellid Co., Ltd.	Replicating Viral Vector	AdCLD-CoV19	ND	ND	IM	Phase 1/2
Gamaleya Research Institute ; Health Ministry of the Russian Federation	Non-Replicating Viral Vector	Gam-COVID-Vac Adeno-based (rAd26-S+rAd5-S)	2	0, 21 days	IM	Phase 3
ReiThera/LEUK OCARE/ Univercells	Non-Replicating Viral Vector	GRAd-COV2	1	Day 0	IM	Phase 1

(Table 2) cont.....

Vaccine Manufacturer	Vaccine Platform	Type of Candidate Vaccine	No. of Doses	Timing of Doses	Route of Administration	Clinical Stage
University of Oxford/ AstraZeneca	Non-Replicating Viral Vector	ChAdOx1-S - (AZD1222) (Covishield)	1/2	0, 28 days	IM	Phase 3
CanSino Biological Inc./Beijing Institute of Biotechnology	Non-Replicating Viral Vector	Adenovirus Type 5 Vector	1	Day 0	IM	Phase 3
Janssen Pharmaceutical Companies	Non-Replicating Viral Vector	Ad26COVS1	1/ 2	Day 0 or 0, 56 days	IM	Phase 3
Vaxart	Non-Replicating Viral Vector	VXA-CoV2-1 Ad5 adjuvanted Oral Vaccine platform	2	0, 28 days	Oral	Phase 1
University of Munich (Ludwig-Maximilians)	Non-Replicating Viral Vector	MVA-SARS-2-S	2	0, 28 days	IM	Phase 1
Shenzhen Geno-Immune Medical Institute	Non-Replicating Viral Vector with APC	LV-SMENP-DC vaccine	1	Day 0	SC & IV	Phase 1/2
ImmunityBio, Inc.	Non-Replicating Viral Vector	hAd5-S-Fusion+N-ETSD vaccine	1	Day 0	Oral	Phase 1
City of Hope Medical Center, National Cancer Institute	Non-Replicating Viral Vector	COH04S1 (MVA-SARS-2-S)	1/2	Day 0 or 0, 28 days	IM	Phase 1
Anhui ZhifeiLongcom Biopharmaceutical/Institute of Microbiology, Chinese Academy of Sciences	Protein Subunit	Recombinant SARS-Co-2 vaccine (CHO Cell)	2/ 3	0, 28 or 0, 28, 56 days	IM	Phase 3
Novavax	Protein Subunit	SARS-CoV-2 rS/Matrix M1-Adjuvant	2	0, 21 days	IM	Phase 3
Kentucky Bioprocessing, Inc.	Protein Subunit	KBP-COVID-19 (RBD-based)	2	0, 21 days	IM	Phase 1/ 2
University of Queensland/CSL/ Seqirus	Protein Subunit	MF59 adjuvanted SARS-CoV-2 S clamp vaccine	2	0, 28 days	IM	Phase 1
Medigen Vaccine Biologics Corporation/NIAID/Dynavax	Protein Subunit	MVC-COV1901 (S-2P protein + CpG 1018)	2	0, 28 days	IM	Phase 1
Instituto Finlay de Vacunas, Cuba	Protein Subunit	FINLAY-FR anti-SARS-CoV-2 Vaccine (RBD + adjuvant)	2	0, 28 days	IM	Phase 1/ 2

Vaccine Manufacturer	Vaccine Platform	Type of Candidate Vaccine	No. of Doses	Timing of Doses	Route of Administration	Clinical Stage
Sanofi Pasteur/GSK	Protein Subunit	SARS-CoV-2 with adjuvant 1 (baculovirus production)	2	0, 21 days	IM	Phase 1/ 2
FBRI SRC VB VECTOR, Rospotrebnadzor Koltsovo	Protein Subunit	EpiVacCorona	2	0, 21 days	IM	Phase 1/ 2
Clover Biopharmaceuticals Inc./GSK/ Dynavax	Protein Subunit	SCB-2019 + AS03 or CpG 1018 adjuvant plus Alum adjuvant	2	0, 21 days	IM	Phase 1
Vaxine Pty Ltd/Medytox	Protein Subunit	COVID19 vaccine	1	Day 0	IM	Phase 1
West China Hospital, Sichuan University	Protein Subunit	RBD (baculovirus production expressed in Sf9 cells)	2	0, 28 days	IM	Phase 2
University Hospital Tuebingen	Protein Subunit	IMP CoVac-1	1	Day 0	SC	Phase 1
COVAXX, United Biomedical Inc.	Protein Subunit	UB-612	2	0, 28 days	IM	Phase 1
Barbara Carlson, University of Oklahoma	Protein subunit	SHINGRIX	2	0, 61 days	IM	Phase 1
Adimmune Corporation	Protein subunit	AdimrSC-2f	ND	ND	ND	Phase 1
Center for Genetic Engineering and Biotechnology (CIGB)	Protein subunit	CIGB-669 (RBD+AgnHB)	3	0, 14,28 or 0, 28,56 days	IN	Phase 1/ 2
Center for Genetic Engineering and Biotechnology (CIGB)	Protein subunit	CIGB-66 (RBD+aluminium hydroxide)	3	0, 14,28 or 0, 28,56 days	IN	Phase 1/ 2
Biological ELimited	Protein subunit	BECOV2	2	0, 28 days	IM	Phase 1/ 2
Medicago Inc.	Virus Like Particle	CoVLP	2	0, 21 days	IM	Phase 2/ 3
Serum Institute of India/ Accelagen Pty	Virus Like Particle	RBD SARS CoV-2 HBsAg VLP Vaccine	2	0, 28 days	IM	Phase 1/ 2
Moderna/NIAID	RNA based Vaccine	mRNA-1273	2	0, 28 days	IM	Phase 3 (Approved by FDA for emergency use)
CureVac AG	RNA based vaccine	CVnCoV Vaccine	2	0,29/ 28 days	IM	Phase 2/ 3

(Table 2) cont.....

Vaccine Manufacturer	Vaccine Platform	Type of Candidate Vaccine	No. of Doses	Timing of Doses	Route of Administration	Clinical Stage
BioNTech + FosunPharma ; Jiangsu Provincial Center for Disease Prevention and Control + Pfizer	RNA based vaccine	BNT162 (3 LNP-mRNAs)	2	0, 28 days	IM	Phase 3(Approved by FDA for emergency use)
Arcturus Therapeutics	RNA based vaccine	ARCT-021	ND	ND	IM	Phase 1/ 2
Imperial College London	RNA based vaccine	LNP-nCoVsaRN A	2	ND	IM	Phase 1
Shulan (Hangzhou) Hospital, Center for Disease Control and Prevention of Guangxi Zhuang Autonomous Region	RNA based vaccine	SARS-CoV-2 mRNA vaccine	2	0, 14 or 0, 28 days	IM	Phase 1
Chulalongkorn University	RNA based vaccine	ChulaCov19 mRNA vaccine	2	0, 21 days	IM	Phase 1
Osaka University/ AnGes/ Takara Bio	DNA based vaccine	AG0301-COVID1 9	2	0, 14 days	IM	Phase 1/ 2
Cadila Healthcare Limited	DNA based vaccine	nCoV vaccine	3	0, 28, 56 days	ID	Phase 1/ 2
Genexine Consortium	DNA based vaccine	GX-19	2	0, 28 days	IM	Phase 1/ 2
Inovio Pharmaceuticals/ International Vaccine Institute	DNA based vaccine	INO-4800+electroporation	2	0, 28 days	ID	Phase 2/ 3
Entos Pharmaceuticals Inc.	DNA based vaccine	Covigenix VAX-001	2	0, 14 days	IM	Phase 1
Providence Health & Services	DNA based vaccine	CORVax	2	0, 14 days	ID	Phase 1
Symvivo Corporation	DNA based vaccine	bacTRL-Spike	1	Day 0	Oral	Phase 1
GeneOne Life Science, Inc.	DNA based vaccine	GLS-5310	2	0, 56 or 0, 84 days	ID	Phase 1/ 2

Reverse Vaccinology Approach in SARS-COV-2 Vaccine Design

To design a vaccine against the target antigen, the conventional approaches generally employed are laborious and time consuming. Bioinformatics and Computational approaches offer boons to the field of vaccine development and especially in the current situation with the SARS-CoV-2 pandemic. The Next

Generation Sequencing technologies enabled the complete sequencing of the SARS-CoV-2 genome and with the advances in immunoinformatics, potential vaccine candidates can be developed *in silico*. The vaccine development for novel viruses needs Sequence Homology studies to reveal the unique regions of these viruses, thereby considering the sequences for the vaccine to prevent cross reactivity and specificity. Multiple Sequence Alignment of Spike protein of the SARS-CoV-2 showed the similarity of 77.38% with SARS-CoV-1 and 31.93% with MERS-CoV genome which revealed the heterogeneity in RBD and NTD regions that are essential for constructing the SARS-CoV-2 specific vaccines. With the help of immunoinformatics 52 B cell epitopes and 77 T cell epitopes in spike protein of SARS-CoV-2 were predicted. Immune simulation studies can be utilized for assessing the efficiency of predicted epitopes in immune response elicitation [48].

Vaccine Platform

The diversity on the vaccine development platforms for vaccine production is overwhelming which includes nucleic acid (DNA and RNA), peptide, virus-like particle (VLP), viral vector (replicating and non-replicating), recombinant protein, live attenuated virus and inactivated virus approaches being studied in pre-clinical and clinical stages (Fig. **4**). Since all of these are not currently in licensed use, many scientists are trying to achieve a breakthrough with these new platforms with next-generation approaches to accelerate the speed of development and manufacture. Some platforms will be helpful in targeting particular subpopulation for vaccines and might offer greater potential and flexibility in terms of designing and production. In some other platforms, the usage of adjuvants can enhance immunogenicity and lower the dosage intake, thereby maintaining the immunity and enabling the availability of vaccines to larger populations without any compromise [49].

Oral Vaccines

Apart from the classical vaccine platforms, for the first time, thermally stable oral COVID-19 vaccine capsules have been developed by ioSBio (earlier known as StabilitechBiopharma Limited) and Vaxart. The oral vaccine capsules offer several advantages over conventional vaccines as they are thermally stable and eliminate the need for injection and trained personnel to administer the vaccine. Interestingly, the Vaxart's VXA-CoV2-1 vaccine which employs adenoviral-vector based adjuvant platform has entered the Phase 1 clinical trials after clearing the IND application in September, 2020. The oral vaccine is shown to induce both mucosal and systemic immunity in Preclinical studies and it is expected to release it's Phase 1 results by early 2021. The Phase 1 trials are aiming to assess the safety, reactogenicity, immunogenicity in 48 healthy adult volunteers by administering the vaccines in varying doses (low or high) at days 1 and 29 [50 - 53]. In addition, Symvivo Corporation and ImmunityBio Inc. are also producing single dose oral vaccines and are currently in the stage of Phase 1 Clinical trials [46]. Similarly, ioSBio'sOra-Pro COVID-19 vaccines are being produced using non-replicating and non-integrating recombinant adenoviral vectors to deliver the genetic code of spike protein as cargo to the mucosal cells in the Gastrointestinal (GI) tract and this vaccine is still in the phase of approval for clinical trials [54 - 56].

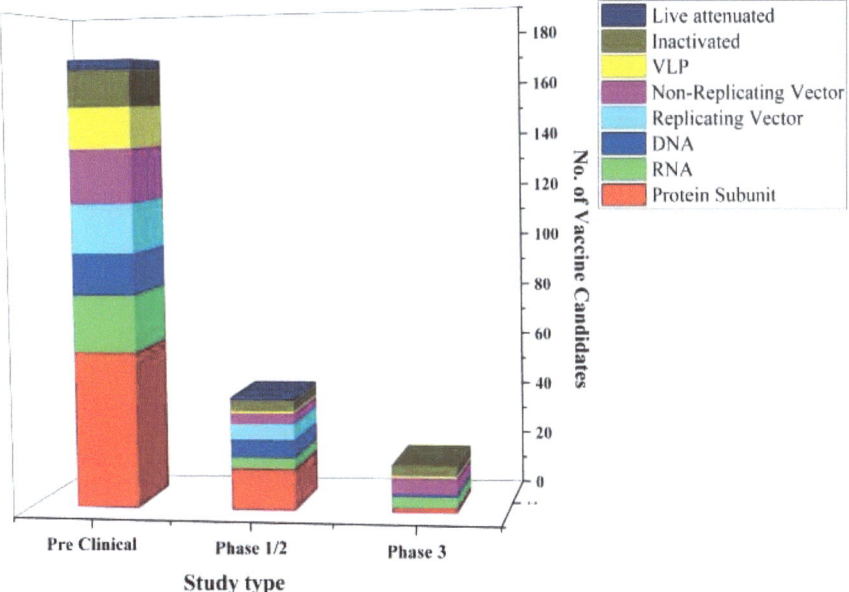

Fig. (4). COVID-19 vaccine candidate platforms [46].

Live Attenuated Vaccines

Live attenuated vaccines are developed by reducing the virulence of a virus without killing the virus. So, the viable virus without virulence is used to provoke immunity. Codagenix/Serum Institute of India is developing a live attenuated vaccine (COVI-VAC) with help of the Synthetic Attenuated Virus Engineering platform which uses synthetic biology to regenerate the genes of SARS-CoV-2 virus. The developed vaccine induces long-lasting and effective cellular immunity in preclinical studies. Therefore, Codagenix entered into Phase 1 trials with 48 volunteers. Single dosage of vaccine administered intranasally to the volunteers at three dosage levels. COVI-VAC does not need a syringe/needle and ultra low temperature conditions for storage [57, 58].

Inactivated Vaccines

Inactivated vaccines are developed from the viruses that are killed or inactivated by the physical or chemical process. Sinovac vaccine (CoronaVac) is one of the chemically inactivated, whole-virus preparations of COVID-19 vaccine candidates that can be administered in a two-dose regimen (at day 0 and day 28). The Sinovac vaccine was granted for emergency use authorization by Chinese government in July, 2020. 90% of the Sinovac company employees were vaccinated after authorization. Phase 1/2 clinical trials enrolled healthy volunteers aged 18–59 years. 143 participants were included in the Phase 1 clinical trial whereas 600 randomly assigned participants in the Phase 2 trial received two intramuscular injections. The trial was designed in such a way that administration of vaccine is either 3 µg per 0·5 mL or 6 µg per 0·5 mL or placebo and the day of administration is either on day 0 and day 14, or on day 0 and day 28. The Sinovac vaccine elicited anti-RBD antibodies which was measured by ELISA, and by a period of 14 days after the second dosage, it was observed to have elicited neutralising antibodies in 92.4% of individuals (0 and 14th day dosage pattern) and in 97.4% individuals (0 and 28th day dosage pattern). The level of neutralizing antibody was higher in the case of younger individuals (aged 18-39 years) than the older individuals (aged 40-59 years) and the immune responses were strongly noted in individuals who were given the second dosage on 28th day than in those, who received the second dosage on 14th day.

Brazil trial showed more than 50% efficiency whereas the Turkey trial showed 91.2% efficiency but the trial was conducted with only 29 participants, where the reliability is uncertain. Brazil's late stage trial included 13,000 participants and suggested the shot was effective and safe. The results of the Phase 3 trial conducted over Brazil, Turkey, Indonesia and Chile are expected to be finalized at the end of December 2020. No major side effects were encountered but the mild adverse effects of the vaccine include fever, mild pain and slight fatigue. This vaccine proves to be successful for mass vaccination in developing countries where it satisfies the minimal conditional requirements like normal refrigeration temperature for storage of vaccines [59 - 61].

Sinopharm developed two inactivated whole-virus vaccines which are alum adjuvanted. Wuhan Institute of Biological Products developed the first vaccine candidate (New Crown COVID-19). The phase 1 trials with 96 participants examined a three-dose series, and the phase 2 trials with 224 participants, studied a 5 µg dose across two study group design: 84 participants with vaccination on day 0 and 14 versus 28 participants with alum only or 84 participants with vaccination on day 0 and 21 versus 28 participants receiving alum only. Phase 1 trials were conducted with adults aged 18-59 years. The phase 2 trials measured neutralising antibody titres which was higher in the case of the participant group vaccinated on days 0 and 21 than the participant group vaccinated on days 0 and 14. Notably, this vaccine didn't induce cellular immunity because the concentrations of leukocyte and cytokines were not changed in the study groups which were measured with flow cytometric assays. Phase 3 clinical trials began in July, 2020 and enrolled 21,000 participants in the United Arab Emirates (UAE), Bahrain, Peru, Morocco, Argentina, and Jordan. The second vaccine candidate that was tested by Sinopharm was developed by the Beijing Institute of Biological Products. Phase 3 trials with 5,000 participants took place in the United Arab Emirates. UAE approved this vaccine for emergency use and the vaccine was administered to thousands of people after the authorization by Chinese Authorities. The phase 3 trials showed 86% efficacy and it was not encountered with any kind of adverse effects and the mild effects were only observed in alum only subgroups of the trials. Sinopharm also targets providing vaccination to developing countries but the reliability in the efficacy of the vaccine has to be considered similar to the case of Sinovac [59, 62 - 64].

Protein Subunit Vaccine

Subunit vaccines consist of synthetic peptides or recombinant antigenic proteins for provoking immune response. This vaccine exhibits low immunogenicity and requires adjuvant to potentiate the effective immune response. In the S Protein of SARS-CoV, S1 subunit has the NTD, RBD and RBM domains and the S2 subunit has FP, HR 1 and HR 2 domains. S proteins, the prime targets for subunit vaccine development, are dynamic proteins which possess two conformational states: pre-fusion and post-fusion state.

Novavax, Inc. (NVX-CoV2373) is developing a subunit vaccine based on the recombinant expression of the stable pre-fusion protein of SARS-CoV-2 using Baculovirus system and then it's post-translationally modified protein is incorporated into a nanoparticle formulation along with Membrane (M) protein adjuvant for enhancing the immune response [2, 65]. Recently, the study has completed the enrollment for the participants in Phase 3 trials in the United Kingdom, U.S./Mexico and Phase 2b trials in South Africa. The primary efficacy data for the vaccine candidate is found to be in harmony with global regulatory standards and the Phase 3 results are expected by the first quarter of 2021 [66].

Anhui ZhifeiLongcom Biopharmaceutical along with the Institute of Microbiology under the Chinese Academy of Sciences are producing China's first recombinant subunit COVID-19 vaccine which has entered for the phase 3 efficacy studies enrolling around 29,000 participants aged above 18 years. With the results of the early-stage trials being promising with safety, efficacy and immunogenicity of the vaccine, the global trials are anticipated to begin in Pakistan, Ecuador and Uzbekistan by the end of the year [67].

University of Queensland collaboration with GSK and Dynavax is developing a stable pre-fusion recombinant viral subunit vaccine using Molecular Clamp technology to maintain the stability of the subunit structure along with AS03 (Squalene, α-tocopherol and Polysorbate 80) adjuvant system. PittCoVacc is developing a Microneedle Array SARS-CoV-2 vaccine based upon recombinant rSARS-CoV-2-S1 and rSARS-CoV-2-S1 fRS09. Premas Biotech is developing a Triple Antigen Vaccine that is a multi-antigenic Virus Like Particle (VLP) vaccine based on co-expression of recombinant spike, membrane, and envelope protein of SARS-CoV-2 to mediate the self-assembly of the these proteins as the VLP [2, 65].

Improvements in the bioinformatics tools and Immunoinformatics approach on prediction of epitopes for SARS-CoV-2 has been studied. It was fortunate that this approach was able to identify 34 linear B-cell epitopes using the IEDB server and 29 epitopes against Major Histocompatibility complex-I (MHC-I) and 8 epitopes against MHC-II using the *ProPred* server [68]. Most of the vaccine candidates have used the RBD for developing viral subunit vaccines [69]. Another study [115], identified two proteins S14P5 and S21P2, respectively, to be present in recovered individuals from both SARS-CoV-1 and SARS-CoV-2 patients. The study also suggested that if the antibodies are targeted against these 2 linear epitopes, it can neutralize the SARS-CoV-2 virus. Extensive immunoinformatics studies on the proteome of SARS-CoV-2 have provided insight about seven epitopes from five immunogenic regions, which cover more than 87% of the world's population (Table **3**). Out of these, three potential immunodominant epitopes each from the region of spike glycoprotein residue 819-918 and from the region of nucleocapsid phosphoprotein residue 292-330 has been proven to have the most coverage in the world's population which can be effective enough for designing potential vaccine candidates against SARS-CoV-2 [70].

Table 3. List of epitopes with more than 85% world population coverage (source from [70]).

Epitopes	Epitope Location	World Population Coverage (%)
PKEITVATSRTLSYYKL	Membrane glycoprotein:165-181	95.82%
QFAPSASAFFGMSRIGM	Nucleocapsid phosphoprotein:306-322	92.81%
FFGMSRIGMEVTPSGTW	Nucleocapsid phosphoprotein:314–330	87.42%
FIEDLLFNKVTLADAGF	Spike glycoprotein: 817-833	94.26%
GAALQIPFAMQMAYRFN	Spike glycoprotein: 891-907	97.46%
PFAMQMAYRFNGIGVTQ	Spike glycoprotein: 897-913	92.52%
EIDRLNEVAKNLNESLIDL QELGKYEQY	Spike glycoprotein: 1182–1209	88.57%

Viral Vector Vaccines

Viral vector vaccines are a promising prophylactic strategy to deliver the genes to the target cells thereby efficiently and specifically inducing the immune response. This type of vaccine offers long term immune response which triggers cytotoxic T cells, ultimately leading to the elimination of the virus infected cells. University of Oxford/Astrazeneca is developing a vaccine based on inserting the SARS-CoV-2 S gene into the E1 locus of ChAdOx1 (Chimpanzee viral vector) adenovirus genome by using the BAC system. The virus is allowed to reproduce in the Human Embryonic Kidney 293 cell lines and purified by the CsCl gradient ultracentrifugation. In a phase 1/2 trial, volunteers received first dose vaccine and second dose vaccine with 5.0×10^{10} viral particles. Additionally, one subset of volunteers received the first dose with 2.5×10^{10} viral particles and the second dose with 5.0×10^{10} viral particles given. The second dose vaccine was administered 28 days after the first dose for testing the immunogenicity and protective efficacy. The results concluded that two standard doses of the vaccine show 62% efficacy in preventing symptomatic COVID-19 disease. In the meantime, volunteers who received a low dose followed by a standard dose of vaccine showed 90% efficacy. After the first dose of administration, humoral responses and IFNγ T-cell responses were observed whereas increase in humoral response was observed in the second dose of administration. The adverse events such as fever, headache, muscle aches and nausea were observed within 4-5 days of vaccination. A large phase 3 trial of the vaccine was performed with 30,000 adults (Vaccine recipients-20,000 and Controls-10,000). The Oxford/AstraZeneca vaccine can be stored at refrigerator temperature and this is a major advantage over the mRNA vaccines being developed by Pfizer and Moderna, so it can be easily transported to many low and middle income countries [59, 71 - 73].

CanSino Biologics Inc. is developing a recombinant, replication defective adenovirus type 5 vector (Ad5) expressing the recombinant spike protein of SARS-CoV-2. This vaccine is prepared by cloning an optimized full length gene of the S Protein along with the plasminogen activator signal peptide gene in the Ad5 vector. The viral vector devoid of E1A and E1B genes, replaced immediately by cytomegalovirus (CMV) early promoter, subsequently drives expression of the target S protein. The phase 1 trials were carried out in Wuhan whereas the phase 3 trials are underway in China and Pakistan. The vaccine was tested for 108 (51% male, 49% female) healthy adults where 38 candidates were aged from 18 to 60 years. The volunteers equally separated to allocate them in three (5×10^{10}, 1×10^{11} and 1.5×10^{11} viral particles) dosage groups to administer the vaccine intramuscularly. The mild adverse effects such as pain, redness, fever, headache and swelling at the injection site were observed after 7 days of the vaccination. Also, the safety of this vaccine was ensured after the 28th day of post vaccination. Humoral responses and neutralizing antibodies level peaked at 28th day of post vaccination whereas T cell specific responses peaked at 14th day of post vaccination. In the phase 3 trials, 40,000 volunteers aged over 18 years participated. Storage conditions for this vaccine could be either at refrigerator temperature or at $-20°C$ [59, 71, 74].

Johnson & Johnson is developing a non replicating adenovirus serotype 26 vector vaccine (Ad26.COV2.S) which encodes stabilized perfusion S protein of SARS-CoV-2 with a wild-type signal peptide. In the phase 1/2 stage, the vaccine is administered either as a single dose or double dose at a dosage level of $5x10^{10}$ or $1x10^{11}$ viral particles in each vaccination. The trials included 402 healthy adults aged between 18-55 years and 394 healthy elderly aged above 65 years. For single dosage, 92% seroconversion rate was observed for $5x10^{10}$ or $1x10^{11}$ viral particles on the 29th day of post vaccination. Th1 cytokine producing S-specific CD4+ T cell responses were measured on the 14th day of post vaccination and neutralizing antibody titre level was increased from the baseline after 28th day of post vaccination. Mild local and systemic adverse effects were observed in volunteers but it resolved within 1 to 2 days after vaccination. The phase 1/2 study analysis indicated that a single dose of vaccine either $5x10^{10}$ or $1x10^{11}$ viral particles induces a highly immunogenic response. So, the lower dosage level is selected for phase 3 trials. Phase 3 studies are planned to assess the efficacy of the vaccine with a two-dose and single dose of $5x10^{10}$ viral particles. This vaccine requires storage at $2-8°C$ [59, 75 - 77].

Institut Pasteur is developing a vaccine to express the membrane-anchored SARS-CoV-1 spike protein or its secreted soluble ectodomain (Ssol) by inserting into additional transcription unit (ATU) of MV (Measles Virus) vector [71, 78]. In another approach, Recombinant Vaccinia Virus used to express SARS-CoV-1 S protein under the control of its hybrid promoters (Poxvirus A-type inclusion body (ATI) late promoter and tandem repeats of mutated 7.5 kDa protein (p7.5) early promoter), strongly induces both humoral and cellular immunity [71].

mRNA Vaccine

mRNA vaccine is an emerging, non-infectious platform where it has potential to mimic the antigen structure and expression for eliciting the immune response. BioNTech or Pfizer is developing a codon optimized mRNA vaccine, which encodes for the trimerized S1 protein (3C-like protease (3CLpro), NSP5, main protease (Mpro)) of SARS-CoV-2 RBD. The vaccine provides an increased immunogenicity due to the addition of T4 fibritin-derived foldon trimerization domain to the RBD antigen. The mRNA is encapsulated in 80 nm ionizable cationic Lipid Nanoparticle (LNP) formulations [2, 65]. Each dose of vaccine contains 30 µg of the mRNA which also include lipids, salts and sucrose for maintaining the stability and pH of the vaccine [79].

The phase 1/2 clinical trials tested two vaccines, BNT162b1 and BNT162b2 in which the BNT162b1 was shown to be effective in individuals with very mild side effects like fever, chills, muscle and joint pain indicating the immune system gearing up for response. These side effects may be caused due to the use of PEG in the formulation. The vaccine was administered *via* intramuscular injection in 2 doses within a period of 21 days. After the second dose of administration, both the vaccines have shown to elicit the neutralizing antibodies in similar dose-dependent SARS-CoV-2 mean titres. However, the BNT162b2 vaccine has shown increased T cell response, thereby offering a safety profile with 95% effectiveness in phase 3 trials involving clinical evaluations with 40,000 participants. The storage of vaccines at subzero temperature, *i.e.* around -70°C while shipping, requires ultra cold freezers which might offer a disadvantage in logistics [59]. Pfizer-BioNTech's vaccine has been sanctioned for emergency use by FDA under Emergency Use Authorization (EUA) in individuals above 16 years of age or older. So Pfizer is planning to distribute 6.4 million doses for the US during the late december of 2020, thereby 3 million people could be vaccinated. Additionally 5,00,000 doses were reserved for unexpected circumstances. More than 28,000 people were administered with this Pfizer vaccine [80, 81].

Moderna TX, Inc. is developing vaccine composed of synthetic mRNA encap-sulated in Lipid Nanoparticle (LNP-cholesterol, 1,2-distearoyl-sn-glycero-3-phos-phocholine (DSPC),and 1,2-dimyristoyl -rac-glycero -3-methoxy polyethylene glycol-2000 (DMG-PEG2000)) which codes for the full-length pre-fusion stabilized Spike (S) protein of SARS-CoV-2 [2, 74]. After Pfizer-BioNTech vaccine, this is the second vaccine to be approved for the EUA by FDA in individuals of 18 years of age or older [82]. The vaccine is administered *via* intramuscular injections in deltoid muscle in 2 doses within 28 days interval [83]. Each dose of vaccine contains 100 μg of mRNA, much larger than Pfizer's vaccine. The phase 3 clinical trials evaluation with around 20,000 participants has shown to be 94.5% effective with mild side effects as in Pfizer's vaccine [84]. The shipping storage of vaccines requires -20° C and it is shown to be stable at normal refrigeration temperature for a month and stable at room temperature for 12 hours unlike Pfizer's vaccine which must be used within 5 days [59, 85].

DNA Vaccines

DNA vaccines are encoded for the antigen along with the adjuvant in the transfected cells which provides steady supply of transgene of specific protein quite similar to live virus. Furthermore, the antigenic material is endocytosed by the immature dendritic cells which ultimately present the antigen to the $CD4^+$ and $CD8^+$ T cells thereby stimulating effective humoral as well as cell-mediated immune responses. AnGes is developing a plasmid DNA vaccine for targeting SARS-CoV-2 spike protein by administering through intradermal gene transfer method. In the phase 1/2 trials, 30 healthy volunteers aged between 20-65 years are selected for vaccination. The candidates were equally divided and were enrolled for the low dose group (1 mg twice at two weeks of interval, 15 individuals) and high dose group (2 mg twice at two weeks of interval, 15 individuals). The adverse effects were observed from week 9 to 53 and raised levels of anti-SARS-CoV-2 spike (S) glycoprotein-specific antibodies were observed from week 3 to week 53 [59, 86, 87].

ZydusCadila is developing a plasmid DNA vaccine for targeting SARS-CoV-2. In the phase 1/2 trials, 1048 Indian healthy volunteers aged between 18-55 years participated in the study. The vaccine administered single time through intradermally using needle or pharmajet at day 0, day 28 and day 58. Either 1 mg or 2 mg dosage were selected for testing. The completed Phase 2 trials were found to be safe and immunogenic and have received an approval from the regulatory authority in India to initiate phase 3 trials with 30,000 volunteers. Zydus Cadila vaccine can be stored at 2-8 °C. The platform simplifies the manufacturing process with minimal biosafety (BSL1) facility. Also, it is designed in such a way that the vaccine can be modified within a couple of weeks if the mutants arise and ensures the vaccine's efficacy and protection [59, 88 - 91].

National Institute of Allergy and Infectious Diseases (NIAID) is developing a vaccine based on full length cDNA expression of SARS-CoV-1 Spike glycoprotein (Urbani strain) by cloning into the expression vector CMV. It has been produced in bacterial cell cultures containing a kanamycin selection medium, and after the growth of bacterial cells harboring the plasmid, it is purified to remove the cellular or viral components [92]. Inovio Pharmaceuticals is developing a vaccine with a codon optimized S protein sequence of SARS-CoV-2, to which an IgE leader sequence is affixed. SARS-CoV-2 IgE-spike sequence was synthesized and digested using BamHI and XhoI restriction enzymes. The digested DNA was incorporated into the expression plasmid pGX0001 to express the S protein of SARS-CoV-2 [2, 65].

Animal Models

Albert Osterhaus and his colleagues from Erasmus University in Rotterdam had identified that cynomolgus macaques developed SARS-like symptoms and found that these macaques had their lungs infected in the same way as humans [94]. Also, it has been reported that the macaques show similar serological responses as humans with respect to viral infections [95] making it an ideal model for study. The virus shedding has been reported in rhesus and macaque species after 2 weeks of infection with SARS-CoV-2. The vaccine studies for animal models included inactivated, DNA and RNA vaccines for different strains of SARS-CoV-2. After vaccination, the infection with SARS-CoV-2 through intranasal, intratracheal, ocular and oral modes were done and the efficacy was determined in assessing the viral loads in upper and lower respiratory tracts. As a result, the viral load was found to be reduced demonstrating the efficacy of the vaccines. However, the macaque species has shown to exhibit natural protective immunity against reinfection with SARS-CoV-2 and it has not developed any severe disease or symptoms upon infection marking as a limitation on using macaques for the study [96, 97]. Also, they cannot be inbred as mice models.

Subbarao from NIAID suggested that mice model can be used because of its reproduction ability, consistent results and the viral replication in them although they couldn't show any clinical sign for SARS virus. Despite its limitations, it has been encouraged to use mice models for better understanding on how vaccines can stop viral replication in them [94]. Studies have shown that immunization of mice with RBD-Fc of SARS virus has induced a long-term immunity against SARS-CoV-1 BJ01 strain [98, 99]. Adeno-associated virus based vaccine containing RBD elicits adequate neutralizing antibodies to inhibit homologous SARS-CoV-1 (GZ50) in the mouse model when administered *via* intramuscular and mucosal pathways [100].

Other animal models like African green monkeys, ferrets, hamsters and transgenic mice are being explored for SARS-CoV-1 studies in preclinical evaluation. The mice model has been improved by the use of transgenic mice with adapted SARS and human ACE-2 receptor protein for testing the efficacy of vaccines despite its certain restrictions [101, 102]. However, the transgenic mice developed a neurologic disease completely irrelevant to SARS virus making it difficult to use for the study [103, 104].

The use of ferrets as a model for study is still under debate as few studies suggest that they show poor clinical signs or symptoms in case of SARS virus. On the other hand, few recent studies suggested that they develop fever upon infection with SARS-CoV-2 which is a commonly observed symptom in human beings, and offers a good model for study [105, 106].

Evidence supports that Gold Syrian hamsters are able to produce symptoms like pneumonitis, pulmonary consolidation and decreased respiratory activity upon infection with SARS-CoV-1 allowing it to employ them for preclinical evaluation [107].

Although several models were discussed for SARS-CoV vaccines, there is no single promising animal model that is proven to replicate the disease exactly as in humans [108]. Nevertheless, the preclinical studies have tried to address the efficacy and potency of vaccine candidates in SARS virus which in turn has shown a certain level of long term protection from infection in at least 75% of mice models after vaccination [99, 109].

CHALLENGES IN VACCINE DEVELOPMENT

Effective development of SARS-CoV vaccines, during the pandemic, is a major challenging process. Typically, it will take decades of basic research on viral biology and the host response to infection. This conventional way of vaccine development is not feasible for a rapidly emerging virulent pathogen. The first major gridlock is the virus itself, as they are vulnerable to mutations which lead to antigenic shift and drift, upon its transmission. Geographical area, environmental conditions and the density of population also have its impact on mutating SARS-CoV. There were 198 mutations identified in 7500 infected patients, which indicate the high mutation rate of SARS-CoV-2 in humans. The result of these mutations produces various subtypes of the virus, which may help the virus to evade the immune mechanisms after vaccination [110]. Handling of highly contagious SARS-CoV during vaccine development requires Biosafety level-3 containment facilities and standardized safety procedures. Secondly, the absence of high-throughput small animal disease models to incorporate vaccine candidates affects the down-selection. Certain animal models lack the hACE-2 receptor, and they are not susceptible to the SARS-CoV infection, which offers a limitation for the preclinical evaluation on vaccine candidates [111]. Thirdly, there is a concern to be addressed about the correlation of neutralizing antibody with immune response and threshold neutralizing antibody level after vaccination which is unanswered [112]. This threshold level acts as an essential factor to determine the booster for vaccination. Immunological assays to evaluate immune responses have not yet been developed and standardized.

The next challenge is about the safety and efficacy of the vaccine candidate in clinical trials that often seem to have been addressed with toxicity, causing adverse effects on the study population. Phase 2/3 Oxford University-AstraZeneca's clinical trials have shown adverse reactions in some volunteers. Generally, these effects are normal in vaccine development, but now it seems to be shown as an exaggerated event due to this short time development.

In some cases, the success of the clinical trials is hindered by insufficient team skills in vaccine administration and inability to comply with the general criteria (such as recruiting participants in low-density regions, variations in age, race or other medical conditions) for clinical study [113].

Speaking of post vaccination challenges, the low threshold of vaccine-induced antibodies leads to Antibody Dependent Enhancement (ADE), which augments the viral entry by conformational change on glycoproteins of the viral envelope, thereby targeting the FcR cells on the host. This ultimately aggravates the disease in the patients causing Vaccine associated Enhanced Respiratory Disease (VAERD) [114]. Having addressed all these challenges, thermal stability of the vaccine candidate, long-term storage and transportation, manufacturing capacity on large scale and worldwide distribution on the eve of pandemic and the cost of production collectively acts as another hurdle for this vaccine race.

CONCLUSION

The recent unlikely event has put pressure on both the scientific community and the biological engineers, and this event has served as both a boon and a bane. In a way, this outbreak projected the importance in the field of science and many researchers are working hard by contributing their knowledge in providing a solution to end this pandemic. In addition to that, a significant number of vaccine candidates in clinical trials show rapid progress when compared to SARS-CoV-1 and MERS vaccine candidates. The number of vaccine candidates developed is relatively high in subunit and viral vector platforms, compared to conventional platforms evidencing the advancements in technology and science. Although these progresses look productive, the reliability of the vaccines for safety and efficacy is still questioned. Evaluation and supporting studies have indirect effects on the formulation of vaccines which signifies the need for a wider perspective on vaccine design. It is still unclear how vaccines target different variants of S protein by relating to each other or how they target the epidemiology of the disease. The high rate of mutation on the SARS-CoV-2 remains a bottleneck for vaccine development. This consideration appeals to the development of broad spectrum vaccines, which might offer a better and improved solution. Developing an organized strategy with worldwide participation of scientific minds could enhance the results in the development of vaccines in the near future.

CONSENT FOR PUBLICATION

Not Applicable.

CONFLICT OF INTEREST

The author declares no conflict of interest, financial or otherwise.

ACKNOWLEDGEMENTS

Declared none.

REFERENCES

[1] Likhacheva A. SARS Revisited. Virtual Mentor 2006; 8(4): 219-22.
[PMID: 23241619]

[2] Funk C, Laferrière C, Ardakani A. A snapshot of the global race for vaccines targeting SARS-CoV-2 and the COVID19 pandemic. Front Pharmacol 2020; 11: 937.

[3] Amanat F, Krammer F. SARS-CoV-2 Vaccines: Status Report. Immunity 2020; 52(4): 583-9.
[http://dx.doi.org/10.1016/j.immuni.2020.03.007] [PMID: 32259480]

[4] International Committee on Taxonomy of Viruses (ICTV). International Committee on Taxonomy of Viruses (ICTV) 2020. https://talk.ictvonline.org/taxonomy/p/taxonomy-history?taxnode_id=20181868

[5] Ge XY, Li JL, Yang XL, et al. Isolation and characterization of a bat SARS-like coronavirus that uses the ACE2 receptor. Nature 2013; 503(7477): 535-8.
[http://dx.doi.org/10.1038/nature12711] [PMID: 24172901]

[6] Woo PC, Huang Y, Lau SK, Yuen KY. Coronavirus genomics and bioinformatics analysis. Viruses 2010; 2(8): 1804-20.
[http://dx.doi.org/10.3390/v2081803] [PMID: 21994708]

[7] Rota PA, Oberste MS, Monroe SS, et al. Characterization of a novel coronavirus associated with severe acute respiratory syndrome. Science 2003; 300(5624): 1394-9.
[http://dx.doi.org/10.1126/science.1085952] [PMID: 12730500]

[8] Snijder EJ, Bredenbeek PJ, Dobbe JC, et al. Unique and conserved features of genome and proteome of SARS-coronavirus, an early split-off from the coronavirus group 2 lineage. J Mol Biol 2003; 331(5): 991-1004.
[http://dx.doi.org/10.1016/S0022-2836(03)00865-9] [PMID: 12927536]

[9] Guan Y, Zheng BJ, He YQ, et al. Isolation and characterization of viruses related to the SARS coronavirus from animals in southern China. Science 2003; 302(5643): 276-8.
[http://dx.doi.org/10.1126/science.1087139] [PMID: 12958366]

[10] Rossi GA, Sacco O, Mancino E, Cristiani L, Midulla F. Differences and similarities between SARS-CoV and SARS-CoV-2: spike receptor-binding domain recognition and host cell infection with support of cellular serine proteases. Infection 2020; 48(5): 665-9.
[http://dx.doi.org/10.1007/s15010-020-01486-5] [PMID: 32737833]

[11] Jiang S, Hillyer C, Du L. Neutralizing antibodies against SARS-CoV-2 and other human coronaviruses. Trends Immunol 2020; 41(5): 355-9.

[12] Shang J, Wan Y, Luo C, *et al.* Cell entry mechanisms of SARS-CoV-2. ProcNatlAcadSci USA 2020; 117(21): 11727-34.

[13] Verdecchia P, Cavallini C, Spanevello A, Angeli F. The pivotal link between ACE2 deficiency and SARS-CoV-2 infection. Eur J Intern Med 2020; 76: 14-20.
[http://dx.doi.org/10.1016/j.ejim.2020.04.037] [PMID: 32336612]

[14] Letko M, Marzi A, Munster V. Functional assessment of cell entry and receptor usage for SARS-CoV-2 and other lineage B betacoronaviruses. Nat Microbiol 2020; 5(4): 562-9.

[15] Chu H, Chan JF, Wang Y, *et al.* Comparative replication and immune activation profiles of SARS-CoV-2 and SARS-CoV in human lungs: An *ex vivo* study with implications for the pathogenesis of COVID-19. Clin Infect Dis 2020; 71(6): 1400-9.
[http://dx.doi.org/10.1093/cid/ciaa410] [PMID: 32270184]

[16] Li YC, Bai WZ, Hashikawa T. The neuroinvasive potential of SARS-CoV2 may play a role in the respiratory failure of COVID-19 patients. J Med Virol 2020; 92(6): 552-5.

[17] Zheng YY, Ma YT, Zhang JY, Xie X. COVID-19 and the cardiovascular system. Nat Rev Cardiol 2020; 175 : 259-60.

[18] Barton LM, Duval EJ, Stroberg E, Ghosh S, Mukhopadhyay S. COVID-19 Autopsies, Oklahoma, USA. Am J ClinPathol 2020; 153(6): 725-33.

[19] Totura AL, Baric RS. SARS coronavirus pathogenesis: host innate immune responses and viral antagonism of interferon. Curr Opin Virol 2012; 2(3): 264-75.
[http://dx.doi.org/10.1016/j.coviro.2012.04.004] [PMID: 22572391]

[20] Huang KJ, Su IJ, Theron M, *et al.* An interferon-gamma-related cytokine storm in SARS patients. J Med Virol 2005; 75(2): 185-94.
[http://dx.doi.org/10.1002/jmv.20255] [PMID: 15602737]

[21] He Y, Li J, Li W, Lustigman S, Farzan M, Jiang S. Cross-neutralization of human and palm civet severe acute respiratory syndrome coronaviruses by antibodies targeting the receptor-binding domain of spike protein. J Immunol 2006; 176(10): 6085-92.
[http://dx.doi.org/10.4049/jimmunol.176.10.6085] [PMID: 16670317]

[22] Grifoni A, Weiskopf D, Ramirez SI, *et al.* Targets of T Cell responses to SARS-CoV-2 coronavirus in humans with COVID-19 disease and unexposed individuals. Cell 2020; 181(7): 1489-1501.e15.
[http://dx.doi.org/10.1016/j.cell.2020.05.015] [PMID: 32473127]

[23] Cao WC, Liu W, Zhang PH, Zhang F, Richardus JH. Disappearance of antibodies to SARS-associated coronavirus after recovery. N Engl J Med 2007; 357(11): 1162-3.
[http://dx.doi.org/10.1056/NEJMc070348] [PMID: 17855683]

[24] Glass WG, Subbarao K, Murphy B, Murphy PM. Mechanisms of host defense following severe acute respiratory syndrome-coronavirus (SARS-CoV) pulmonary infection of mice. J Immunol 2004; 173(6): 4030-9.
[http://dx.doi.org/10.4049/jimmunol.173.6.4030] [PMID: 15356152]

[25] Peiris JSM, Guan Y, Yuen KY. Severe acute respiratory syndrome. Nature News 2004.
https://www.nature.com/articles/nm1143

[26] Li T, Xie J, He Y, *et al.* Long-term persistence of robust antibody and cytotoxic T cell responses in recovered patients infected with SARS coronavirus. PLoS One 2006; 1(1): e24.
[http://dx.doi.org/10.1371/journal.pone.0000024] [PMID: 17183651]

[27] Gudbjartsson DF, Norddahl GL, Melsted P, *et al.* Humoral Immune Response to SARS-CoV-2 in Iceland. N Engl J Med 2020; 383(18): 1724-34.
[http://dx.doi.org/10.1056/NEJMoa2026116] [PMID: 32871063]

[28] Long QX, Tang XJ, Shi QL, *et al.* Clinical and immunological assessment of asymptomatic SARS-CoV-2 infections. Nat Med 2020; 26(8): 1200-4.
[http://dx.doi.org/10.1038/s41591-020-0965-6] [PMID: 32555424]

[29] Le Bert N, Tan AT, Kunasegaran K, *et al.* SARS-CoV-2-specific T cell immunity in cases of COVID-19 and SARS, and uninfected controls. Nature 2020; 584(7821): 457-62.
[http://dx.doi.org/10.1038/s41586-020-2550-z] [PMID: 32668444]

[30] Dong C, Ni L, Ye F, Chen ML, Yu F, *et al.* Characterization of anti-viral immunity in recovered individuals infected by SARS-CoV-2. medRxiv 2020.

[31] Hung IF, Cheng VC, Wu AK, *et al.* Viral loads in clinical specimens and SARS manifestations. Emerg Infect Dis 2004; 10(9): 1550-7.
[http://dx.doi.org/10.3201/eid1009.040058] [PMID: 15498155]

[32] Oran DP, Topol EJ. Prevalence of Asymptomatic SARS-CoV-2 Infection : A Narrative Review. Ann Intern Med 2020; 173(5): 362-7.
[http://dx.doi.org/10.7326/M20-3012] [PMID: 32491919]

[33] Grant MC, Geoghegan L, Arbyn M, *et al.* The prevalence of symptoms in 24,410 adults infected by the novel coronavirus (SARS-CoV-2; COVID-19): A systematic review and meta-analysis of 148 studies from 9 countries. PLoS One 2020; 15(6): e0234765.
[http://dx.doi.org/10.1371/journal.pone.0234765] [PMID: 32574165]

[34] Larsen JR, Martin MR, Martin JD, Kuhn P, Hicks JB. Modeling the onset of symptoms of COVID-19. Front Pub Health 2020; 8: 473.
[http://dx.doi.org/10.3389/fpubh.2020.00473] [PMID: 32903584]

[35] Guo L, Ren L, Yang S, *et al.* Profiling early humoral response to diagnose novel coronavirus disease (COVID-19). Clin Infect Dis 2020; 71(15): 778-85.
[http://dx.doi.org/10.1093/cid/ciaa310] [PMID: 32198501]

[36] Van Kasteren PB, van der Veer B, van den Brink S, Wijsman L, de Jonge J, van den Brandt A, *et al.* Comparison of seven commercial RT-PCR diagnostic kits for COVID-19. J Clin Virol 2020 07;128:104412 2020; 128: 104412.

[37] Jin YH, Cai L, Cheng ZS, Cheng H, Deng T, Fan YP, *et al.* A rapid advice guideline for the diagnosis and treatment of 2019 novel coronavirus (2019-nCoV) infected pneumonia (standard version). Mil Med Res 2019; 7(1): 4.

[38] Piechotta V, Chai KL, Valk SJ, *et al.* Convalescent plasma or hyperimmune immunoglobulin for people with COVID-19: a living systematic review. Cochrane Database Syst Rev 2020; 7: CD013600.
[PMID: 32648959]

[39] Mire CE, Geisbert JB, Agans KN, *et al.* Passive immunotherapy: Assessment of convalescent serum against ebola virus makona infection in nonhuman primates. J Infect Dis 2016; 214 (Suppl. 3): S367-74.
[http://dx.doi.org/10.1093/infdis/jiw333] [PMID: 27571900]

[40] Ye M, Fu D, Ren Y, *et al.* Treatment with convalescent plasma for COVID-19 patients in Wuhan, China. J Med Virol 2020; 92(10): 1890-901.
[http://dx.doi.org/10.1002/jmv.25882] [PMID: 32293713]

[41] Chowdhury MA, Hossain N, Kashem MA, Shahid MA, Alam A. Immune response in COVID-19: A review. J Infect Public Health 2020; 13(11): 1619-29.
[http://dx.doi.org/10.1016/j.jiph.2020.07.001] [PMID: 32718895]

[42] de Wit E, van Doremalen N, Falzarano D, Munster VJ. SARS and MERS: recent insights into emerging coronaviruses. Nat Rev Microbiol 2016; 14(8): 523-34.
[http://dx.doi.org/10.1038/nrmicro.2016.81] [PMID: 27344959]

[43] Song Z, Xu Y, Bao L, *et al.* From SARS to MERS, Thrusting Coronaviruses into the Spotlight.

Viruses 2019; 11(1): 59.
[http://dx.doi.org/10.3390/v11010059] [PMID: 30646565]

[44] Coronavirus N. WHO R&D Blueprint https://www.who.int/blueprint/priority-diseases/ke--action/Outline_CoreProtocol_vaccine_trial_09042 020.pdf

[45] Lurie N, Saville M, Hatchett R, Halton J. Developing Covid-19 Vaccines at Pandemic Speed. N Engl J Med 2020; 382(21): 1969-73.
[http://dx.doi.org/10.1056/NEJMp2005630] [PMID: 32227757]

[46] Draft landscape of COVID-19 candidate vaccines 2020. https://www.who.int/publications/m/item/draft-landscape-of-covid-19-candidate-vaccines

[47] Wrapp D, Wang N, Corbett KS, Goldsmith JA, Hsieh CL, Abiona O, *et al.* Cryo-EM structure of the 2019-nCoV spike in the prefusion conformation. Science 2019; 367(6483): 1260-3.

[48] Rahman MS, Hoque MN, Islam MR, *et al.* Epitope-based chimeric peptide vaccine design against S, M and E proteins of SARS-CoV-2, the etiologic agent of COVID-19 pandemic: an in silico approach. PeerJ 2020; 8: e9572.
[http://dx.doi.org/10.7717/peerj.9572] [PMID: 33194329]

[49] Thanh Le T, Andreadakis Z, Kumar A, *et al.* The COVID-19 vaccine development landscape. Nat Rev Drug Discov 2020; 19(5): 305-6.
[http://dx.doi.org/10.1038/d41573-020-00073-5] [PMID: 32273591]

[50] Vaxart's oral COVID-19 tablet vaccine to enter clinical trials 2021. https://www.biopharma-reporter.com/Article/2020/09/15/Vaxart-First-tablet-COVID-19-vaccine-to-entbiopharma-reporter.com

[51] Parkinson J. First Oral COVID-19 Vaccine in Phase 1 Trial. Contagion Live 2020. https://www.contagionlive.com/view/vaxart-has-developed-the-first-oral-investigational-covid-19-vacc

[52] Vaxart COVID-19 Oral Vaccine. Precision Vaccinationscom 2020. https://www.precisionvaccinations.com/vaccines/vaxart-covid-19-oral-vaccine

[53] Vaxart, Inc. Press Releases | Vaxart, Inc 2020. https://investors.vaxart.com/press-releases?page=0

[54] Iosbio.com.. iosbiocom | iosbiocom 2020. https://iosbio.com/

[55] Stabilitech.com. OraPro-COVID-19 | Home 2020. https://www.stabilitech.com/orapro-covid-19/

[56] Ltd S. Prnewswire.com. Stabilitech's COVID-19 vaccine intended to be delivered in a disruptive thermally stable oral capsule 2020. https://www.prnewswire.com/news-releases/stabilitechs-covid-19-vaccine-intended-to-be-delivered-in- a-disruptive-thermally-stable-oral-capsule-301026531.html

[57] Codagenix and Serum Institute of India Initiate Dosing in Phase 1 Trial of COVI-VAC, a Single Dose, Intranasal, Live Attenuated Vaccine for COVID-19 | BioSpace. BioSpace 2021. https://www.biospace.com/article/releases/codagenix-and-serum-institute-of- india-initiate-dosing-in-phase-1-trial-of-covi-vac-a-single-dose-intranasal -live-attenuated-vaccine-for-covid-19/

[58] Codagenix I. Prnewswire.com. Codagenix and Serum Institute of India Announce Commencement of First-in-Human Trial of COVI-VAC, A Single Dose, Intranasal Live Attenuated Vaccine for COVID-19 2021. https://www.prnewswire.com/news-releases/codagenix-and-serum-institute-of-india-announce-commencement-of-first-in-human-trial-of-covi-vac-a-single-dose--ntranasal-live-attenuated-vaccine-for-covid-19-301191756.html

[59] Poland GA, Ovsyannikova IG, Kennedy RB. SARS-CoV-2 immunity: review and applications to phase 3 vaccine candidates. Lancet 2020; 396(10262): 1595-606.
[http://dx.doi.org/10.1016/S0140-6736(20)32137-1] [PMID: 33065034]

[60] Sinovac vaccine shot's efficacy uncertain despite Brazil, Turkey result 2020.https://www.hindustantimes.com/world-news/sinovac-vaccine-sht-s-efficacy-uncertain-despite-brazil- turkey-results/story-oapZWFIBXB4pU22RHv4WdM.html

[61] NDTV.com.. Turkey Says China's Sinovac Covid-19 Vaccine, CoronaVac, 9125% Effective In Late

Trials 2020.https://www.ndtv.com/business/turkish-researchers-say-china-s-sinovac-covid-19-vaccine-91-25-effect

[62] Aa.com.tr. China begins procedure to approve Sinopharm vaccine 2021. https://www.aa.com.tr/en/asia-pacific/china-begins-procedure-to-approve-sinopharm-vaccine/2087541

[63] Sinopharm Covid-19 vaccine undergoing regulatory review, report says 2020. https://www.scmp.com/news/china/science/article/3115309/coronavirus-sinopharm-vaccine-undergoin

[64] Globaltimes.cn.. Chinese drug regulators accept application for Sinopharm vaccine rollout - Global Times 2020.https://www.globaltimes.cn/content/1210872.shtml

[65] Kaur SP, Gupta V. COVID-19 Vaccine: A comprehensive status report. Virus Res 2020; 288: 198114.
[http://dx.doi.org/10.1016/j.virusres.2020.198114] [PMID: 32800805]

[66] Announces N. Novavax Inc. - IR Site. Novavax Announces COVID-19 Vaccine Clinical Development Progress | Novavax Inc - IR Site 2020.https://ir.novavax.com/news-releases/news-relea-e-details/novavax-announces-covid-19-vaccine-clinic

[67] Chinese COVID-19 vaccine enters third-stage human trial 2020. https://economictimes.indiatimes.com/news/international/world-news/chinese-covid-19- vaccine-enters-third-stage-human-trial/articleshow/79325744.cms?from=mdr

[68] Bhattacharya M, Sharma AR, Patra P, *et al.* Development of epitope-based peptide vaccine against novel coronavirus 2019 (SARS-COV-2): Immunoinformatics approach. J Med Virol 2020; 92(6): 618-31.
[http://dx.doi.org/10.1002/jmv.25736] [PMID: 32108359]

[69] Liu C, Zhou Q, Li Y, *et al.* Research and development on therapeutic agents and vaccines for COVID-19 and related human coronavirus diseases. ACS Cent Sci 2020; 6(3): 315-31.
[http://dx.doi.org/10.1021/acscentsci.0c00272] [PMID: 32226821]

[70] Mukherjee S, Tworowski D, Detroja R, Mukherjee SB, Frenkel-Morgenstern M. Immunoinformatics and structural analysis for identification of immunodominant epitopes in SARS-CoV-2 as potential vaccine targets. Vaccines (Basel) 2020; 8(2): 290.
[http://dx.doi.org/10.3390/vaccines8020290] [PMID: 32526960]

[71] Escriou N, Callendret B, Lorin V, *et al.* Protection from SARS coronavirus conferred by live measles vaccine expressing the spike glycoprotein. Virology 2014; 452-453: 32-41.
[http://dx.doi.org/10.1016/j.virol.2014.01.002] [PMID: 24606680]

[72] Knoll MD, Wonodi C. Oxford–AstraZeneca COVID-19 vaccine efficacy. Lancet 2020; (Dec): 1-3.
[PMID: 33306990]

[73] STAT. AstraZeneca-Oxford Covid-19 vaccine has moderate efficacy, data show 2020. https://www.statnews.com/2020/12/08/detailed-data-on-astrazeneca-oxford-covid-19-vaccine-show -it-has-moderate-efficacy/

[74] Zhu FC, Li YH, Guan XH, *et al.* Safety, tolerability, and immunogenicity of a recombinant adenovirus type-5 vectored COVID-19 vaccine: a dose-escalation, open-label, non-randomised, first-in-human trial. Lancet 2020; 395(10240): 1845-54.
[http://dx.doi.org/10.1016/S0140-6736(20)31208-3] [PMID: 32450106]

[75] Clinicaltrials.gov. A Study of Ad26COV2S in Adults (COVID-19) - Full Text View - ClinicalTrialsgov 2020. https://clinicaltrials.gov/ct2/show/study/NCT04436276?term= Johnson+%26+Johnson%3B+Beth+Israe

[76] Bos R, Rutten L, van der Lubbe J, Bakkers M, *et al.* Ad26 vector-based COVID-19 vaccine encoding a prefusion-stabilized SARS-CoV-2 Spike immunogen induces potent humoral and cellular immune responses. npj. Vaccines (Basel) 2020; 5: 1.

[77] Comeaux C, Bastian A, Paepe E, *et al.* Safety and immunogenicity of a seasonal influenza vaccine and Ad26.RSV.preF vaccine with and without co-administration: A randomized, double-blind, placebo-

controlled phase 2a study in adults aged ≥ 60 years. Open Forum Infectious Diseases 2019; 6(Supplement_2): S979-9.

[78] He Y, Jiang S. Vaccine design for severe acute respiratory syndrome coronavirus. Viral Immunol 2005; 18(2): 327-32.
[http://dx.doi.org/10.1089/vim.2005.18.327] [PMID: 16035944]

[79] What's in Pfizer's vaccine? A look at the ingredients. Global News 2020.https://globalnews.ca/news/7525406/covid-vaccine-ingredients-pfizer/

[80] Pfizer.com.. COVID-19 Vaccine US Distribution Fact Sheet | Pfizer 2020.https://www.pfizer.com/news/hot-topics/covid_19_vaccine_u_s_distribution_fact_sheet

[81] FDA authorizes Pfizer-BioNTech vaccine for emergency use 2020.https://www.raps.org/news-an--articles/news-articles/2020/12/fda-authorizes-pfizer-biontech-vaccine-f

[82] Takes Additional Action FDA. FDA Takes Additional Action in Fight Against COVID-19 By Issuing Emergency Use Authorization for Second COVID-19 Vaccine 2020. https://www.fda.gov/news-events/press-announcements/fda-takes-additional-action-fight-against-covid-19 -issuing-emergency -use-authorization-second-covid

[83] Cdc.gov. Moderna COVID-19 Vaccine Vaccine Preparation and Administration Summary 2021.https://www.cdc.gov/vaccines/covid-19/info-by-product/moderna/downloads/prep-and--dmin-summar y.pdf

[84] Modernatx.com. Moderna's Work on a COVID-19 Vaccine Candidate | Moderna, Inc 2020.https://www.modernatx.com/modernas-work-potential-vaccine-against-covid-19

[85] STAT. A side-by-side comparison of the Pfizer/BioNTech and Moderna vaccines 2020. https://www.statnews.com/2020/12/19/a-side-by-side-comparison-of-the-pfizer-biontech-and-moderna -vaccines/

[86] Japan-made coronavirus vaccines may not be available until 2022 2020. https://www.japantimes.co.jp/news/2020/12/04/national/japanese-coronavirus-vaccines-2022/

[87] Go.drugbank.com. AG0301-COVID19 | DrugBank Online 2020.https://go.drugbank.com/drugs/DB15856

[88] Umarji V. Business-standardcom ZydusCadila seeks nod for phase three clinical trials of Covid vaccine 2020.https://www.business-standard.com/article/current-affairs/zydus-cadila-seeks-nod -fo--phase-three-clinical-trials-of-covid-vaccine-120122401233_1.html

[89] ZydusCadila Plans To Test Its COVID-19 Vaccine On 30,000 Volunteers In Late Stage Trial 2020. https://www.moneycontrol.com/news/coronavirus/zydus-cadila-plans-to-test-its-covid-19-vaccine-on -30000-volunteers-in- late-stage-trial-6268991.html

[90] Ctri.nic.in. Clinical Trial Details 2021. http://ctri.nic.in/Clinicaltrials/pdf_generate.php?trialid=45306&EncHid=&modid=&compid=%27,%27

[91] Zyduscadila.com. Zydus Cadila Announces Completion of Dosing in Phase I Clinical Trial of ZyCoV-D 2021.https://www.zyduscadila.com/public/pdf/pressrelease/Press-Release-ZyCoV-D.pdf

[92] Buchholz UJ, Bukreyev A, Yang L, et al. Contributions of the structural proteins of severe acute respiratory syndrome coronavirus to protective immunity. Proc Natl Acad Sci USA 2004; 101(26): 9804-9.
[http://dx.doi.org/10.1073/pnas.0403492101] [PMID: 15210961]

[93] Who.int. List of candidate vaccines developed against SARS-CoV 2021. https://www.who.int/blueprint/priority-diseases/key-action/list-of-candidate-vaccines-developed-agai nst-sars.pdf

[94] Marshall E, Enserink M. Medicine. Caution urged on SARS vaccines. Science 2004; 303(5660): 944-6.

[http://dx.doi.org/10.1126/science.303.5660.944] [PMID: 14963300]

[95] David WV, Stephen SW, Anna PD. Dengue.Vaccines for Biodefense and Emerging and Neglected diseases. 1st ed. London, UK: Academic Press 2009; pp. 287-785.

[96] Chandrashekar A, Liu J, Martinot AJ, *et al.* SARS-CoV-2 infection protects against rechallenge in rhesus macaques. Science 2020; 369(6505): 812-7.
[http://dx.doi.org/10.1126/science.abc4776] [PMID: 32434946]

[97] Rockx B, Kuiken T, Herfst S, *et al.* Comparative pathogenesis of COVID-19, MERS, and SARS in a nonhuman primate model. Science 2020; 368(6494): 1012-5.
[http://dx.doi.org/10.1126/science.abb7314] [PMID: 32303590]

[98] He Y, Zhou Y, Liu S, *et al.* Receptor-binding domain of SARS-CoV spike protein induces highly potent neutralizing antibodies: implication for developing subunit vaccine. Biochem Biophys Res Commun 2004; 324(2): 773-81.
[http://dx.doi.org/10.1016/j.bbrc.2004.09.106] [PMID: 15474494]

[99] Du L, Zhao G, He Y, *et al.* Receptor-binding domain of SARS-CoV spike protein induces long-term protective immunity in an animal model. Vaccine 2007; 25(15): 2832-8.
[http://dx.doi.org/10.1016/j.vaccine.2006.10.031] [PMID: 17092615]

[100] Du L, He Y, Wang Y, *et al.* Recombinant adeno-associated virus expressing the receptor-binding domain of severe acute respiratory syndrome coronavirus S protein elicits neutralizing antibodies: Implication for developing SARS vaccines. Virology 2006; 353(1): 6-16.
[http://dx.doi.org/10.1016/j.virol.2006.03.049] [PMID: 16793110]

[101] Roberts A, Lamirande EW, Vogel L, *et al.* Animal models and vaccines for SARS-CoV infection. Virus Res 2008; 133(1): 20-32.
[http://dx.doi.org/10.1016/j.virusres.2007.03.025] [PMID: 17499378]

[102] Yang XH, Deng W, Tong Z, *et al.* Mice transgenic for human angiotensin-converting enzyme 2 provide a model for SARS coronavirus infection. Comp Med 2007; 57(5): 450-9.
[PMID: 17974127]

[103] McCray PB Jr, Pewe L, Wohlford-Lenane C, *et al.* Lethal infection of K18-hACE2 mice infected with severe acute respiratory syndrome coronavirus. J Virol 2007; 81(2): 813-21.
[http://dx.doi.org/10.1128/JVI.02012-06] [PMID: 17079315]

[104] Tseng CT, Huang C, Newman P, *et al.* Severe acute respiratory syndrome coronavirus infection of mice transgenic for the human Angiotensin-converting enzyme 2 virus receptor. J Virol 2007; 81(3): 1162-73.
[http://dx.doi.org/10.1128/JVI.01702-06] [PMID: 17108019]

[105] See RH, Petric M, Lawrence DJ, *et al.* Severe acute respiratory syndrome vaccine efficacy in ferrets: whole killed virus and adenovirus-vectored vaccines. J Gen Virol 2008; 89(Pt 9): 2136-46.
[http://dx.doi.org/10.1099/vir.0.2008/001891-0] [PMID: 18753223]

[106] Martina BE, Haagmans BL, Kuiken T, *et al.* Virology: SARS virus infection of cats and ferrets. Nature 2003; 425(6961): 915.
[http://dx.doi.org/10.1038/425915a] [PMID: 14586458]

[107] Roberts A, Vogel L, Guarner J, *et al.* Severe acute respiratory syndrome coronavirus infection of golden Syrian hamsters. J Virol 2005; 79(1): 503-11.
[http://dx.doi.org/10.1128/JVI.79.1.503-511.2005] [PMID: 15596843]

[108] Subbarao K, Roberts A. Is there an ideal animal model for SARS? Trends Microbiol 2006; 14(7): 299-303.
[http://dx.doi.org/10.1016/j.tim.2006.05.007] [PMID: 16759866]

[109] Kapadia SU, Rose JK, Lamirande E, Vogel L, Subbarao K, Roberts A. Long-term protection from SARS coronavirus infection conferred by a single immunization with an attenuated VSV-based vaccine. Virology 2005; 340(2): 174-82.

[http://dx.doi.org/10.1016/j.virol.2005.06.016] [PMID: 16043204]

[110] van Dorp L, Acman M, Richard D, *et al.* Emergence of genomic diversity and recurrent mutations in SARS-CoV-2. Infect Genet Evol 2020; 83: 104351.
[http://dx.doi.org/10.1016/j.meegid.2020.104351] [PMID: 32387564]

[111] Bao L, Deng W, Huang B, *et al.* The pathogenicity of SARS-CoV-2 in hACE2 transgenic mice. Nature 2020; 583(7818): 830-3.
[http://dx.doi.org/10.1038/s41586-020-2312-y] [PMID: 32380511]

[112] Diamond MS, Pierson TC. The Challenges of Vaccine Development against a New Virus during a Pandemic. Cell Host Microbe 2020; 27(5): 699-703.
[http://dx.doi.org/10.1016/j.chom.2020.04.021] [PMID: 32407708]

[113] Cohen J. Pandemic vaccines are about to face the real test. Science 2020; 368(6497): 1295-6.
[http://dx.doi.org/10.1126/science.368.6497.1295] [PMID: 32554572]

[114] Wang SF, Tseng SP, Yen CH, *et al.* Antibody-dependent SARS coronavirus infection is mediated by antibodies against spike proteins. Biochem Biophys Res Commun 2014; 451(2): 208-14.
[http://dx.doi.org/10.1016/j.bbrc.2014.07.090] [PMID: 25073113]

[115] Poh CM, Carissimo G, Wang B, *et al.* Two linear epitopes on the SARS-CoV-2 spike protein that elicit neutralising antibodies in COVID-19 patients. Nat Commun 2020; 11(1): 2806.
[http://dx.doi.org/10.1038/s41467-020-16638-2] [PMID: 32483236]

CHAPTER 3

Potassium Permanganate, the Vikut® Formula, an Innovation using non-antibiotic Antimicrobial Agents to Treat both Chronic and Non-chronic Wounds: A Clinical Approach with Scientific Evidence

Agustín Lara-Esqueda[1],[*], Iván Delgado-Enciso[2], Agustín D. Lara-Basulto[3] and Margarita Balayan[4]

[1] *Department of Psychology and Human Communication Therapy, University of Durango, Durango, CO 81301, United States*

[2] *Department of Medicine, University of Colima, 28040 Colima, Mexico*

[3] *Consultant in "Consultoria LARBAS S.A de C.V", Mexico*

[4] *Chemist in Salipro Group S.A of C.V., Mexico*

Abstract: The increase in antibiotic resistance is an imminent and mainly silent threat, which would lead to an unprecedented situation with multivariable implications. It is challenging to solve due to having nuances in the regulatory, health-related, financial, and administrative aspects. The skin is one of the most common areas where antimicrobial-resistant infections develop; such is the case with MRSA (Methicillin-Resistant Staphylococcus aurcus), which is capable of causing deep painful boils. Besides, the chronic wounds, whose healing processes become aberrant, add complexity, yet these occur with features, such as aberrant cellular profile, persistent inflammation, and the formation of biofilms. The former issues make crucial the use of non-antibiotic antimicrobial agents, such as topical antiseptics for their treatment. In the present writing, we have introduced an innovative formula with relatively familiar ingredients to most people. One of those compounds is the potassium permanganate, a strong oxidative, astringent, and antimicrobial agent. This chapter consists of five sections: (1) the first section presents a general review of the antibiotics, their types and mechanism of action, and resistance caused in response to them from bacteria; this section also describes causes for this resistance, the bacterial strategies to achieve it, and possible solutions; (2) the second section highlights the approach to healing processes both acute and chronic, exploring the stages of the former, and both the abnormal features and possible therapies for the latter; (3) the third section discusses the non-antibiotic antimicrobial agents and the antiseptics in general, and then a brief

---

[*] **Correspondence author Agustín Lara-Esqueda:** Department of Psychology and Human Communication Therapy, University of Durango, Durango, CO 81301, United States; E-mail: alaraemx@gmail.com

Parvesh Singh, Vipan Kumar & Rajshekhar Karpoormath (Eds.)
All rights reserved-© 2021 Bentham Science Publishers

description is provided for the healing properties of each of the component of Vikut®, and finally, hypotheses for its performance have been proposed; (4) the fourth section presents the results of the clinical cases using the potassium permanganate-based formula obtained by healthcare professionals in the treatment of both chronic and non-chronic wounds. Two main subsections have discussed wound treatment using Vikut® formula; (4.1) the first subsection presents a 21 days-long comparative analysis between the usual treatment (neutral pH super-oxidation solutions) and the potassium permanganate-based formula for diabetic patients with chronic, 3 month-duration, Wagner I & II ulcers (average area 5-6cm2), where potassium permanganate-based formula has shown an average percentage reduction of 73% and a percentage of patients with area reduction greater or equal to 50% of 86%, in contrast to the usual treatment with ratios below 40% and 40% respectively, and (4.2) the second subsection is an exposition with respect to the clinical cases of both chronic and non-chronic wounds of different natures making use of the potassium permanganate-based formula; and (5) finally, the fifth section demonstrates an economical study performed on the public health condition in Mexico where several topical treatments are compared including the Vikut® formula, showing it as a viable option in terms of both the cost per se and the wound-reductive effect, which can be interpreted with respect to both time and resources available for the treatment of other afflictions in the public health domain.

Keywords: Antiseptic, Antibiotic resistance, Benzoic acid, BEB, Chronic wound, Clinical trial, Local oxygenation, Non-antibiotic antimicrobial agents, Potassium permanganate, Salicylic acid, Wound healing.

INTRODUCTION

Our ancestors attributed the ailments that afflicted them to the gods and supernatural entities. However, the medical area had witnessed a high development, and it was not until the beginning of the 20th century that medicine began to look more like today's science.

However, according to James Le Fanu, the development of contemporary medicine slowed down if compared with the period between the post-war and 1970 [1].

One of the branches where this trend is very noticeable is that of antibiotics. Since, in 1909, Paul Ehrlich invented Salvarsan to treat syphilis, and in 1928, a serendipity led Alexander Fleming to discover penicillin. These discoveries were the first milestones and served as a spearhead for others to search for substances with bactericidal and bacteriostatic activities, unleashing the "antibiotic revolution" [2].

However, after this era of medical bonanza regarding the treatment of bacterial infectious diseases, a strong decline began with resistance to antibiotics. Although this had been in sight since the first half of the 20th century, this started a fierce arms race between humans and bacteria until recent years when a wide variety of factors began to wane the fight for bacteria and antibiotic resistance [3].

This situation makes a necessity to improve the management of the resources that we have prepared to treat diseases related to bacteria [3, 4], as is the case of dermal wounds, particularly those called chronic [5]. Various factors, such as chronic diseases, impede these wounds that do not go through the usual wound healing process, making them aberrant and developing varied complications [6, 7].

Due to the properties of chronic wounds, including constant inflammation, lack of cell proliferation, and bacterial biofilms [6], their treatment is quite challenging and, even though the use of systemic antibiotics is recommended by international consensus and practical guidelines [8], there is no concise evidence that such treatments are effective. However, there is evidence that topical treatment may be beneficial [9].

Due to the growing need for innovation regarding the treatment against infections, non-antibiotic antimicrobial agents (NAAA) are a viable option to treat dermal infections with minimal risk of developing resistance to antibiotics. Vikut®, a preparation based on potassium permanganate, has proven to have properties that contribute to the healing of both chronic and non-chronic wounds [10 - 12]; in turn, it represents economic advantages over other options in the market [13], not counting the benefits described in the time saved in working hours by health workers.

THE ADVENT OF THE ANTIBIOTIC RESISTANCE

Antibiotics: What are They, and How do They Work?

Infectious diseases have been a prevalent and long-lived issue until the first half of the twelfth century when antibiotics were introduced to the world, providing usable weapons against them that only have increased since penicillin discovery [2, 14]. The antibiotics are microorganism-produced substances which inhibit growth or kill other microorganisms, whose selective toxicity allows them to affect specific microorganism groups while minimizing its effect in human [15].

According to Ebimieowei Etebu and Ibemologi Arikekpar [14], there are two classifications, the first by their molecular structure and the second by their mechanism of action:

CLASSIFICATION BASED ON THE MOLECULAR STRUCTURE

According to their molecular similarities, Etebu and Arikekpar classified them into nine categories:

β-lactams

These are compounds with a highly reactive ring (see Fig. **1**) that interferes with cell wall-assembler enzymes known as penicillin-binding proteins (PBP). The latter synthesize peptidoglycan through peptide cross-linking, and its inhibition results in the lysis and death of bacteria [14].

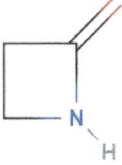

Fig. (1). β-lactam ring's structure.

According to the location and conformation of the β-lactam ring, there are four classes of these antibiotics:

- Penicillins, have cores of penicillanic amino acid.
- Cephalosporins have cores of 7-aminocephalosporanic acid.
- Monobactams have a single β-lactam ring without another ring.
- Carbapenems have penicillin-like rings but substitute the sulfur atom with a carbon one [14].

Macrolides

These are compounds with a highly reactive ring (see Fig. **2**) that interferes with cell wall-assembler enzymes known as penicillin-binding proteins (PBP). The latter synthesize peptidoglycan through peptide cross-linking, and its inhibition results in the lysis and death of bacteria [14].

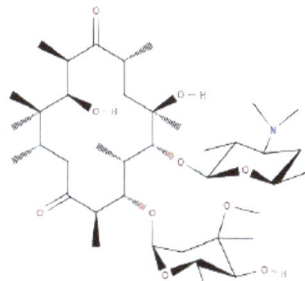

Fig. (2). Macrolides' structure.

They are structurally macrocyclic lactose rings with L-cladinose and Ddesosamine (see Fig. **2**) and have either a bactericidal or bacteriostatic effect. They inhibit the protein synthesis by binding to the ribosome and preventing amino acids' addition to the polypeptide, having a greater spectrum than the penicillins [14].

Tetracycline

They have a structure of four hydrocarbon rings (see Fig. **3**), which disrupts the amino acid's addition to the polypeptides in the ribosome. First (natural), second (semi-synthetic), and third-generation (fully synthetic) of these antibiotics are found [14].

Fig. (3). Tetracycline's structure.

Quinolones

Discovered as an impurity during quinine development in the sixties, they have shown to be effective despite their basic two-rings structure (see Fig. **4**). Another ring has been added to broaden its spectrum in once resistant bacteria in more recent generations [14].

Fig. (4). Quinolone's structure.

Aminoglycosides

Their structure is three amino sugars connected by a glycosidic bond (see Fig. **5**); they inhibit protein synthesis by binding to bacterial ribosomal units and have a broad antimicrobial spectrum. However, streptomycin (its first member) is highly toxic [14].

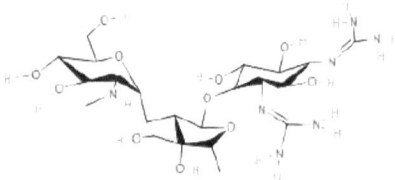

Fig. (5). Aminoglycosides' structure.

Sulfonamides

The first therapeutically-used antibiotic (see Fig. **6**) is a competitive antagonism of para-aminobenzoic acid (PABA), a folic acid precursor. Despite its efficacy, it has specific toxicity and side effects, such as urinary tract disorders, hemolytic anemia, porphyria, and hypersensitivity reactions [14].

Fig. (**6**). Sulfonamides' structure.

Glycopeptides (GPA's)

Once naturally produced and with improved synthetic variants, GPAs consist of 7 amino acids linked with two sugars (hence their name) and inhibit cell wall formation [14].

Polymyxins

These are cationic lipopeptides, also known as non-ribosomal peptides, a decapeptide with an intramolecular cycle conformed by seven of its peptides. They are amphoteric, which permits them to interact with the lipid A component of lipopolysaccharide [16, 17].

Oxazolidinones

New synthetic broad-spectrum antibiotics with unknown action mechanisms (see Fig. **7**) have been observed to bind to the 50 S ribosomal subunit P site [14].

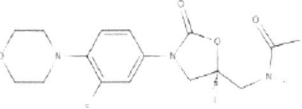

Fig. (**7**). Oxazolidinone's structure.

CLASSIFICATION BASED ON ITS MECHANISM OF ACTION

Depending on how they work, the groups of antibiotics are [14]:

Inhibition of cell wall synthesis

The bacterial cell wall of bacteria made up of peptidoglycan protects the cell and provides consistent osmotic pressure due to the peptide cross-linking in its structure. β-lactams and glycopeptides inhibit the action of the PBPs and peptidoglycan, respectively [14].

Disruption of the structure or function of the cell membrane

Antibiotics, such as daptomycin and polymyxins, break the cell membrane, either by depolarizing or disintegrating it, respectively [14].

Inhibition of nucleic acid structure or function

Quinolones interfere with bacterial helicase, topoisomerases and disrupting RNA production without affecting their human homologous [14], and with this blocking both replication and protein transcription.

Inhibition of protein synthesis

Macrolides, tetracyclines, and aminoglycosides disrupt the protein synthesis by binding to the ribosomes by blocking translation, which is lethal due to the high importance of the proteins to life [14].

Blocking key metabolic pathways

The sulfonamides impede the folic acid synthesis, an essential nutrient for bacteria for producing nucleotides and amino acids, which disrupts homeostasis and leads to cell death [14].

The bacteria strike back: mechanisms of resistance to antibiotics

Evolution is inexorable. The discovery of selectively toxic substance occasion a selective pressure which force bacteria to adapt or die and the survivors both replicate and spread their resistance among other populations through horizontal gene transfer.

On one side, some bacteria, such as Pseudomonas, are inherently resistant, which endure the triclosan due to an additional enoyl-ACP enzyme [18]. On the other hand, however, bacteria have developed ways of dealing with antibiotics. Here are the four main strategies:

Enzyme inhibition

The most common strategy consists of modifying the antibiotic's molecular structure to disable their properties, which is achieved by hydrolysis, functional group transfer, redox reactions, and bond breaking. One problematic example is the β-lactams resistance, for which bacteria have evolved enzymes, such as penicillinases, cephalosporinases or carbapenemases, the latter capable of disabling all the β-lactams excepting aztreonam [18, 19].

Modification of molecular targets

Another strategy is to change the lock rather than break the key, which is achieved by changing the site where the antibiotics act, and there are two mechanisms. The first one is by altering the polypeptide sequence (by mutation) [18 - 20], and the second one is by protecting the susceptible site with non-protein molecules addition (by post-translational modifications) [18, 19, 21, 22].

Efflux pumps

Some bacteria take a different approach and take the antibiotics out of their internal environment. For this, they produce proton-dependent efflux pumps to actively remove antibiotics, which is an efficient mechanism of resistance by preventing the compound from staying long enough to act. There are several types of membrane efflux proteins, which many of them can carry multiple dissimilar substrates and, due to mutation, some species such as *P. aeruginosa* and *S. aureus* start to overexpress these pumps, enhancing their resistance [18, 19].

Porin modification

Porins (such as *OmpF*, *OmpC*, or *OmpE*) are required for hydrophilic antibiotics to pass Gram-negative bacteria outer lipid membrane. The development of reduced permeability due to the decreasing and even loss of expression contributes to resistance [18, 19].

LOOKING FOR ANSWERS: THE CAUSES OF ANTIBIOTIC RESISTANCE

Antibiotics have increased life length and quality by treating and preventing infections even in people with cancer, chronic diseases, and those undergoing transplants. However, their success may be the cause of their diminishing effectiveness due to their misusage leading to urgent situations respecting health, finances, and regulations.

INTRINSIC RESISTANCE IN NATURE

Some bacteria have a resistant phenotype (a quasi-resistance) to antibiotics due to specific genes and other strategies such as gene amplification. Unsurprisingly, specific resistances have been tracked to individual species, such as *Streptomycetes* and specific beta-lactamases, *Kluyvera* and the CTM-X enzyme, or the efflux pump-related resistances certain antibiotic-producing bacteria which tend to be multi-resistant. The dissemination of the resistance mechanisms is partially due to horizontal genetic transfer, such as conjugation, translation, and transformation [2, 3, 23].

EXCESSIVE AND INAPPROPRIATE USE

The use of antibiotics and the development of resistance is correlated, and the former has been inadequate. The length and the choice of therapy are incorrect between 30% to 50%, and antibiotics usage was found unnecessary, inappropriate, or suboptimal between the 30% and the 60% of cases in the ICU. Subinhibitory and suboptimal concentrations stimulate resistance development, promoting mutagenesis generation and proteomic alteration induction. The anthropogenic activities induce selective pressure, which increases, even more, the resistance development [3, 23 - 25].

EXTENSIVE USE IN THE AGRICULTURAL SECTOR

Farming antibiotic use represents 80% of the sold antibiotics in the USA, used in cattle to promote growth and prevent infection, limiting its intestinal flora and increasing its nutrient absorption. The presence of antibiotics in feces and meat promotes resistance development and dissemination due to manure being used as fertilizer, producing crop antibiotic bioaccumulation [3, 26, 27].

UNAVAILABILITY OF NEW ANTIBIOTICS

New antibiotics development is stalled because they are unsuitable investments and a decreasing research budget due to short periods and perceived as low-value drug compared to other drugs. On the other hand, the fear of resistance development impedes the swift use of new antibiotics as the first-line drug, making the health insurance companies reluctant to include them in their policies [3, 28].

REGULATORY BARRIERS

These are also obstacles that inhibit financial incentive for antibiotics development; including bureaucracy, procedural opacity, clinical requirement differences between countries, changes in licensing and regulatory standards, and ineffective communication channels. Despite this, a new clinical model, such as the limited population antibiotic drug (LPAD) [3, 28].

POSSIBLE SOLUTIONS: HOW CAN WE DEAL WITH ANTIBIOTIC RESISTANCE?

Acknowledging the current antibiotics situation shows us ways to deal with, mitigate, and reduce it. The CDC has outlined four key actions to reduce antibiotic-resistant bacterial infections [29]:

PREVENTION OF TRANSMISSION OF BACTERIAL INFECTIONS

Preventing infections reduces resistance by eliminating the need for antibiotics; therefore, we must avoid cross-contamination by implementing infection control guidelines, maintaining hand hygiene between interactions, and disinfecting health facilities and patient care equipment [29].

TRACKING METHODOLOGIES

It is necessary to trace data of antibiotics use in health and farming and the regions where resistance in development. Even if it has not been done systematically, gathering this information is desirable and valuable for strategizing and preventing [4].

IMPROVING THE USES OF EXISTING ANTIBIOTICS

Antibiotic Stewardship Programs

Antibiotic Stewardship Programs (ASP) are systematic institutional efforts to manage antibiotics respecting correct usage, dosage, therapeutic period, and necessity, which has proven to be effective by diminishing its use between 11% - 38% and decreasing non-guide-based therapy, stay time, mortality and cost. The former is achieved with the support of diagnosis, antibiotic rotation, and determination of minimum inhibitory concentration, along with other strategies, and by prioritizing health quality instead of cost-effectiveness, which is ironically more cost-effective and self-sustaining [4, 30].

IMPROVEMENT OF PRESCRIPTION PRACTICES AND THERAPEUTIC TIME LENGTH

Antibiotic prescription is improvable by up to 37% by implementing diagnostic tests, documentation of symptoms, and optimizing antimicrobial therapies. One example is the viral respiratory infections, for which between 40% - 75% of the patients due to the latter expectation. Additionally, the therapy's length may be shortened without losing effectiveness, and the use of bioindicators such as procalcitonin may reduce antibiotic consumption by 51% [4].

PROMOTION OF THE DEVELOPMENT OF NEW ANTIBIOTICS AND DIAGNOSTIC TESTS

Improvement of Diagnostic Tools

Diagnosis is possibly the most effective way to reduce antibiotic inappropriate use. In contrast with former diagnostic techniques that take days or weeks, the current ones, such as real-time multiplex PCR or mass spectrometry, can diagnose in minutes or hours. However, most of these techniques require a certain level of infrastructure and equipment lacking in the developing countries; for this, the development of the ASSURED test is desirable. Furthermore, diagnosing resistance may allow a Search and Destruction (S&D) approach, easing a correct and specific prescription [4, 31, 32].

INCREASE THE VARIETIES OF ANTIMICROBIAL TREATMENTS

Developing new antibiotics is essential due to resistance inevitability. Institutional intervention and public and international initiatives are needed to achieve it. In turn, non-antibiotic-based therapies are arising, such as silver and copper nanoparticles, the use of bacteriophages as treatment, the discovery of the antimicrobial properties of essential oils and phytochemicals. Additionally, topical antiseptics have been used for preventing and treating surgical and chronic wounds as an ASP strategy [4, 33 - 39].

Conclusion: Persist or Perish

Bacterial resistance is a challenging yet inevitable situation due to the anthropogenic selective pressure. However, its inadequate management, antibiotic sanitary misuse, non-therapeutical uses in farming have led to resistance to the most common antibiotics. Therefore, critical actions include infection prevention, resistance monitoring, improving antibiotics management, and developing new antimicrobial compounds.

Antibiotic intensive use has led to the emergence of multi-resistant and pan-resistant strains. Alternative therapeutic strategies, such as phytochemicals, nanoparticles, bacteriophages, or topical antiseptic agents represent viable alternatives to mitigate and decelerate antibiotic resistance.

UNDERSTANDING THE WOUND HEALING PROCESS AND ITS RELATION TO THE CHRONICITY OF WOUNDS

Wounds and their Normal Healing Process

Even though wounds can be defined as rupture of tissue continuity by any external agency, the term usually refers to disruption of the skin [40, 41].

Complex interactions between skin cellular and matrix occur during wounding. In healthy individuals, acute healing proceeds with coordinated and regulated cell processes, such as phagocytosis, chemotaxis, mitogenesis, and matrix synthesis; differentiated in four coupled phases [6, 41, 42]:

Hemostasis: Vasoconstriction occurs to stop bleeding and easing clot formation and aggregation of platelet, which have multiple growth factors that promote several cells activation (fibroblasts, endothelial cells and macrophages) and amines that produce oedema through microvascular permeability and fluid exudation [41].

Inflammation: between 24-48 hours, immune cell infiltration begins with granulocytes or polymorphonuclear leukocytes (PMNLs) attracted by multiple compounds, adhering to epithelial cells and moving *via* diapedesis engulfing pathogens to later be removed *via* macrophage phagocytosis and extrusion as slough [41].

Between 48-72 hours, compounds, such as matrix components, clotting components, and growth factors attract monocytes that convert into macrophages. The latter may act as crucial regulatory cells for repair, releasing cell-migration cytokines and tissue-cleaning proteases. Both PMNL and macrophages secrete additional growth factors to stimulate inflammation and antimicrobial Reactive Oxygen Species (ROS) [41].

After 72 hours, lymphocytes arrive at the injury, and evidence suggests its involvement in extracellular remodeling, although their role is yet to be defined [41].

Recent observations suggest that inflammation may lead to fibrosis in wounds, leading to scar formation [6].

Proliferation

Between the third day and over two weeks, cell proliferation and extracellular matrix construction occur, increasing the nutrients and gas requirements, and angiogenesis is produced due to PMNL and macrophage promotion. Vascular sprouting is essential to adult wound healing, for which endothelial progenitor cells (EPC) are required. Later, epithelialization occurs at the edges through migration and mitosis. Genetically, usually disable genes related to cell proliferation and migration, such as *Ap1*, *Fos* and *Jun*, and became active during wound healing [6, 41, 44]

Remodeling

After granular tissue formation, the matrix matures by decomposing fibronectin and hyaluronan and increasing collagen bundles, and metalloproteases action decrease as tissue inhibitors of metalloproteases (TIMPs) increase. Collagen became organized through wounds contraction, cell density decreases through apoptosis, and blood flow and metabolic activity diminish through growth stagnation. This process results in a scar devoid of cells and vascularity [41].

Chronic Injuries: When Things Go the Wrong Way

Chronic wounds are injuries with an interrupted healing process usually stagnant in the inflammatory or proliferative phases.

Types of Chronic Wounds

Ageing and chronic diseases, such as diabetes, cause the skin's acute healing process to deviate. Chronic wounds can be classified as [43]:

Venous Vascular Ulcers: The veins' vascular incompetence increases pressure due to the blood backflow and leakage of fibrin and other plasmatic compounds that inhibit correct oxygenation and delay wound healing [43, 44].

Arterial Vascular Ulcers: Ischemic arterial insufficiency induces atherosclerosis or embolism, and resolve the subjacent wound issues is required [43, 44].

Diabetic ulcers: Hyperglycemia-related chronic wounds are developed due to diabetes complications such as vasculopathy and neuropathy, characterized by cell and metabolic abnormalities [43].

Pressure ulcers: Prolonged and unrelieved pressure applied to an area that leads to hypoxia, an ischemia-derived injury, reperfusion, and tissue necrosis [43, 44].

Chronic Wound Profile: What Went Wrong?

Chronic wounds present various aberrant features such as [6,41,42]:

Alteration of proteolytic activity: Higher proteases concentration and diminished protease inhibitors, causing the degradation of fibronectin, collagen, and growth factors and a defective ECM composition and rearrangement, the inability of the fibroblast population to contract, the reduction in the production of laminin 332 and haptotactic subtract for the motility of post-traumatism keratinocytes [6, 41, 43 - 45].

Alteration in cytokine profiles and the inflammatory response: there are increased proinflammatory cytokines, which results in growth inhibition and induction of morphological changes in fibroblasts. Moreover, chronic and persistent inflammation in chronic wounds is perceived, observing an increase in the innate cell immune system populations; furthermore, the cell populations profile in chronic wounds is aberrant, such as a reduced capacity for bactericidal and phagocytic activity in macrophages [6, 41].

Alterations in cell profiles: Morphological changes and proliferation patterns are observed in fibroblasts with decreasing proliferative capability is also observed [41].

Another vital cell alteration is the diminished migration capacity, as in keratinocytes, with reduced integrin $\alpha5\beta1$ expression and suppressing both control regulators and p53 despite retaining partial proliferative activity. Also, fibroblasts in chronic wounds become senescent, irresponsive to growth factors, and reduced migratory activity [6].

Key intermediates concerning both the regulation and coordination signaling of the angiogenesis and vasculogénesis are defective in diabetes patients. The former is probably due to the deficiencies of EPCs release from the bone marrow or the impaired capability of homing and engraftment of the injured tissue [45].

It has shown that hyperglycemia may be one of the main factors, both promoting senescence and decreasing the proliferative capabilities of the EPCs, in addition to changing its cell profile, making it less angiogenic and more proinflammatory [45, 46].

The Presence of ROS and Other Metabolic By-Products

The presence of ROS has been implicated in the development and persistence of chronic wounds such as venous, arterial wounds. The former is released by both PMNC and macrophages during the persistent inflammation, which is usual in chronic wounds [41, 48]. The presence of NO, which can react with hydroxyl free radical forming peroxynitrite, a potent free radical capable of tissue destruction [41].

In normally healing wounds, the ROS induce wound healing through cell signaling. Ironically, both hypoxia and hyperoxia increase ROS production, which in significant quantities is harmful to the wound, causing additional tissue damage [42, 47]. Persistent hypoxia is pivotal in chronic wounds due to its incapability of angiogenesis to ongoing [6].

An Increased Presence of Slough and Necrotic Tissue

Due to aberrant and pathogenic characteristics in both their histology and their biochemistry, the presence of necrotic tissue and slough production as usual. Due to the hypoxic and nutrient-depleted environment derived from the lack of an appropriate blood supply, the cells die, and their remains become necrotic tissue and slough, which promotes bacterial colonization preventing wound healing even further. The presence of necrotic tissue and slough perpetuate the inflammation and impede both contraction and epithelization of the wound [41].

The Occupation of Microorganism: Unwanted Visitors

The process of microorganism appearance can be divided into four categories based on the induced response of the host: the first is contamination, where there is a non-replicating microorganism in the wound; the secondly is colonization, where the microorganism is self-replicating, but there is not damaged tissue; the third is a local infection or critical colonization, where the bacterial burden is increasing, and it is the intermediate category between colonization and infection; and the fourth is the invasive wound infection, where there is both the presence of self-replicating microorganism and subsequent host response, leading to delay healing [41].

There is still debate regarding if either the bacterial infection produces the chronic suboptimal inflammation or the latter facilitates the former; whatever is the causality of events, the result is a vicious cycle usually resulting in a formation of a biofilm, from which its importance would be thoroughly described later [6].

Due to the persistent yet inefficient inflammatory response on the wound, further complications caused by microorganisms are observed. One of the essential bacterial presence features in the chronic wound is their biofilm production [6, 41 - 44, 48 - 50]. The former allows them to be altering their own phenotypical and genotypical characteristics, the presence of multiple strains, and even aiding in the development of antibiotic resistance [41, 48].

The Biofilm: The Invaders' Fortress

The biofilm is a structure formed for bacteria for inhabitation composed by glycocalyx, a polysaccharide-rich exopolymer (also known as *exo-polysaccharide* or EPS). The structure alone conforms to about 80% of its volume, where the other 20% are bacteria [48]. It is particularly resistant to even more aggressive treatments due to its structural characteristics.

Another of its pivotal characteristic is its microbial diversity. There is evidence that in a sole wound, there could be a myriad of species. A study of analyses samples of 13 patients with chronic wounds, where 249 bacteria species were found, including bacteria from the genera *Staphylococcus, Streptococcus, Clostridium, Proteus,* and *Pseudomonas* [51]. A study even links the presence of yeast to biofilms [52]. All the previous features make the management of chronic wounds through antibiotics seldom successful [9, 48].

The complexity and organization within the biofilm can generate concentration gradients and microenvironments, which allow heterogeneity of bacterial species to exist within the biofilm, even anaerobic ones, due to the presence of oxygen-deprived places deeper in the biofilm [48]. Furthermore, another study indicates that the bacteria species, such as *P. aeruginosa,* produce microcolonies embedded in the self-produced matrix [53].

The biofilm structure also facilitates the development of antibiotic resistance due to two factor: the first one is because the phenotype of the biofilm-encased bacteria (BEB) is sessile (non-motile) and presents a reduced metabolic rate, which produces a tolerant profile to the bacteria due to the activity of multiple antibiotics act during cell division, such as the β-lactams, aminoglycosides, and quinolones [50]; the second one is because the EPS serves as a mechanical barrier which prevents the antibiotics for crossing it, leading to a suboptimal concentration of antibiotics and the generation of selective pressure toward the resistance [48, 50].

The mechanism with which the BEB develops its sessile phenotype is through a process called *quorum sensing*, which permits the cell-to-cell communication with autoinductors, allowing the bacteria to coordinate activities based on its population size. A link between biofilm formation and the quorum sensing mechanisms was observed in bacteria such as *P. aeruginosa, S. aureus,* and *V. cholera* [50].

The biofilm formation can be separated into five stages: the first is the arrival of the planktonic free-living actively-growing bacteria which attach reversibly to the surface; the second is the irreversible attachment to the surface and the inception of the EPS matrix formation; the third is the early biofilm development with the microcolony formation, where the planktonic bacteria become BEB and proliferate; the fourth is the growth and differentiation, where the BEB generate complex matrix architecture, channels, pores, and the bacterial cells redistribute; the fifth and last stage is the dispersion stage, where some cells acquire more planktonic profiles and prepare themselves for new colonization [50, 54].

In addition to the formerly exposed, the BEB had been observed to have the ability to manipulate the immune response to their advantage, disrupting the three laws of immunity of universality, tolerance, and appropriateness. That disruption is achieved due to the incapacity of both the leucocytes and the antibodies to penetrate the biofilm structure, inhibiting the immune response's downregulation, perpetuating the inflammation, and using the host's response for the disruption of its tissue [50].

The Treatment of Chronic Wounds: Untying a Gordian Knot

There is significant complexity of chronic wounds, involving both features of each chronic wound-causing diseases, such as diabetes and atherosclerosis, and general features respecting the undergoing abnormal healing process, such as impaired angiogenesis non-migratory and senescent cells, and biofilm formation.

Despite the significant challenge regarding this aberrant skein of processes, some proposals have been made by numerous researchers:

Patient and Wound Assessment

Knowing both the patient situation and the wound condition is essential to determine the treatment to follow. Patient information such as the presence of similar affliction like diabetes and atherosclerosis, the registration of the medical history, the laboratory studies, the nutrition, and the patient's reliability must be considered, regarding the wound, features such as previous diagnosis, physical characteristic like wound extension or even odor, vascular examination, and the ascertainment of infection [5].

Topical Wound Therapy

While many topical therapies/antimicrobials and dressings are available, research respecting its efficacy is needed. There are multiple types of options with different approaches, such as hydrogels, hypochlorous acid, honey, povidone-iodine solutions, cadexomer iodine, silver-containing products, collagenase, and super-oxidative agents had been tested [5]. The use of natural agents such as honey [55 - 58] and phytochemicals [38] and both super oxidant and antimicrobial agents has been proposed [11, 59]. Regarding diabetic ulcers, topical wound therapy resulted in being more effective than systemic antibiotics [11] due to the nature of biofilms developed on chronic wounds [48, 50].

New Therapies

Although basic tenets regarding chronic wounds exist, discovering and assessing new treatments is crucial to afford this sizeable issue. Some of the proposed therapies are:

- Negative pressure wound therapy
- Hyperbaric oxygen therapy
- Biophysical modalities, such as electrical stimulation
- Biological and bioengineering therapies, such as platelet-rich plasma, growth factors, acellular therapies, bioengineered cellular therapies, stem cell therapies [5]

Conclusion: Thinking Out of the Box

International guidelines respecting the management and prevention of diabetic foot ulcers had established the use of antibiotics for the treatment of the diabetic foot due to the subjacent infection which use to develop [8], despite that had proven to be ineffective and seldom successful on the treatment of chronic disease [9].

Due to its infective nature, biofilms associated with chronic wounds had been treated as systemic infection. Still, its nature as a complex microbial gathering has proven to overcome the issue regarding antibiotics.

That is why to achieve a successful wound healing, we have to think respecting the chronic wounds as a skein of processes like the knot of Gordius, which leave us with two possible approaches, we can try to untie the knot, or we can cut it, as Alexander the Great did it.

THE APPLICATION OF NON-ANTIBIOTIC ANTIMICROBIAL AGENTS FOR THE TREATMENT OF WOUNDS: THE EMERGENCE OF VIKUT®

Non-antibiotic Antimicrobial Agents: A Possible Solution?

As indicated in its name, the Non-Antibiotic Antimicrobial Agents (NAAA) are substances that have an antimicrobial property despite not being an antibiotic. This definition is overly broad, including a myriad of compounds that can have antimicrobial activity. A study gives us two categories of NAAAs used as a topical treatment, the antimicrobial nanoparticles such as those made of silver, zinc oxide, and titanium dioxide, and the antimicrobial peptides [60].

However, another type of NAAAs is antiseptics, which represents a large number of compounds. An antiseptic is an antimicrobial agent that kills, inhibits, or reduces the number of microorganisms [61]. According to Janos Cambiaso-Daniel and his colleagues [62], the classifications of antiseptics of clinical use are:

Emulsifiers

These are compounds with various natures whose mechanism of action is the disruption of the cell wall and cytoplasmic membrane through acting, as their name indicates, as emulsifiers that their amphoteric nature makes them capable of dissolving the cellular barriers, provoking the pathogen's lysis. The most ubiquitous members of this class are soaps and detergents consisting of sodium or potassium salts of saponified lipid acids [62].

They are a powerful resource against biofilms, disrupting their layers and decreasing the microbial burden. They can cause a 99% reduction of the colony count for 48 hours [62].

Other emulsifiers are available such as non-ionic detergents like the hydrogel PluroGel® are used clinically. Biguanides like chlorhexidine or polyhexamethylene biguanide (PHMB) are cationic emulsifiers with biocide properties.

Oxidizers

These agents act through a free radicals' mediator, which disrupts biofilm EPS, cell walls, cytoplasmic membranes, proteins, nucleic acids, and even intracellular metals. They have broad-spectrum activity, but their therapeutic use is limited due to their high reactivity and high host toxicity [62].

These groups include hydrogen peroxide, potassium permanganate, and some oxidative halides such as sodium hypochlorite, hypochlorous acid, povidone-iodine, and caxomer iodine. Bacteriotoxic foam dressing such as gentian violet and methylene blue dyes was recently approved for chronic and burned wounds [62].

The increase of antibiotic resistance has made the reemergence of compounds such as sodium hypochlorite as an adjunct of wound cares [62]

Acids

Weak acids, such as acetic acid, honey, and boric acid, have been used since ancient times. The acetic acid is helpful in eradicating biofilms of multiple bacteria species, being capable of eliminating biofilm containing *Pseudomonas* spp., *Acinetobacter* spp., *Escherichia coli,* MRSA, *Proteus* spp., *Enterobacter* spp. and *Klebsiella* spp. However, due to its fibroblast's cytotoxicity, its therapeutic use is limited [62].

Boric acid, despite its limited antimicrobial activity, may have a protective effect by reducing DNA damage due to oxidative stress [62].

Honey has been used as a topical agent since antiquity and presents surprising beneficial features such as a broad-spectrum antimicrobial activity, the maintenance of the moisture in the wound, which is crucial to its healing and is less toxic than silver [62].

Heavy Metals

Four metals are used as antiseptics: ionic silver, bismuth, copper, and mercury. While the latter has been fallen out of use due to concerns respecting systemic toxicity, and both bismuth and copper have limited use, the silver's antimicrobial activity has been well established [62].

The use of silver nitrate has a bacteriostatic effect in *P. aeruginosa*, *S. aureus,* and *E. coli*, while silver sulfadiazine has been proven effective against *Pseudomonas* spp., *Candida albicans*, enteric bacteria, and fungi. Acting by binding to both DNA and proteins and destroy them *via* the oxidative pathway. It is considered less toxic than oxidative halides, but recent studies have questioned its non-toxic nature [62].

The inception of Vikut®: a synergetic surprise.

Vikut® is a wound healing adjuvant that was first produced as a topical antiseptic for chronic wounds. Regardless of that, its effectiveness in both acute and chronic wounds [10 - 12].

Vikut® is composed of four substances: potassium permanganate, ethanol, salicylic acid, and benzoic acid. In this section, the healing properties of each of the components will be discussed.

Potassium Permanganate: an Unexpected ally

The potassium permanganate is a potent oxidizing and astringent agent. Its chemical features display specific properties that make it useful in the treatment of wounds.

The first one is its chemical cauterization capability, produced due to the oxidation of organic matter in the tissue. This property's clinical application had been observed in veterinary [63, 64] and medical areas, despite that the latter one was recorded in 1933 [65].

The second is its antimicrobial activity against bacteria, fungi, and viruses [66,

67]. As an oxidizer, the potassium permanganate presents the capacity to disrupt the bacteria's organic material, including the cell wall, the cytoplasmic membranes, the proteins, and the DNA [62]. Even though it is supposed, its capacity to break down the biofilm has not been proved yet.

The third is its capacity for wound healing. Its administration has been linked with wound healing [10 - 12] and ingrown toenails' repairment [68].

The potassium permanganate is included in the WHO model formulary, a source of references of essential medicines for the use of guidelines writers. It is used to treat impetigo, suppurating superficial wounds, and tinea pedis [69].

There is disagreement respecting its use as a topical treatment. While some authors consider the obsolete [70], others use it as topical antiseptic collaboratively with other wound treatment methods such as vacuum sealing draining and dressings based on polyvinyl alcohol and polyurethane [71].

Due to the antibiotic-resistant bacteria emergence, topical treatment such as potassium permanganate and silver particles is crucial for the prevention and therapy of wounds developed in hospitals [39.72,73].

Ethanol: the perfect mixer

Ethanol, also known as ethyl alcohol, is the second simplest alcohol and has multiple uses. It is considered a suitable solvent. Used at a concentration between 70 and 85%, it is a disinfectant of surfaces and a skin antiseptic. The former is due to its capacity to denaturalize protein and inhibit its synthesis. Ethanol is effective against most bacteria and fungi, and this is also true for many viruses. However, it is ineffective against endospores. It has a broad spectrum of activity, particularly sessile bacteria such as the BEB [74].

Salicylic and Benzoic Acids: An Old but good team

Salicylic acid is a type of phenolic acid identified as antipyretic and anti-inflammatory, decreasing the formation of pro-inflammatory prostaglandins modulating the expression of COX 2 [75, 76]. It also has an exfoliant and peeling ability, making it a useful cosmetic ingredient [77]. In addition to the former, salicylic acid presents bacteriostatic activity [79], and there is evidence indicating that both salicylic and acetylsalicylic acid can break down biofilms [79 - 82]. However, there is disagreement regarding the capacity of biofilm disruption, and other studies suggest that the opposite might occur [83]. Regarding benzoic acid, it has shown that it also presents bacteriostatic activity [78, 84]

Both the salicylic and the benzoic acids are included in the WHO model formulary. The salicylic acid is indicated mainly for topical use and, in combination with another substance, its molecular cousin, the acetylsalicylic acid, is more used as an ingested drug. It is described as having keratolytic and antimicrobial activities and it's prescribed to treat ringworm, mild dermatitis infections, seborrheic dermatitis, and ichthyosis, acne vulgaris, and warts. Respecting the benzoic acid, it appears only in conjunction with salicylic acid on ointment or cream presentation with the proportion of benzoic and salicylic acids of 6% and 3%, respectively. The former is denominated "Whitfield ointment" and is used to treat mild dermatophyte infections, such as tinea [69].

Concerning other applications, both compounds of debriding wounds' capability by dissolving the necrotic material are known [85, 86].

Comparison Between Topical Antiseptics and Topical Antibiotics

Despite their apparent similarities, the mechanism of action of the antibiotic and the antiseptics are quite different. The reason is that because the former acts through mechanisms and structures which are distinctive of bacteria [15], while the latter relies upon more disruptive methods such as emulsify and denaturalize the microorganism, and because of this, its spectrum of action is broader, as shown in Table **1** [15, 62].

Table 1. Comparison between a topical antibiotic and Vikut®, a topical antiseptic.

-	Antibiotic Topical Ointment	Vikut®
Active Ingredients	• Polymyxin B • Bacitracin	• Potassium Permanganate • Ethanol • Salicylic and benzoic acid
Excipient	Zinc oxide	Water
Against microorganisms	Antibiotic Effect (specific to bacteria)	Microbicidal Effect (broad spectrum of microorganism)
Analgesic	Maybe added	No
Astringent	No	Yes
Protection against infections	Yes	Yes
Form	Semisolid / Cream	Liquid
Antibiotic resistance development	Due to its antibiotic content, it promotes the antibiotic resistance	Due to its chemical action, do not contribute to the antibiotic resistance
Pain	No	Yes
Anti-inflammatory	Maybe added	Yes

	Antibiotic Topical Ointment	Vikut®
Chemical Scar	No	Chemical cauterization *via* oxidation, providing a temporary barrier against external agents.

Furthermore, the antibiotics, even the topical ones, have proven to be ineffective in treating chronic wounds due to biofilm, which presents low-metabolically active BEB and the protecting barrier of EPS.

The Synergies within the Vikut® Formula

There have not been studies regarding the interaction of the components of the Vikut® beside the clinical cases, but the latter only showed the wound progress.

However, knowing its features and chemical properties, hypotheses regarding the mechanism of action can be made.

Turning the Alcohol into Acetic Acid

The potassium permanganate is a highly oxidative compound, especially regarding organic compounds. It reacts with the ethanol contained in the Vikut® formula, as is expressed in the following equations [87]:

Oxidation **(i)**: $H_3C-CH_2OH + H_2O \rightarrow H_3C-CO_2H + 4H^+ + 4e^-$

Reduction **(ii)**: $MnO_4^- + 4H^+ + 3e^- \rightarrow MnO_2(s) + 2H_2O$

Overall: 3 **(i)** + 4x **(ii)**

$3H_3-CH_2OH + 4MnO_4^- + 4H^+ \rightarrow 3H_3C-CO_2H + 4MnO_2(s) + 5H_2O$

This reaction transforms both components; the ethanol becomes acetic acid due to its acidity having particular antimicrobial activity [62]. On the other hand, potassium permanganate converts into manganese dioxide (MnO_2).

The former reaction may lead to two hypotheses concerning the manganese dioxide, which would be exposed here below:

Hypothesis I: Transforming the Oxidizer in Oxygen

The MnO_2 is a catalyst for hydrogen peroxide (H_2O_2), allowing it to make the H_2O_2 react unlimitedly and produce oxygen continuously [88]. These could lead to an increase in the oxygen level in the wound. Due to the chronic non-healing wound's hypoxic nature, this could lead to a temporal improvement that could add up gradually. The improvement of chronic wounds with treatments related to improving oxygenation either *via* hyperbaric oxygen therapy [89] or *via* local oxygenation of the wound has been observed [90].

However, despite that the presence of MnO_2 would catalyze the biogenic H_2O_2 produced continuously by the PMNLs and the macrophages into oxygen, doubts emerge regarding if the biogenic H_2O_2 quantity would be enough to provide the tissue of enough oxygen.

Hypothesis II: The ROS Thief

On the other hand, maybe it is due to the lack of ROS in the wound. Even though if the quantities of H_2O_2 could not produce enough oxygen to alleviate the tissue's hypoxia, the MnO_2 may be eliminating enough H_2O_2 to reduce the oxidative stress. The use of antioxidants to scavenging free radical appears to expedite the healing of chronic wounds [41, 91].

Conclusion: Toward Unknown Waters

We are confronting unprecedented problems such as the increment of age mean and the escalating number of deceases, leading to chronic wounds. Besides the former, the antibiotic resistance is conducting us in an increasingly complex battle with gradually diminishing tools and weapons to deal with them.

That is why the innovation respecting the discovery of new antibiotics and new antimicrobial agents, such as the NAAAs, is essential.

Sometimes, we do not even have to reinvent the wheel. There are old tools that, with minor modifications, can lead to remarkable achievements.

The proposed formula of Vikut® does not have new compounds. It just uses them in a new way. On the other hand, the knowledge respecting the mechanism of action of the NAAAs and the undergoing processes of both acute and chronic wounds will be handy to attack the chronic wound's critical aspects.

However, even though the course of our journey may be clear, there still are obstacles to overcome. The continuous and persistent research and development of both compounds and strategies is the spearhead that will facilitate this journey.

CLINICAL EVIDENCE OF THE FORMULA BASED ON POTASSIUM PERMANGANATE FOR THE TREATMENT OF BOTH ACUTE AND CHRONIC WOUNDS

Despite the unknown mechanism of Vikut®, its efficacy has been proven on several occasions, being effective with both acute and chronic wounds. In the next section, a description of the comparative analysis between the Vikut® and the conventional treatment shows a satisfactory result respecting its efficacy.

Comparative Analysis Between Vikut® and the Conventional Treatment

A study was performed by the Delgado-Enciso and its colleagues [11] to compare the formula of Vikut® based on potassium permanganate and the traditional treatment. The executed study was a simple-blind, randomized, and controlled clinical trial.

Patients' Selection

There were 25 patients selected for participation in the study. Specific characteristics were required for being selected [11]:

- Previous diagnosis of diabetes Mellitus 2.
- The presence of diabetic foot ulcers. These also have to fulfill specific requirements:
    - Early wound development stage, such as Wagner I (uninfected superficial ulcer) or Wagner II (deep ulcer, often infected, no bone involvement or abscesses).
    - Previous history of progression of the wound greater than three months.

The patients ended up having an age range between 18 and 65 years and a male-female ratio of 1:1.5. Then, these were randomly divided into two groups [11]:

- The control group (n=10) which received the standard treatment consisting of:
    - Measures for reducing pressure on the ulcerated area.
    - Daily wound cleansing.
    - Topical application of a super oxidizing disinfectant solution (Microdacyn™, TeArai BioFarma Auckland, New Zealand) to all the wound area.

- The experimental group (n=15) which received the experimental treatment consisting of:
    - Measures for reducing pressure on the ulcerated area.
    - Daily wound cleansing.

- Topical application of a 5% potassium permanganate solution (Vikut®) to all the wound area.

The mean of the clinical features of the participants is shown in Table **2**:

Table 2. Clinical characteristics of the study subjects.

Clinical Characteristics	Treatment		P-value
	Standard	(n=10)	
Men (%)	50	35.71	0.5
Age (years)	58±4.70	53.50±2.34	0.36
Diabetes duration (years)	12.81±3.78	12.14±3.43	0.9
High blood pressure (%)	50	21.4	0.1
Hyperlipidemia (%)	10	21.4	0.54
Alcoholism (%)	10	21.4	0.54
Smoking (%)	10	7.14	0.75
Fasting glucose (mg/dl)	140.11±19.81	161.50±15.40	0.4
HbA1c (%)	6.65±0.42	7.83±1.35	0.38
Body mass index (kg/m2)	30.61±1.74	28.02±1.09	0.2
Ulcer area (mm2)	5.38±1.24	6.20±1.23	0.65
Days with ulcer	114.00±61.95	169.16±58.39	0.56
Wagner stage I (%)	50	50	0.82
Wagner stage II (%)	50	50	0.82
Local infection (%)	20	64.28	0.03
HbA1c, glycated hemoglobin [as] Of the 15 patients initially included, 1 was withdrawn from the trial due to potassium permanganate intolerance; this patient's clinical data was not included in analysis.			

Once all the measures were obtained, the statistical analysis was done.

Statistical Analysis

Once the normal distribution was confirmed *via* the Shapiro-Wilk test, the groups were compared using a Student's test. Categorical values were compared using Fisher's exact test. The relative risk (RR) was calculated to determine the probability of an ulcer area reduction equal to 50% at day 21 of the experimental group compared to the control group. Besides, the number-needed-to-treat (NNT) was obtained, which is an epidemiological measure expressing the effectiveness of an intervention and is defined as the necessary number of individuals receiving the experimental treatment to increase in one the benefited persons in comparison with the control group [92], being, in this case, the beneficial effect a decrease equal or greater to 50% on ulcer's area on day 21. The confidence interval was calculated for both the RR and the NNT [11].

RESULTS

Regarding the treatment, intolerance to the Vikut® formula was observed in a patient, which was withdrawn from the trial without further complication or follow-up [11].

The experimental group showed superior ulcer reduction compared to the control group in both Percentual Mean Reduction in Ulcer Size (see Fig. **8**) and Population percentage achieving ulcer reduction equal to or greater than 50%. Additionally, the experimental group was the only one to accomplish some complete ulcer closure. The results can be observed in Table **3** [11].

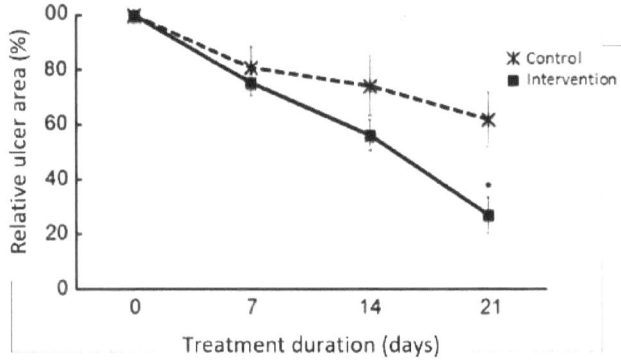

Fig. (8). Ulcer area progression in the control and intervention groups. The mean ulcer area of patients treated with 5% potassium permanganate solution was significantly lower compared with those receiving the standard treatment for 21 days.

Table 3. Comparative Table of Results.

-	Experimental Group n=14	Control Group n=10
Percentual Mean Reduction in Ulcer Size	73%	38%
Population percentage achieving ulcer reduction equal or greater than the 50%	86%	40%
Population percentage achieving complete ulcer closure	29%	0%
Relative Risk	3, CI 95% [1.1-7.6]	
Number-Needed-to-Treat	2.18, CI 95% [1.26-8.25]	

DISCUSSION

This trial results reveal that the Vikut® 5% potassium permanganate-based formula is superior, respecting its capacity for wound closure in diabetic foot ulcers. Previous studies have shown the efficacy of potassium permanganate in a myriad of different wounds, including varicose eczema [93, 94], *Clostridium perfringes*-caused gas gangrene [71], and oncogenic ulcers [95, 97]. Additionally, the potassium permanganate's antiseptic activity remains effective even in mixed infections [71].

The benefits regarding the use of Vikut® 5% potassium permanganate-based formula include the economical. A market study compares the Vikut® with other wound-related products, show that the former is one of the cheaper respecting of cost [13]. It is worth mentioning that other indirect costs, such as healthcare worker time and the facilities' use, were not included, so it is plausible that the Vikut® may save additional costs, resources, and time due to its efficacy.

Another usually unobserved complication regarding chronic wounds is the risk of amputations, which diminish the life quality of those who suffer them [71] in addition to the implicated economic repercussions [96].

The previous data indicate Vikut® formula's effectiveness as a topical antiseptic and antibiotics alternative.

The Use of Vikut® 5% Potassium Permanganate-based Formula in Both Acute and Chronic Wounds: Several Clinical Cases

There have been sundry reported cases where the use of Vikut® 5% potassium permanganate-based formula had been a support in the treatment of wounds of multiple natures, including acute and chronic wounds.

Cases of Acute wounds

Clinical Case 1: Neglected Post- caesarian Wound

The present case is regarding a 24-years old female patient with normal arterial pressure (110/80 mmHg) and without diabetes. She was attended on "Dr. Vikut" Wound Clinic on Morelos (Mexico). The wound inception was caused due to the exert of force (carrying her 5-years old daughter) one month after been subjected to a cesarean, opening the wound.

The wound (see Fig. 9) presented a small area between 0.7 and 1.0 cm^2 in the trunk area. It presents epithelial tissue and light exudated without neither bleeding nor odor.

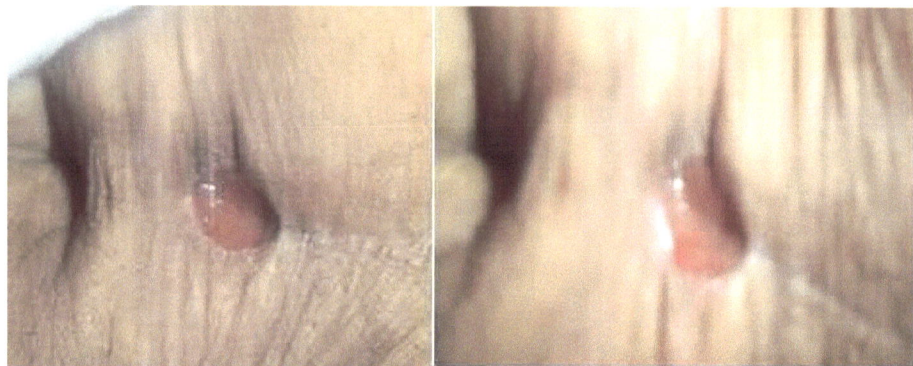

Fig. (9). Clinical case 1, initial time.

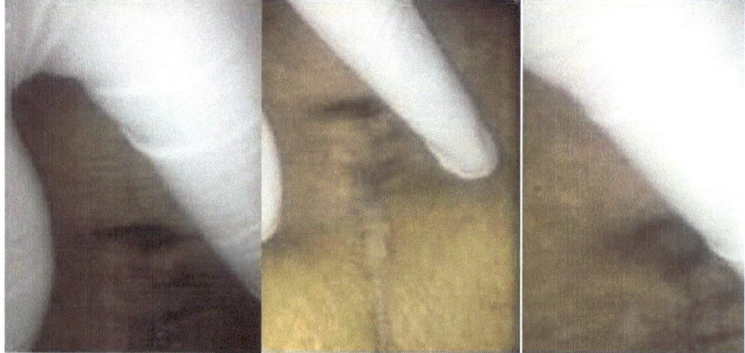

Fig. (10). Clinical case 1, after seven days.

The wound was first cleaned, and then the Vikut® 5% potassium permanganate-based formula was applied.

After seven days and only one application, the wound was completely closed (see Fig. **10**).

Clinical Case 2: Post-surgical Wound

In this case, a 48-years old male patient without any subjacent affliction such as diabetes or hypertension. He was subjected to a hernia surgery in the ISSSTE hospital in Colima (Mexico). At the end of it, Vikut® formula after cleaning the tissue and notify his doctor. After five days, during which the formula had been applied three times a day, the scar formation appears to have been accelerated (see Fig. **11**).

Fig. (11). Clinic case 2, initial time (left), and after five days.

Cases of Chronic Wounds

Clinical Case 3: Diabetic Foot Ulcer on the Big Toe

This case is regarding a 64-years old male patient, with normal arterial pressure but with diabetes (post-prandial blood sugar of 176 $^{mg}/_{mL}$). He was attended in High Specialty Hospital "Centenario de la Revolución Mexicana ISSSTE" in Mexico City. The Wound inception causes are unknown.

The wound (see Fig. **12**), after multiple infructuous attempts, the injury had an area between 3.1 and 4.0 cm^2. There was the presence of necrotic tissue at the edges of the wound and light exudated. There was a deep wound on the big toe and another more superficial wound between the toes. The tissue was classified as Wagner stage 2.

The wound was first cleaned, and then the Vikut® formula was applied.

After the seventh weeks, the wound appeared to have diminished to between 1.5 and 2.0 cm^2, new epithelial tissue had appeared, and the necrotic tissue had diminished. However, both the exudated and the Wagner classification remains (see Fig. **13**).

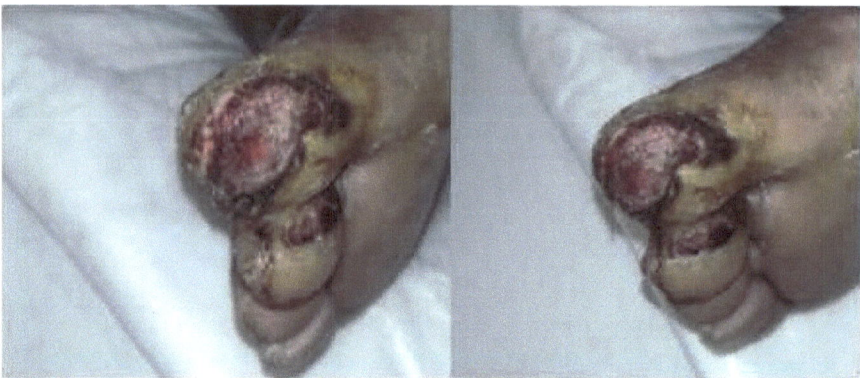

Fig. (12). Clinic case 3, initial time.

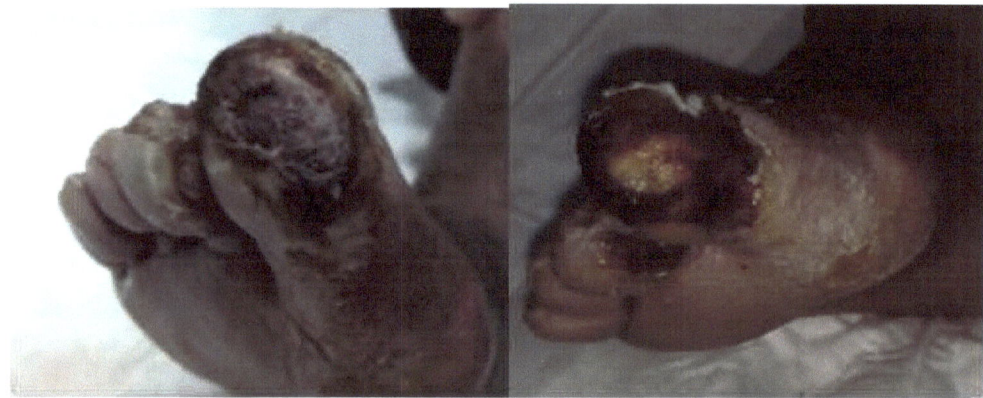

Fig. (13). Clinic case 3, after seven weeks.

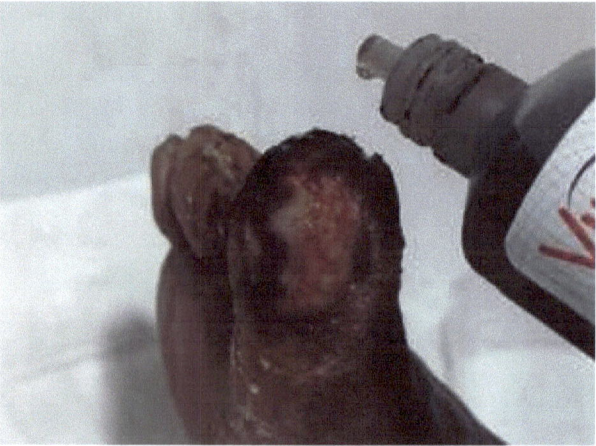

Fig. (14). Clinic case 3, after nine weeks.

After the ninth week, the affected area remains within an extension between 1.5 and 2.0 cm², a light exudate, and its classification as Wagner stage 2. However. The necrotic tissue appears to have diminished even more (see Fig. **14**).

Clinical Case 4: Diabetic Ulcer in the Leg

This case describes a 64-years old male patient with normal arterial pressure (110/80 mmHg) but with diabetes (pre-prandial blood sugar of 136 $^{mg}/_{mL}$). He was attended in High Specialty Hospital "Centenario de la Revolución Mexicana ISSSTE" in Mexico City. The Wound inception causes are unknown.

The wound (see Fig. **15**), after various infructuous attempts, the injury had an area between 8.1 and 12.0 cm². There was a slough tissue presence, moderate exudated, and hyperproliferation sign on the edges of the wound.

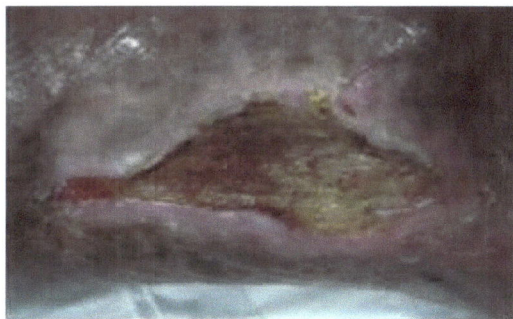 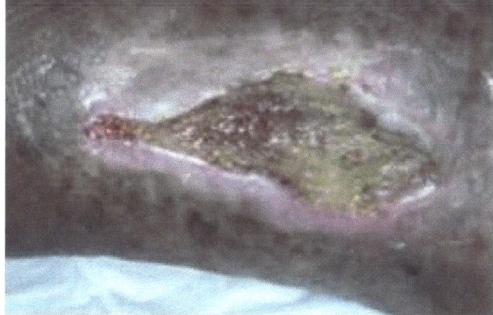

Fig. (15). Clinic case 4, initial time.

The wound was first cleaned, and then the Vikut® formula was applied, which continued to be applied daily for 49 days.

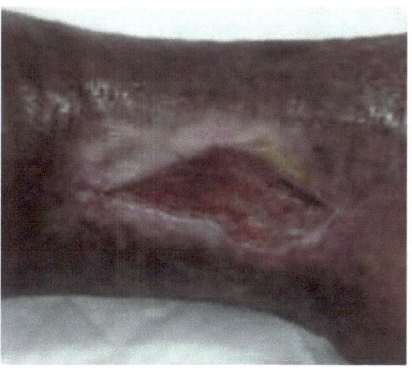 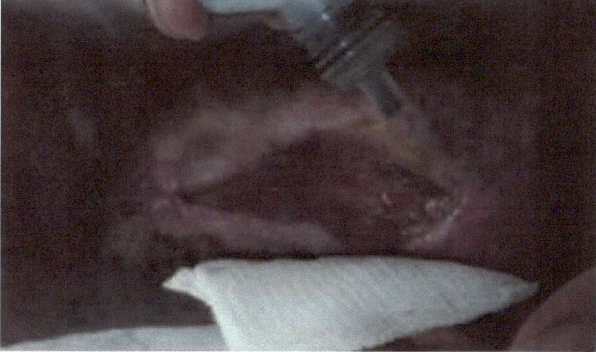

Fig. (16). Clinic case 4 after three weeks.

After the third week, the ulcer area remained between 8.1 and 12.0 cm and with moderated exudates. However, there was new epithelial tissue while the slough had diminished (see Fig. **16**).

After the seventh week, the ulcers had diminished to a range between 1.1 and 2.0 cm and with light exudates. Also, the tissue had become both epithelial and superficial (see Fig. **17**).

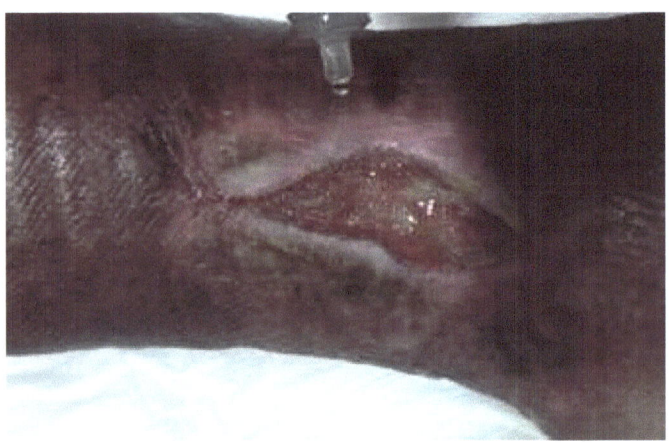

Fig. (17). Clinic case 4, after seven weeks.

Clinical Case 5: Osteomyelitis-caused Injury

This case describes a 64-years old female patient with normal arterial pressure (120/80 mmHg) but with diabetes (post-prandial blood sugar of 176 $^{mg}/_{mL}$). She was attended in High Specialty Hospital "Centenario de la Revolución Mexicana ISSSTE" in Mexico City. The Wound inception causes are unknown.

After several unsuccessful treatment attempts, there was an osteomyelitis-caused wound between 3.1 and 4.0 cm^2 but deep, slough, and moderate exudation (see Fig. **18**).

The wound was first cleaned, and then the Vikut® formula was applied, which continued to be applied daily for 63 days.

After the third week, the ulcer area remained between 3.1 and 4.0 cm and moderated exudates. However, there was new epithelial tissue while the slough had diminished (see Fig. **19**).

After the ninth week, the ulcer area keeps its same range but now presents light exudates. Besides, the epithelial tissue has increased (see Fig. **20**).

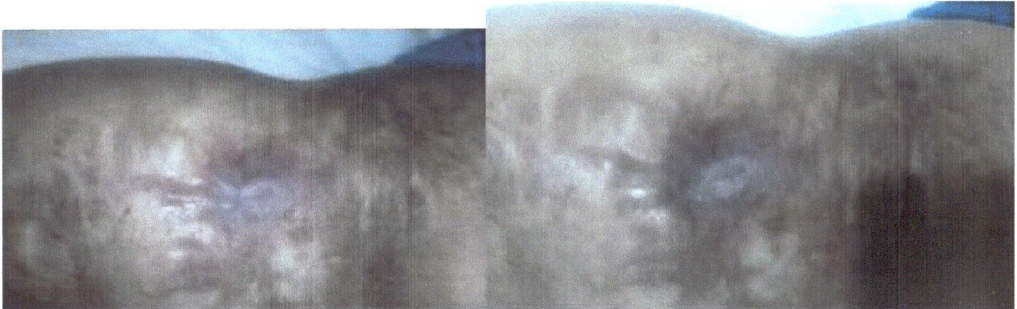

Fig. (18). Clinic case 5, initial time.

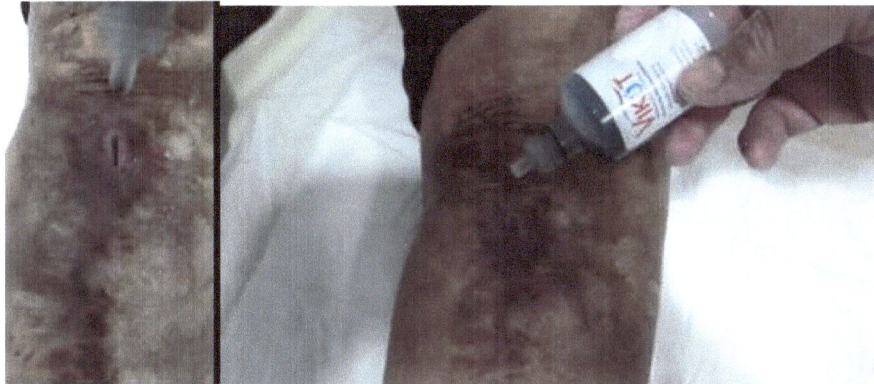

Fig. (19). Clinic case 5, after three weeks.

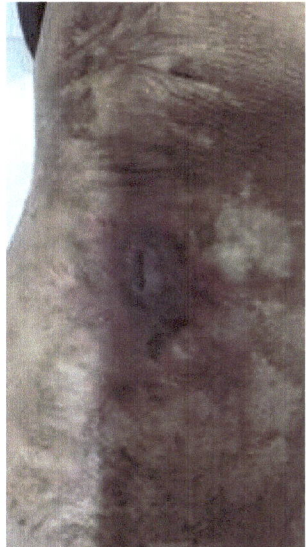

Fig. (20). Clinic case 5, after nine weeks.

CONCLUSION: GATHERING THE INFORMATION

There are several proofs regarding the Vikut® 5% potassium permanganate-based formula's effectiveness in acute and chronic wounds. However, there is still crucial information, such as the molecular mechanism underlying the product's composition, which is unknown. Obtaining that knowledge is pivotal for improving the formulation of wound-related products such as Vikut® and for the development of therapeutic substances and strategies that help us overcome problems such as bacterial resistance or the chronicity of wounds in general.

The use of topical antiseptics such as Vikut® 5% potassium permanganate-based formula could be a tipping point respecting the treatment of wounds. Every day, new NAAAs such as antimicrobial peptides are discovered and tested, while other substances, ancient and previously forgotten, are now being reassessed, such as the honey or the potassium permanganate.

The health situation respecting microorganism management has become complicated. The problem is often like fighting like a hydra with many heads that every time one of them is cut, two more emerge. The use of tools such as the clinic trials help us unravel this situation, letting us understand how a wound interacts with certain substances or specific environments and giving us one of the more valuable resources of this era, which is knowledge.

ECONOMIC AND FUNCTIONAL COMPARATIVE ANALYSIS BETWEEN THE FORMULA BASED ON POTASSIUM PERMANGANATE AND OTHER TOPICAL TREATMENTS

An assessment study was done by Grupo Salipro de México S.A de C.V. regarding the cost-benefit of using Vikut® 5% potassium permanganate-based formula. For this, a cost comparison was performed between five wound-related solutions, including Vikut®. The names, characteristics, and prices would be exposed in Table **4** [13]:

Table 4. Price comparison between wound-related products.

Product's Name	Presentation	Unit Cost Without IVA (MXN)	Unit Cost Including IVA (MXN)
14 pH Antiseptic/Astringent Solution (Vikut®)	40 mL	$450.00	$522.00
Broad-spectrum Antiseptic Solution, electrolyzed with neutral pH superoxydant (BSAS)	250 mL	$50.68	$58.79

Product's Name	Presentation	Unit Cost Without IVA (MXN)	Unit Cost Including IVA (MXN)
Wound Treatment in Aerosol (WTA)	20 mL aluminum flask	$339,928.00	$394,316.48
Tixothrophic Solution (TS)	30 g containing flask	$885.00	$1,026.68
Hydrocolloid Apposite (HA)	Piece	$ 35.29	$40.94

Which is the goal?

The study's main objective was to prove that the use of the Vikut® formula was advantageous both clinically due to the product's capacity to treat wounds more effectively than its comparable, and economically so it could become attractive to be acquired for the public sector.

Vikut® formula offers two main advantages in contrast with the other wound-related products [13]:

- Efficacy, since the study shows a better ratio of wound healing and wound closure than the other products.
- Use for multiple purposes, since its intrinsic characteristics, Vikut® acts as both antiseptic and healing promotor compared to other products that only do one of those. Such is the case of hemoglobin-containing solutions such as the WTA, promoting wound healing but are useless respecting bacterial infection.

One of the Vikut® formula's key features is shortening healthcare facilities' use due to reduced actions. Although Vikut® is more expensive than the broad-spectrum antiseptic solution, its effectiveness leads to a shorter period of staying in hospitals, which could either reduce indirect costs or decrease resource consumption use regarding the hours used by the healthcare workers and the availability of hospital rooms.

RESULTS OBTAINED REGARDING VIKUT®

The analysis concludes that there are potential benefits both pharmaceutical and economical regarding the use of Vikut® 5% potassium permanganate-based formula as an alternative for patients with chronic diabetic foot ulcers under the perspective of several Mexican healthcare institutions such as the IMSS, the ISSTE, the SSA, PEMEZ, SEDENA, and SEMAR [13].

The complete economic assessment presented in the study, including cost-effectivity analysis, was considered valid, respecting its demographic features.

Those correspond to a data-constructed hypothetical patient cohort. Both effectiveness rates and resource consumption were attributed through literature review from the topic and applying healthcare costs for patients of the Mexican healthcare institutions previously mentioned [13].

It is emphasized that the results presented in the different tables and figures meet the study's objectives since the results respecting the effectiveness of the model were obtained and the average cost estimates. Similarly, the ICERs of the issue management alternatives were estimated from the target population of a particular condition and within the Mexican Public Health Sector (IMSS, ISSTE, SSA, PEMEX, SEDENA, and SEMAR) [13].

The estimates' results are robust, according to the deterministic and univariate sensitivity analysis developed for the most relevant ICERs. The ICER estimated in the study corresponds to clinical parameters percentage reduction of ulcers' size). The analysis context found that Vikut® is a cost-effective and dominant strategy respecting its comparators, mainly because it can significantly reduce the ulcer size, issue particularly relevant due to this type of patient's propensity to worsen its complications. The results of this economic evaluation indicate that a cost of MXN$ 522.00 for the 40 ml presentation of Vikut® incurs the following ICER [13]:

Likewise, it can be observed that patients treated with Vikut® incur higher costs, only respecting the BSAS due to its acquisition cost, which is repeated with neither the WTA nor the TS (see Table **5**). Furthermore, Vikut® showed a better rate of wound size reduction compared to its comparators. Finally, in the results of the budget impact, it was observed that the greater the market share of the Vikut®, there will be more significant reduction in both the health budget and the percentage of current health spending. The different market penetration scenarios show that the factor that significantly impacts budgets is the percentual share of the Vikut®. This model used specific epidemiological data, such as the prevalence of PD ulcers, obtained from national sources. To predict the market share of the different alternatives in comparison, the model used various scenarios. This model was built using the best assumptions, data, and hypotheses available [13].

Table 5. ICER in the relationship of both the alternative product and the institution.

Alternative	ICER					
Vikut®	**IMSS**	**ISSSTE**	**SSA**	**PEMEX**	**SEDENA**	**SEMAR**
BSAS	$764.05	$767.50	$759.74	$755.41	$757.00	$756.51
HA	-$1,703.48	-$1,703.12	-$1,705.97	-$1,685.13	-$1,706.49	-$1,704.75
TS	-$868.72	-$866.02	-$867.77	-$868.51	-$871.33	-$872.51

CONCLUSION: LOOKING AT THE FOREST

The Vikut® 5% potassium permanganate-based formula seems cost-effective but not the cheapest topical antiseptic. Regardless of this, it is crucial to look beyond the mere price and look at its wound closing ability, which avoids the need for a prolonged stay and even more drastic solutions, such as amputation.

Treating chronic wounds is a challenge, and it will become both a more severe and more common threat. Complications associated with chronic wounds are rather unpleasant for patients and their relatives. It is exhausting for the companies with workers suffering chronic injuries, and for both public and private health, institutions are costly [97].

That is why when approaching an issue, sometimes the one which does not seem to be the best is the long-term optimal, and vice versa.

CONSENT FOR PUBLICATION

Not applicable.

CONFLICT OF INTEREST

These researchers are partially sponsored by "Grupo Salipro de México S.A de C.V." and may lead to the development of products that may be licensed to the company mentioned earlier, in which the participants of the present document have a business and financial interest.

ACKNOWLEDGEMENTS

Declared none.

REFERENCES

[1] Le Fanu J. The Rise and Fall of Modern Medicine. 1st ed., London: Little, Brown & Co 1999.
[http://dx.doi.org/10.1016/S0140-6736(05)75559-8]

[2] Borghi L. Breve historia de la medicina. Madrid: EDICIONES RIALP 2018.

[3] Ventola CL. The antibiotic resistance crisis: part 1: causes and threats. P&T 2015; 40(4): 277-83.
[PMID: 25859123]

[4] Ventola CL. The antibiotic resistance crisis: part 2: management strategies and new agents. P&T 2015; 40(5): 344-52.
[PMID: 25987823]

[5] Frykberg RG, Banks J. Challenges in the Treatment of Chronic Wounds. Adv Wound Care (New Rochelle) 2015; 4(9): 560-82.
[http://dx.doi.org/10.1089/wound.2015.0635] [PMID: 26339534]

[6] Martin P, Nunan R. Cellular and molecular mechanisms of repair in acute and chronic wound healing. Br J Dermatol 2015; 173(2): 370-8.

[http://dx.doi.org/10.1111/bjd.13954] [PMID: 26175283]

[7]   Enoch S, Price P. Cellular, molecular and biochemical differences in the pathophysiology of healing between acute wounds, chronic wounds and wounds in the aged. World Wide Wounds 2004; 13: 1-17.

[8]   Apelqvist J, Bakker K, van Houtum WH, Nabuurs-Franssen MH, Schaper NC. International Working Group on the Diabetic Foot. International consensus and practical guidelines on the management and the prevention of the diabetic foot. Diabetes Metab Res Rev 2000; 16 (Suppl. 1): S84-92.
[http://dx.doi.org/10.1002/1520-7560(200009/10)16:1+<::AID-DMRR113>3.0.CO;2-S] [PMID: 11054895]

[9]   O'Meara S, Cullum N, Majid M, Sheldon T. Systematic reviews of wound care management: (3) antimicrobial agents for chronic wounds; (4) diabetic foot ulceration. Health Technol Assess 2000; 4(21): 1-237.
[PMID: 11074391]

[10]   Lara Basulto AD, Delgado González M, Delgado Enciso I, Sánchez González JM, Lara Esqueda A. Wound closure in inferior extremities, using topical 5% potassium permanganate solution, about two cases. Diabetes Hoy 2018; 67: 22-7.

[11]   Delgado-Enciso I, Madrigal-Perez VM, Lara-Esqueda A, *et al.* Topical 5% potassium permanganate solution accelerates the healing process in chronic diabetic foot ulcers. Biomed Rep 2018; 8(2): 156-9.
[http://dx.doi.org/10.3892/br.2018.1038] [PMID: 29435274]

[12]   Lara-Basulto AD, Delgado-Enciso I, Lara-Esqueda A, Inzunza-Barragán P, Fregoso-Sotres OM. Closing of complicated postoperative wound by negligence, by means of the topical use of solution of 5% Potassium Permanganate; presentation of a case. Diabetes Hoy 2019; 20(1): 18-21.

[13]   Navarro-Rodriguez R, Luna-Casas G. Estudio de evaluación del uso de la solución antiséptica y astringente con ph 14 (vikut®) como auxiliar en el tratamiento de pacientes con úlceras crónicas de pie diabético bajo la perspectiva del sistema de salud público mexicano. (IMSS, ISSSTE, SSA, PEMEX, SEDENA y SEMAR). Grupo Salypro de México, S.A de C.V. 2017. 71 Report No. 1.

[14]   Etebu E, Ibemologi A. Antibiotics: Classification and mechanisms of action with emphasis on molecular perspectives. Int J Appl Microbiol Biotechnol 2016; 2016(20): 90-101.

[15]   Denyer SP, Hodges NA, German SP. Introduction to pharmaceutical microbiology.Hugo and Russell "s Pharmaceutical Microbiology. 7th ed. UK: Blackwell Science 2004; pp. 3-8.
[http://dx.doi.org/10.1002/9780470988329.ch1]

[16]   Velkov T, Roberts KD, Nation RL, Thompson PE, Li J. Pharmacology of polymyxins: new insights into an 'old' class of antibiotics. Future Microbiol 2013; 8(6): 711-24.
[http://dx.doi.org/10.2217/fmb.13.39] [PMID: 23701329]

[17]   Vattimo MdeF, Watanabe M, da Fonseca CD, Neiva LB, Pessoa EA, Borges FT. Polymyxin B nephrotoxicity: from organ to cell damage. PLoS One 2016; 11(8): e0161057.
[http://dx.doi.org/10.1371/journal.pone.0161057] [PMID: 27532263]

[18]   Blair JM, Webber MA, Baylay AJ, Ogbolu DO, Piddock LJ. Molecular mechanisms of antibiotic resistance. Nat Rev Microbiol 2015; 13(1): 42-51.
[http://dx.doi.org/10.1038/nrmicro3380] [PMID: 25435309]

[19]   de Sousa Oliveira K, de Lima LA, Cobacho NB, Dias SC, Franco OL. Antibiotic Resistance: Mechanisms and New Antimicrobial Approaches. 1st ed. London: Elsevier 2016; pp. 19-35.
[http://dx.doi.org/10.1016/B978-0-12-803642-6.00002-2]

[20]   Ray MD, Boundy S, Archer GL. Transfer of the methicillin resistance genomic island among staphylococci by conjugation. Mol Microbiol 2016; 100(4): 675-85.
[http://dx.doi.org/10.1111/mmi.13340] [PMID: 26822382]

[21]   Zhang WJ, Xu XR, Schwarz S, *et al.* Characterization of the IncA/C plasmid pSCEC2 from Escherichia coli of swine origin that harbours the multiresistance gene *cfr*. J Antimicrob Chemother 2014; 69(2): 385-9.

[http://dx.doi.org/10.1093/jac/dkt355] [PMID: 24013193]

[22] Leclercq R. Mechanisms of resistance to macrolides and lincosamides: nature of the resistance elements and their clinical implications. Clin Infect Dis 2002; 34(4): 482-92.
[http://dx.doi.org/10.1086/324626] [PMID: 11797175]

[23] Davies J, Davies D. Origins and evolution of antibiotic resistance. Microbiol Mol Biol Rev 2010; 74(3): 417-33.
[http://dx.doi.org/10.1128/MMBR.00016-10] [PMID: 20805405]

[24] Luyt CE, Bréchot N, Trouillet JL, Chastre J. Antibiotic stewardship in the intensive care unit. Crit Care 2014; 18(5): 480.
[http://dx.doi.org/10.1186/s13054-014-0480-6] [PMID: 25405992]

[25] Viswanathan VK. Off-label abuse of antibiotics by bacteria. Gut Microbes 2014; 5(1): 3-4.
[http://dx.doi.org/10.4161/gmic.28027] [PMID: 24637595]

[26] Gaskins HR, Collier CT, Anderson DB. Antibiotics as growth promotants: mode of action. Anim Biotechnol 2002; 13(1): 29-42.
[http://dx.doi.org/10.1081/ABIO-120005768] [PMID: 12212942]

[27] Zhao F, Yang L. Bioaccumulation of antibiotics in crops under long-term manure application: Occurrence, biomass response and human exposure. Chemosphere 2019; 219: 882-95.

[28] Jacobs A. Crisis looms in antibiotics as drug makers go bankrupt. The New York Times 2019 Dec; Sect. A: 1 (col 1).

[29] Lushniak BD. Antibiotic resistance: a public health crisis. Public Health Rep 2014; 129(4): 314-6.
[http://dx.doi.org/10.1177/003335491412900402] [PMID: 24982528]

[30] Hsieh L, Amin A. Antimicrobial Stewardship: Hospital Strategies to Curb Antibiotic Resistance.Antibiotic Resistance: Mechanisms and New Antimicrobial Approaches. 1st ed. London: Elsevier 2016; pp. 1-18.
[http://dx.doi.org/10.1016/B978-0-12-803642-6.00001-0]

[31] Okeke IN, Peeling RW, Goossens H, *et al.* Diagnostics as essential tools for containing antibacterial resistance. Drug Resist Updat 2011; 14(2): 95-106.
[http://dx.doi.org/10.1016/j.drup.2011.02.002] [PMID: 21398170]

[32] McAdams D, Wollein Waldetoft K, Tedijanto C, Lipsitch M, Brown SP. Resistance diagnostics as a public health tool to combat antibiotic resistance: A model-based evaluation. PLoS Biol 2019; 17(5): e3000250.
[http://dx.doi.org/10.1371/journal.pbio.3000250] [PMID: 31095567]

[33] Rai M, Kon K, Gade A, *et al.* Antimicrobial Resistance: Can nanoparticles tackle the problem?Antibiotic Resistance: Mechanisms and New Antimicrobial Approaches. 1st ed. London: Elsevier 2016; pp. 121-35.
[http://dx.doi.org/10.1016/B978-0-12-803642-6.00006-X]

[34] Bragg RR, Boucher CE, van der Wasthuizen WA, *et al.* The Potential Use of Bacteriophage Therapy as a Treatment Option in a Post-Antibiotic Era.Antibiotic Resistance: Mechanisms and New Antimicrobial Approaches. 1st ed. London: Elsevier 2016; pp. 309-135.
[http://dx.doi.org/10.1016/B978-0-12-803642-6.00015-0]

[35] Chávez-González ML, Rodríguez-Herrera R, Aguilar CN. Essential Oils: A natural alternative to combat antibiotics resistance.Antibiotic Resistance: Mechanisms and New Antimicrobial Approaches. 1st ed. London: Elsevier 2016; pp. 227-37.
[http://dx.doi.org/10.1016/B978-0-12-803642-6.00011-3]

[36] Horvath G, Bencsik T, Acs K, Kocsis B. Sensitivity of ESBL-producing Gram-negative bacteria to essential oils, plant extracts, and their isolated compounds.Antibiotic Resistance: Mechanisms and New Antimicrobial Approaches. 1st ed. London: Elsevier 2016; pp. 239-69.
[http://dx.doi.org/10.1016/B978-0-12-803642-6.00012-5]

[37] Kon K, Rai M. Antibiotic Resistance: Mechanisms and New Antimicrobial Approaches. 1st ed. London: Elsevier 2016; pp. 271-89.

[38] Beoletto VG, de las Mercedes-Oliva M, Marioli JM, Carezzano ME, Demo MS. Antimicrobial Natural Products against Bacterial Biofilms.Antibiotic Resistance: Mechanisms and New Antimicrobial Approaches. 1st ed. London: Elsevier 2016; pp. 291-307.
[http://dx.doi.org/10.1016/B978-0-12-803642-6.00014-9]

[39] Roberts CD, Leaper DJ, Assadian O. The Role of Topical Antiseptic Agents Within Antimicrobial Stewardship Strategies for Prevention and Treatment of Surgical Site and Chronic Open Wound Infection. Adv Wound Care (New Rochelle) 2017; 6(2): 63-71.
[http://dx.doi.org/10.1089/wound.2016.0701] [PMID: 28224049]

[40] The Editors of Encyclopaedia Britannica. Wounds: Encyclopædia Britannica. [cited: 20th September 2020] Available from. https://www.britannica.com/science/wound

[41] Enoch S. Price Cellular, molecular and biochemical differences in the pathophysiology of healing between acute wounds, chronic wounds and wounds in the aged. World Wide Wounds 2014; 13: 1-17.

[42] Guo S, Dipietro LA. Factors affecting wound healing. J Dent Res 2010; 89(3): 219-29.
[http://dx.doi.org/10.1177/0022034509359125] [PMID: 20139336]

[43] Zhao R, Liang H, Clarke E, Jackson C, Xue M. Inflammation in Chronic Wounds. Int J Mol Sci 2016; 17(12): 1-14.
[http://dx.doi.org/10.3390/ijms17122085] [PMID: 27973441]

[44] Demidova-Rice TN, Hamblin MR, Herman IM. Acute and impaired wound healing: pathophysiology and current methods for drug delivery, part 1: normal and chronic wounds: biology, causes, and approaches to care. Adv Skin Wound Care 2012; 25(7): 304-14.
[http://dx.doi.org/10.1097/01.ASW.0000416006.55218.d0] [PMID: 22713781]

[45] Kuki S, Imanishi T, Kobayashi K, Matsuo Y, Obana M, Akasaka T. Hyperglycemia accelerated endothelial progenitor cell senescence *via* the activation of p38 mitogen-activated protein kinase. Circ J 2006; 70(8): 1076-81.
[http://dx.doi.org/10.1253/circj.70.1076] [PMID: 16864945]

[46] Loomans CJM, van Haperen R, Duijs JM, *et al.* Differentiation of bone marrow-derived endothelial progenitor cells is shifted into a proinflammatory phenotype by hyperglycemia. Mol Med 2009; 15(5-6): 152-9.
[http://dx.doi.org/10.2119/molmed.2009.00032] [PMID: 19295918]

[47] Wlaschek M, Scharffetter-Kochanek K. Oxidative stress in chronic venous leg ulcers. Wound Repair Regen 2005; 13(5): 452-61.
[http://dx.doi.org/10.1111/j.1067-1927.2005.00065.x] [PMID: 16176453]

[48] Omar A, Wright JB, Schultz G, Burrell R, Nadworny P. Microbial biofilms and chronic wounds. Microorganisms 2017; 5(1): 1-15.
[http://dx.doi.org/10.3390/microorganisms5010009] [PMID: 28272369]

[49] Wolcott RD, Rhoads DD, Dowd SE. Biofilms and chronic wound inflammation. J Wound Care 2008; 17(8): 333-41.
[http://dx.doi.org/10.12968/jowc.2008.17.8.30796] [PMID: 18754194]

[50] Clinton A, Carter T. Chronic wound biofilms: pathogenesis and potential therapies. Lab Med 2015; 46(4): 277-84.
[http://dx.doi.org/10.1309/LMBNSWKUI4JPN7SO] [PMID: 26489671]

[51] Kalan L, Zhou M, Labbie M, Willing B. Measuring the microbiome of chronic wounds with use of a topical antimicrobial dressing - A feasibility study. PLoS One 2017; 12(11): e0187728.
[http://dx.doi.org/10.1371/journal.pone.0187728] [PMID: 29155834]

[52] Leake JL, Dowd SE, Wolcott RD, Zischkau AM, Sun Y. Identification of yeast in chronic wounds

using new pathogen-detection technologies. J Wound Care 2009; 18(3): 103-104, 106, 108.
[http://dx.doi.org/10.12968/jowc.2009.18.3.39810] [PMID: 19247230]

[53] Kirketerp-Møller K, Jensen PØ, Fazli M, *et al.* Distribution, organization, and ecology of bacteria in chronic wounds. J Clin Microbiol 2008; 46(8): 2717-22.
[http://dx.doi.org/10.1128/JCM.00501-08] [PMID: 18508940]

[54] Stoodley P, Sauer K, Davies DG, Costerton JW. Biofilms as complex differentiated communities. Annu Rev Microbiol 2002; 56(1): 187-209.
[http://dx.doi.org/10.1146/annurev.micro.56.012302.160705] [PMID: 12142477]

[55] Cooper R. Honey as an effective antimicrobial treatment for chronic wounds: is there a place for it in modern medicine? Chronic Wound Care Management and Research 2014; 1: 15-22.
[http://dx.doi.org/10.2147/CWCMR.S46520]

[56] Mandal MD, Mandal S. Honey: its medicinal property and antibacterial activity. Asian Pac J Trop Biomed 2011; 1(2): 154-60.
[http://dx.doi.org/10.1016/S2221-1691(11)60016-6] [PMID: 23569748]

[57] Shenoy VP, Ballal M, Shivananda P, Bairy I. Honey as an antimicrobial agent against pseudomonas aeruginosa isolated from infected wounds. J Glob Infect Dis 2012; 4(2): 102-5.
[http://dx.doi.org/10.4103/0974-777X.96770] [PMID: 22754244]

[58] Al-Maaini RAS. Honey as an antimicrobial agent against multi-drug resistant Gram negative bacterial rods. PhD. Dissertation. University of Wales 2012.

[59] Piaggesi A, Goretti C, Mazzurco S, *et al.* A randomized controlled trial to examine the efficacy and safety of a new super-oxidized solution for the management of wide postsurgical lesions of the diabetic foot. Int J Low Extrem Wounds 2010; 9(1): 10-5.
[http://dx.doi.org/10.1177/1534734610361945] [PMID: 20207618]

[60] Cao Y, Naseri M, He Y, Xu C, Walsh LJ, Ziora ZM. Non-antibiotic antimicrobial agents to combat biofilm-forming bacteria. J Glob Antimicrob Resist 2020; 21(1): 445-51.
[http://dx.doi.org/10.1016/j.jgar.2019.11.012] [PMID: 31830536]

[61] Atiyeh BS, Dibo SA, Hayek SN. Wound cleansing, topical antiseptics and wound healing. Int Wound J 2009; 6(6): 420-30.
[http://dx.doi.org/10.1111/j.1742-481X.2009.00639.x] [PMID: 20051094]

[62] Cambiaso-Daniel J, Boukovalas S, Bitz GH, Branski LK, Herndon DN, Culnan DM. Topical Antimicrobials in Burn Care: Part 1-Topical Antiseptics. Ann Plast Surg 2018; 10: 1-26.
[http://dx.doi.org/10.1097/SAP.0000000000001297] [PMID: 29319571]

[63] Sagar RS, Maruthi ST, Prasad CK, Chethan GN, Belakeri P. Surgical Management of Interdigital Hyperplasia-A Report of Four Dairy cows. Intas Polivet 2017; 18(2): 465-7.

[64] Kubiak M. Handbook of Exotic Pet Medicine. 1st ed. New Jersey: Wiley, 146.
[http://dx.doi.org/10.1002/9781119389934]

[65] Duemling WW, Elston RW. Postoperative Gangrenous Ulcer of the Abdominal Wall: Report of a Case with Special Notes on Treatment. Arch Derm Syphilol 1933; 27(4): 624-30.
[http://dx.doi.org/10.1001/archderm.1933.01450040631007]

[66] Anderson I. Should potassium permanganate be used in wound care? Nurs Times 2003; 99(31): 61.
[PMID: 13677127]

[67] Sánchez-Saldaña L, Sáenz-Anduaga E. Antisépticos y desinfectantes. Dermatol Peru 2015; 2005(15): 82-103.

[68] Erdogan FG. A simple, pain-free treatment for ingrown toenails complicated with granulation tissue. Dermatol Surg 2006; 32(11): 1388-90.
[PMID: 17083593]

[69] Stuart. MC, Kouimtzi M, Hill SR. WHO model formulary 2008. WHO. 2019. 2019.

[70] Kujath P, Michelsen A. Wounds - from physiology to wound dressing. Dtsch Arztebl Int 2008; 105(13): 239-48.
[PMID: 19629204]

[71] Hu N, Wu XH, Liu R, *et al.* Novel application of vacuum sealing drainage with continuous irrigation of potassium permanganate for managing infective wounds of gas gangrene. J Huazhong Univ Sci Technolog Med Sci 2015; 35(4): 563-8.
[http://dx.doi.org/10.1007/s11596-015-1471-9] [PMID: 26223928]

[72] Howell-Jones RS, Wilson MJ, Hill KE, Howard AJ, Price PE, Thomas DW. A review of the microbiology, antibiotic usage and resistance in chronic skin wounds. J Antimicrob Chemother 2005; 55(2): 143-9.
[http://dx.doi.org/10.1093/jac/dkh513] [PMID: 15649989]

[73] Wright JB, Lam K, Burrell RE. Wound management in an era of increasing bacterial antibiotic resistance: a role for topical silver treatment. Am J Infect Control 1998; 26(6): 572-7.
[http://dx.doi.org/10.1053/ic.1998.v26.a93527] [PMID: 9836841]

[74] National Center for Biotechnology Information. PubChem Compound Summary for CID 702, Ethanol. PubChem; [cited: 27 September, 2020]. Available from. https://pubchem.ncbi.nlm.nih.gov/compound/Ethanol

[75] Itami T, Kanoh S. [Mechanism of the antipyretic effect of acetylsalicylic acid and salicylic acid in rabbits (author's transl)]. Nippon Yakurigaku Zasshi 1977; 73(6): 683-90.
[http://dx.doi.org/10.1254/fpj.73.683] [PMID: 303603]

[76] Higuchi S, Osada Y, Shioiri Y, Tanaka N, Otomo S, Aihara H. [The modes of anti-inflammatory and analgesic actions of aspirin and salicylic acid]. Nippon Yakurigaku Zasshi 1985; 85(1): 49-57.
[http://dx.doi.org/10.1254/fpj.85.49] [PMID: 3921440]

[77] Arif T. Salicylic acid as a peeling agent: a comprehensive review. Clin Cosmet Investig Dermatol 2015; 8: 455-61.
[http://dx.doi.org/10.2147/CCID.S84765] [PMID: 26347269]

[78] Bosund I. The bacteriostatic action of benzoic and salicylic acids. Acta Chem Scand 1959; 13(0): 803-13.
[http://dx.doi.org/10.3891/acta.chem.scand.13-0803]

[79] Cattò C, Grazioso G, Dell'Orto S, *et al.* The response of Escherichia coli biofilm to salicylic acid. Biofouling 2017; 33(3): 235-51.
[http://dx.doi.org/10.1080/08927014.2017.1286649] [PMID: 28270055]

[80] Stepanović S, Vuković D, Jesić M, Ranin L. Influence of acetylsalicylic acid (aspirin) on biofilm production by Candida species. J Chemother 2004; 16(2): 134-8.
[http://dx.doi.org/10.1179/joc.2004.16.2.134] [PMID: 15216946]

[81] Stathopoulou MK, Banti CN, Kourkoumelis N, Hatzidimitriou AG, Kalampounias AG, Hadjikakou SK. Silver complex of salicylic acid and its hydrogel-cream in wound healing chemotherapy. J Inorg Biochem 2018; 181: 41-55.
[http://dx.doi.org/10.1016/j.jinorgbio.2018.01.004] [PMID: 29407907]

[82] Park WB, Kim SH, Cho JH, *et al.* Effect of salicylic acid on invasion of human vascular endothelial cells by Staphylococcus aureus. FEMS Immunol Med Microbiol 2007; 49(1): 56-61.
[http://dx.doi.org/10.1111/j.1574-695X.2006.00170.x] [PMID: 17094786]

[83] Dotto C, Lombarte Serrat A, Cattelan N, *et al.* The Active Component of Aspirin, Salicylic Acid, Promotes *Staphylococcus aureus* Biofilm Formation in a PIA-dependent Manner. Front Microbiol 2017; 8(4): 4.
[http://dx.doi.org/10.3389/fmicb.2017.00004] [PMID: 28167931]

[84] Goshorn RH, Degering F, Tetrault PA. Antiseptic and Bactericidal Action of Benzoic Acid and Inorganic Salts Effect of PH. Ind Eng Chem 1938; 30(6): 646-8.

[http://dx.doi.org/10.1021/ie50342a009]

[85] O'Brien M. O'Brien M. (2002). Exploring methods of wound debridement. Br J Community Nurs. 2002; 7(Sup3), 10-18.
[http://dx.doi.org/10.12968/bjcn.2002.7.Sup3.10906]

[86] Shai A, Maibach HI. Shai A, Maibach HI. Debridement. Wound Healing and Ulcers of the Skin: Diagnosis and Therapy—The Practical Approach, 119-134.

[87] Roberts JD, Caserio MC. Alcohol, and ethers.Basic principles of organic chemistry WA Benjamin, Inc. 2nd ed. California: W.A. Benjamin, Inc 1977; pp. 599-670.

[88] Broughton DB, Wentworth RL, Laing ME. Mechanism of decomposition of hydrogen peroxide solutions with manganese dioxide. J Am Chem Soc 1947; 69(4): 744-7.
[http://dx.doi.org/10.1021/ja01196a004] [PMID: 20292459]

[89] Kanta J. The role of hydrogen peroxide and other reactive oxygen species in wound healing. Acta Med (Hradec Kralove) 2011; 54(3): 97-101.
[http://dx.doi.org/10.14712/18059694.2016.28] [PMID: 22250477]

[90] Ochoa M, Rahimi R, Zhou J, *et al.* Integrated sensing and delivery of oxygen for next-generation smart wound dressings. Microsyst Nanoeng 2020; 6(1): 1-16.
[http://dx.doi.org/10.1038/s41378-020-0141-7]

[91] Salim AS. The role of oxygen-derived free radicals in the management of venous (varicose) ulceration: a new approach. World J Surg 1991; 15(2): 264-9.
[http://dx.doi.org/10.1007/BF01659062] [PMID: 2031364]

[92] Porta M. A Dictionary of Epidemiology. 6th ed., Oxford: University Press 2014.
[http://dx.doi.org/10.1093/acref/9780199976720.001.0001]

[93] Quartey-Papafio CM. Lesson of the week: importance of distinguishing between cellulitis and varicose eczema of the leg. BMJ 1999; 318(7199): 1672-3.
[http://dx.doi.org/10.1136/bmj.318.7199.1672] [PMID: 10373173]

[94] Biswas M, Gibby O, Ivanova-Stoilova T, Harding K. Cushing's syndrome and chronic venous ulceration--a clinical challenge. Int Wound J 2011; 8(1): 99-102.
[http://dx.doi.org/10.1111/j.1742-481X.2010.00746.x] [PMID: 21078130]

[95] Dulciné-Roque R, Pullés-González V, Gutierrez-González L. Eficiencia del Permanganato de Potasio aplicado en las heridas sépticas en el servicio de cirugía cérvico-facial. Centro Provincial de Información de Ciencias Médicas de Santiago de Cuba 1995; 1: 1-10.

[96] Danmusa UM, Terhile I, Nasir IA, Ahmad AA, Muhammad HY. Prevalence and healthcare costs associated with the management of diabetic foot ulcer in patients attending Ahmadu Bello University Teaching Hospital, Nigeria. Int J Health Sci (Qassim) 2016; 10(2): 219-28.
[http://dx.doi.org/10.12816/0048814] [PMID: 27103904]

[97] Sen CK, Gordillo GM, Roy S, *et al.* Human skin wounds: a major and snowballing threat to public health and the economy. Wound Repair Regen 2009; 17(6): 763-71.
[http://dx.doi.org/10.1111/j.1524-475X.2009.00543.x] [PMID: 19903300]

CHAPTER 4

Approaches to Anti Infective Therapies

Sonia Sethi[1,*]

[1] *Dr. B. Lal Institute of Biotechnology Malviya Industrial Area, Malviya Nagar, Jaipur, India*

Abstract: With the increase in the prevalence of chronic microbial infections and disorders associated with it, the incidence of antibiotic resistance among microorganisms has continued to rise. Due to this, resistance against conventional antibiotic therapy is also increasing, which has become a public health concern. It is necessary to make clinical trials better, improve the idea of research plans, and take into account the cutting-edge drug safety approaches for the development of anti-infective drugs. In this regard, biofilm development and quorum sensing associated virulence approach appears insufficient for the use of traditional antibiotics. The exploitation of different synthetic and natural compounds for their efficacy in combating microbial infections associated with QS has been done, but the compatibility and availability of these compounds limit their applications. Therefore, for the diagnosis and treatment of infectious diseases, particularly resistant to antibiotics, nanotechnological interventions offer various biomedical applications. Nanomaterials exhibit intrinsic anti-infective properties towards the MDR phenomenon and also can be used as carriers for targeted and site-specific delivery of potential drugs.

Keywords: Anti-biofilm activity, Bacteriophage, Innate modulators, Microbial peptide, Microbial biofilms, Nanotechnology systems.

INTRODUCTION

Diseases related to infection have been a prime cause of death over a while in human history. Bacterial diseases are decreasing nowadays due to the awareness of hygiene, nutrition, use of antimicrobial drugs, and immunization. A collective effort has been made globally to stop the transmission of infectious diseases, resulting in the loss of DALY, *i.e.*, quantifying the burden of disease from mortality and morbidity [1]. Unfortunately, the use of antimicrobial drugs is disintegrating gradually over a period of time as resistance against antibiotics

---

[*] **Corresponding author Sonia Sethi:** Dr. B. Lal Institute of Biotechnology Malviya Industrial Area, Malviya Nagar, Jaipur, India; E-mail:soniakaura198@gmail.com

Parvesh Singh, Vipan Kumar & Rajshekhar Karpoormath (Eds.)
All rights reserved-© 2021 Bentham Science Publishers

allows pathogens to rush over it. A bacteria called super-bacteria has recently been developed, which is multidrug-resistant due to a super resistance gene called NDM-1 [2]. Antibiotics mainly target three bacterial processes: DNA replication process, cell wall synthesis, and translational machinery. Unfortunately, resistance among bacteria can develop against any of these processes. Mechanisms behind the resistance include the expression of enzymes that modify or degrade antibiotics [3]. Modifications in cell components result in resistance against cell walls (*e.g.*, Vancomycin) and ribosomes (Tetracycline) [4].

The ability to cure infections is reducing, threatening us to impair our medical practices, weakening global economic growth, and intensifying the mortality rates at all stages of life. Society has met with self-satisfaction through the imminent crisis, which comes from two factors. First, the risk is shared by everyone, and second, those who suffered from untreatable bacterial infections are not generally familiar with the infection before and, once they get infected, they die quickly.

Although new antibiotics, antifungal, and antiviral agents have been developed in recent years, which have shown positive impacts on the health of human beings, still infectious diseases are a major patron for mortality to human health systems globally. Reports from WHO indicated that one-third of global deaths were due to HIV, Malaria, TB, and lower respiratory tract infections in 2004 [5]. Due to the development of MDRs throughout the world, the single-agent and combination therapies development against infections has become a challenge for scientists as well as clinicians to seek a multi-disciplinary approach; one that circumscribes drug development, microbiology, and clinical expertise. To provide a rationale and scientific structure in the process of drug development and clinical applications, pharmacometrics acts as an alarming tool and bridge between key concepts of these disciplines [6].

Along with the prevalence of antibiotic-resistant bacteria, new and other pathogens are also increasing, highlight the need to develop strategies against them immediately. For nanoparticles, antibiotic resistance is not relevant because of their mode of action and also because they are in direct contact with the bacterial cell wall, without penetrating the cell. Therefore, nanoparticles do not promote resistance in bacteria in comparison to antibiotics, and hence new and exciting NP-based materials with antibacterial activity have been focused on.

History of Antibiotics and their Resistance Mechanism

Antibiotics are used since ancient civilizations for the treatment of bacterial infections. Traditional medicines include remedies for malaria; the best known anti malarial drug named artemisinin or "qinghaosu with potent anti-infective properties [7]. From the concept of 'magic bullet given by Paul Erlich, the modern antibiotic era begins. Arsenic dye Arsphenamine (Salvarson) was discovered by Paul Erlich together with Alfred Bertheim and Sahachiro Hata as a potent anti-syphilis drug [8]. Sulfonamidochrysoidine (Prontosil) was introduced for the treatment against bacteria and was the first antibiotic available in 1935, with potent activity. It was a precursor of p-aminophenyl sulfonamide, modified derivatives of sulfonamide antibiotics [9]. One best-known antibiotic was discovered by Alexander Fleming in 1928, but its mass production started during World War II by Howard Florey and Ernest Chain. In 1944, Selman Waksman isolated an aminoglycoside antibiotic from Streptomyces griseus and named it streptomycin [10]. This further led to the discovery of different groups of antibiotics: macrolides, sulfonamides, cyclic peptides, β-lactams, tetracyclines, aminoglycosides, lipopeptides, and lipoglycopeptides, quinolones, dihydrofolate reductase (DHFR) inhibitors, amphenicols, *etc.* Antibiotics have saved billions of lives worldwide and also have changed the journey of medicine. They have also led to the treatment of those Infectious diseases whose treatment was not possible previously.

Traditional medicines prepared from herbs possess antimicrobial activity and active components present in them can be used for medicine preparation [11]. But the long-term use of traditional medicines imposes a selective pressure that contributes to the development of antibiotic resistance genes in human populations. In past years, the advent and dispersal of antibiotic-resistant pathogens, especially multi- drug-resistant, reveal our unawareness about the evolution and processes occurring in microbial eco- systems.

Various mechanisms of protection in microbes allow them to withstand the pressures which are due to changes in the environment and interventions of human beings. This capability of microbes against antibiotics and pressure imposed by the antibiotics during long-term activity have led to the emergence of antibiotic-resistant pathogens. Antibiotic-resistant pathogens carry genes responsible for resistance mechanisms to various antibiotics whose analysis explains the phylogenetic [12]. Recently, the emergence and dissemination of antibiotic-resistant pathogens (MDR) make us undefended against the microbial processes of evolution. Microbes develop protective mechanisms from their metabolic activity which allows them to withstand the unfavorable conditions and pressure imposed by human interventions.

Shortly after the initial isolation of Penicillin antibiotic, resistance to it among *Staphylococcus* was already developed but resistance toward methicillin occurred only two years after its introduction. Some antibiotics were believed to be resistance-proof, but later they developed resistance. For example, vancomycin was believed to be resistance-proof, but, a resistance among Enterococcus and Staphylococci emerged. The emergence of Multi drug resistance (MDR), Pan Drug resistance (PDR), or extensively drug-resistant strains (XDR) are of great concern nowadays. For example, Mycobacterium tuberculosis develops resistance to fluoroquinolones and all second-line injectable drugs (capreomycin, kanamycin, or amikacin) [13]. Every year millions of people are getting affected by different infections and ultimately dying because of them. For this, novel antibiotics development and investigations are in pace, but there are limitations in their mode of action as compared to previously approved drugs.

Therefore, action to prevent the presence of large gaps in existing surveillance of global crisis in health care and an improved, coordinated global effort to contain AMR are imperative. After recognizing this need, the World Health Organization (WHO) in 2001, developed a Global Strategy for Containment of Antimicrobial Resistance, which has provided a framework of national and international surveillance network interventions to slow the emergence and reduce the spread of antimicrobial-resistant microorganisms [14]. In 2012, WHO published "The Evolving Threat of Antimicrobial Resistance – Options for Action," [15] proposing a combination of interventions that include: strengthening health systems and surveillance, improving the use of antimicrobials in hospitals and the community, preventing infection and its control, encouraging the development of appropriate new drugs and vaccines, and political commitment. Following the indication of a primary role for surveillance, in April 2014, WHO published the first global report on surveillance of AMR [16]. This helps for orienting treatment choices, understanding the trends of AMR, interventions area identification, and their impact.

Antibiotics Resistance Mechanisms

The antibiotics show resistance by various mechanisms and, can be classified as a target or bullet-related. Targets include (i) modifications leading to protection (mutations), (ii) use of enzyme for modification (*e.g.* methylation) (iii) replacement (for example, *Klebsiella pneumoniae* bacteria produce enzymes called carbapenemases, which break down carbapenem drugs and most other beta-lactam drugs), and (iv) protection at cellular or population levels (Tet(M) and Tet(O) proteins commonly encoded by genes located on MGEs in *S. aureus*. These proteins are homologous to the elongation factors EF-G and EF-Tu, and their binding to the ribosome facilitates removal of tetracycline in a GTP-ase activity-dependent manner). The bullet includes (i) loss of efficiency by modification, as in the case of acetylation of aminoglycosides, (ii) destruction (as the β-lactam antibiotics by the action of β- lactamases), and (iii) pumping out from the cell as in efflux pump mechanisms of resistance.

This mechanism of resistance is dominant among antibiotics, like quinolones, rifampin, and fosfomycin, and it directs the evolution of horizontally transferred antibiotic resistance genes structurally, such as extended-spectrum beta-lactamases (ESBLs). Mutation-directed antibiotic resistance occurs mainly during in-host evolution [17].

Phylogenetic analysis of several groups of antibiotic resistance genes has suggested that genetic material for present-day antibiotic resistance has had a long history of selection and diversification [12]. Other antibiotic resistance mechanism uses the "kin selection" concept, which operates at the population/system level.

Moreover, in complex biofilm consortia, all community members are protected against antibiotics, irrespective of the kinship, which requires a conceptual framework operating at the system level. Therefore, the base of microbe–antibiotic interaction has been broadened the bullet-target model to reflect complex interactions [18].

Impact of Antibiotic Resistance

Antimicrobial use reduces morbidity and mortality from infectious disease, but the emergence and spread of organisms with resistance against antimicrobials have become a widespread problem in the whole world. Every year, so many people get affected by infections related to antibiotic resistance and die [19]. In Europe, the estimated number of infections and death due to MDR infections is approximately 400000 and 25000. The MDR bacterium includes *S. aureus, Escherichia coli, Enterococcus faecium, Streptococcus pneumonia*e, Klebsiella pneumonia, and Pseudomonas [20].

The availability of drugs for various treatments, including chemotherapy, cancer treatment, organ transplantation, hip replacement surgery, intensive care, make these activities possible but the main factor influencing mortality and morbidity in patients undergoing these procedures are the infections caused by MDR strains.

Factors Contributing to the Emergence of Antibiotic Resistance

There are three main sectors that are involved in the development of antibiotic resistance:

a. Human medicine in the community and hospital
b. Animal production and agriculture

c. Environmental compartment.

Antibiotic Resistance in Human Medicine

In a community, the development of antibiotic resistance is the inappropriate use of antibiotics due to the prescriptions given by general practitioners. One more factor that plays an important role is self-medication, which involves the availability of drugs without prescription. In the case of hospitals, the continued use of antimicrobial drugs leads to the emergence and spread of highly antibiotic-resistant nosocomial infections. Also, other factors like the presence of the highly susceptible immunosuppressed patient and fragile elderly patients result in the failure to control infections spread from patient to patient [21].

Use of Antibiotics in Food-producing Animals and Agriculture

Another factor of spreading resistance is the use of antibiotics in animal feedstock and agriculture for growth promotion and disease treatment or prevention [22]. An increase in the frequency of antibiotic resistance genes in bacteria and transferring those genes of resistance into clinically important bacteria has resulted in tighter restrictions on the use of antibiotics in plant agriculture [23].

Resistance Spread and The Environment

During the last years, the environment is also responsible for the spread of antibiotic resistance. Antibiotic resistance is disseminated from soil microorganisms and water contaminated with fecal microorganisms. Water is an important source of dissemination of resistance among microorganisms between different environmental compartments. Due to incomplete metabolism in human beings or due to the disposal of unused antibiotics, large amounts of antibiotics are released into municipal wastewater. Antibiotic-resistant bacteria and antibiotic-resistant genes can be detected in wastewater samples because the conditions in wastewater treatment plants (WWTPs) are favorable for the proliferation of resistant bacteria [24].

Prevention of Antibiotic Resistance

As new antibiotics are developing, the main problem is resistance to it sooner or later. The level of antibiotic consumption is related to the level of antibiotic-resistant [25]. It is, therefore, urgently required to fight against, multi-drug resistant bacteria which show alternative modes of action against antimicrobial agents. Worldwide many scientists are trying to solve this crisis [26] by searching and selecting the various alternatives against conventional antibiotics with therapeutic uses, which have a relatively low potential to elicit resistance [27]. There is a need to develop effective blockers of bacterial drug efflux pumps to reduce heritable antibiotic resistance and knowledge about antibiotic persistence, adaptive resistance, and phenotypic tolerance is required for nonheritable tolerance. A target such as transcriptional regulators mediates a downshift in the metabolism of microorganisms due to slow replication which is accompanied by nonheritable resistance [28].

How phenotypic and induced tolerance is related to nonreplicative and replicative states, stress responses and DNA damage should be initiated. Researchers should also initiate studies related to tolerance residing in biofilms, inoculum density, oxidative stress, and antibiotics exposure [29]. Biofilms are a major contributor to antibiotic resistance and tolerance, so there is a need to investigate the ways by which biofilm formation is discouraged in tissues and implanted devices [30] and how to generate the anti-infective activity from endogenous host precursors [31]. Also, blocking the synthesis of components involved in the synthesis of biofilms resistant to some compounds and interrupting signaling pathways for the biofilm formation and their dispersal. To prevent or avoid antibiotic resistance, virulence mechanism and bacterial membrane should be targeted [32]. Also, the development of a prodrug should be emphasized so that a bacteria-restricted enzyme would be inactivated with diverse targets.

Two classes of anti- infective drugs with multiple targets, ROI and RNIs, have been developed for antibiotic resistance. For example, nitroimidazole PA824, a drug for tuberculosis: mycobacterial nitroreductase results in the generation of RNI by the use of mycobacterial flavin as a cofactor to metabolize the drug. The generation of intrabacterial RNI controls infection with its ability to interfere with the pathogens and neutralize host-derived ROI and RNI.

APPROACHES FOR ANTIINFECTIVE THERAPIES

Role of Reactive Oxygen and Nitrogen Species

Free radicals derived from nitrogen and molecular oxygen can act as intercellular and intracellular messengers. The most commonly generated ones are superoxides, hydroxyl species, hydrogen peroxides, singlet oxygen, nitric oxide, and peroxynitrite [33]. These free radicals are termed reactive oxygen intermediates and reactive nitrogen intermediates. This ROI and RNI can damage DNA and other chemical moieties [34]. ROI and RNI are mainly generated by mammalian phagocytes, with polymorphonuclear leukocytes, and thus can produce their destructive product peroxynitrite. Hence, a microbe cannot easily evade in their targets and interfere with host cell production of ROI and RNI, catabolize them, or repair their damage [35]. Both of them are immunoregulatory, can inhibit G proteins, kinases, caspases, transcription factors, lymphocyte proliferation, alter cytokine and prostaglandin production and prevent apoptosis of host cells.

Microbes are killed not only by oxidants but also by phagocytosis and the release of antimicrobial compounds. ROI in the immune system utilizes macrophages, dendritic cells, and neutrophils for the determination (Toll receptors) and phagocytosis of a foreign body. Microbes are bounded by the toll-like receptors-4, followed by ingestion by phagosomes, and the process of killing is triggered by NADPH oxidase action, releasing cytoplasmic granules which cause a decrease in pH and hence results in microbial destruction [36]. Production of ROS, such as H_2O_2 and ozone, can be brought about by the activation of a chemical by the light source of narrowband wavelengths in photodynamic antimicrobial chemotherapy (PACT) and can be used for the treatment of root canal infections and killing of other cells too [37].

Another type of therapy that involves the generation of free radicals (ROS), is antimicrobial photodynamic therapy (PDTa) used for carcinogenic biofilms. It involves either of two processes; the first process involves the interaction of the photosensitizer with the substrate *via* electron transfer and in the second process the photosensitizer reacts with oxygen [38]. This therapy is beneficial for the periodontal treatment for scaling and root planning. Similar to reactive oxygen intermediates (ROI), reactive nitrogen intermediates (RNI), including nitric oxide, are also involved in the antimicrobial activity of activated macrophages against a variety of intracellular microorganisms, *e.g.*, Leishmania major, *Toxoplasma gondii*, Legionella pneumophila, Mycobacterium tuberculosis, Mycobacterium Bovis BCG, and L. monocytogenes.

Mechanism of ROI and RNI against various microbes

Reactive oxygen intermediates (ROI) and reactive nitrogen intermediates (RNI) have the ability to cause DNA damage and other chemical moieties on which its propagation and protection depend. Mammalian phagocytes with polymorphonuclear leukocytes lead to high output ROI production which leads to immunologically activated macrophages and mammalian cells in response to appropriate inflammatory stimuli, macrophages considerably outpacing polymorphonuclear leukocytes are capable of generating high RNI. Also, macrophages can produce superoxide (O_2-) and nitric oxide ($\cdot NO$) and thus can be prolific generators of destructive product, peroxynitrite ($OONO-$).

RNI are used as antimicrobial agents in gastric juice, a key component of the innate immune system of the epithelium (Fig. 1) [39]. For example, M. tuberculosis is killed by RNI in its liquid and gaseous form. 2 days' exposure to 90 ppm of ·NO gas kills more than 99% of M. tuberculosis in culture. Therefore, concentrations (80 ppm) have been administered to patients for days or weeks to dilate the pulmonary vasculature. M. tuberculosis is sensitive to nitrogen dioxide but is much more resistant than other mycobacteria to peroxynitrite [40].

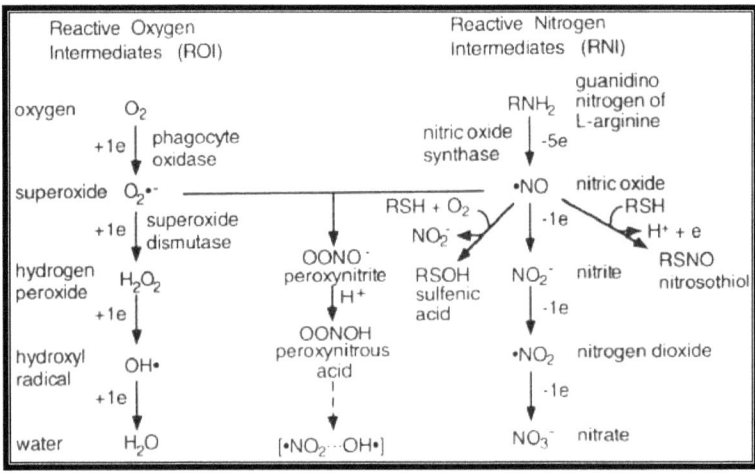

Fig. (1). Mechanism of ROI and RNI.

Host Innate Immunity Defense Systems

Towards the development of novel strategies interest in the modulation of our immune system has increased. Our immune system shows the multi-facetted response to the infection caused by pathogenic microorganisms through different recognition receptors patterns with host cells. Therefore, different therapies are either under development or available for stimulation of the immune system without overtly stimulating harmful inflammation. This technique of modulating immunity as an ant -infective strategy is an emerging technology for understanding the host defense system.

Stimulation of pathogen sensing mechanism and intracellular signaling pathways has occurred through the discovery of pathogen recognition receptors which may be membrane-bound or cytosolic receptors like Toll-like receptors, Nod-like receptors, and RIGI-like receptors resulting in rapid and effective clearance of pathogens [41]. This leads to valuable insights into the role of immunity against the pathogenesis of infectious diseases and the intervention of therapeutics. Some pathogens cause damage directly by releasing their factors or indirectly as a result of immune response; some enhance pro-inflammatory response but some result in insufficient response [42]. Hence, immunomodulation offers the potential either to boost or inhibit the elements of immune response and effectors mechanisms for pathogen clearance so can be used as an anti-infective strategy. It also forms the basis for therapeutics against a diverse array of pathogens including bacterial, viral, fungal, or parasitic.

Immune Modulators Expression and Secretion

The Central interface between pathogen and host is the external surface of pathogens (bacteria/viruses). The immune system recognizes the exposed surface of pathogens which provides the host a pathway to initiate the removal of microbes. Pathogen becomes opportunistic to show mimics of host immune modulators to avoid host immune response, to express adhesions for anchoring pathogen on host surface, and present fusion proteins for uptake in host cells [43]. Impingement of a virus on the host immune system is *via*molecules that are present on the external surface. It is studded with immunomodulatory proteins and host-derived [44]. These act as immunoregulators, receptors, inhibitors, ligand molecules that transform the virus particle that can enhance immunomodulatory responses in host cells. For example, gp env glycoprotein of HIV [45].

The surface of bacteria shows diverse antigenic targets which protects them from immune vigilance and TLR recognition molecules like adhesions. Expression of carbohydrate capsules on surfaces of bacteria masks them from antibody and complement deposition in turn prevents opsonization and phagocytosis. Microorganisms having capsules often have adhesions like pili on them that enable them to bind host receptors and keep them hidden. For example, Streptococcus pyogenes having Cytolysin (that makes it host-specific) need to deliver a NAD glycohydrolase in host cells to trigger cytotoxicity [46]. Different bacteria use their fragments/ molecules as a driving force in host cells (Table 1).

Table 1. Anti-immune strategies of viruses and bacteria.

S. No.	Strategy	Viral Examples	Bacterial Examples
1.	Secreted modulators or toxins	Ligand mimics virokines Receptor mimics viroreceptors	Many toxins Proteases
2.	Modulators on the pathogen surface	Complement inhibitors Coagulation regulators Immune receptors Adhesion molecules	Lipid A of LPS Carbohydrates such as capsules Outer membrane proteins Adhesion and invasion

(Table 1) cont.....

S. No.	Strategy	Viral Examples	Bacterial Examples
3.	Hide from immune surveillance	Latency Infect immune-privileged tissues	Avoid phagolysosomal fusion Inhibit phagocytosis
4.	Antigenic hypervariability	Express error-prone replicase Escape from antibody recognition "outrun" T Cell recognition	Vary many surface structures Pili, outer membrane proteins, LPS Strain to strain variation
5.	Subvert or kill immune cells/phagocytes	Infect and kill immune cells (DCs, APcs, lymphocytes, macrophages, *etc*) Inhibit CTL/NK cell killing pathways Alter immune cell signaling, effector functions, or differentiation Express superantigens	Superantigens Avoid phagolysosomal fusion Block inflammatory pathways by injecting effectors Replicate within and overrun immune cells
6.	Block acquired immunity	Downregulate MHC I/II Block antigen presentation/proteosome Prevent induction of immune response genes	IgA proteases Block antigen presentation
7.	Inhibit complement	Soluble inhibitors of the complement cascade Viral Fc receptors	Proteases to degrade complement Produce capsules and long-chain LPS to avoid complement deposition and MAC attack
8.	Inhibit cytokines/ interferons/ chemokines	Inhibit ligand gene expression Ligand/receptor signalling inhibitor Block secondary antiviral gene induction Interfere with effector protein	Block inflammatory pathways Activate alternate pathways Secrete proteases to degrade
9.	Modulate apoptosis/autophagy	Inhibit or accelerate cell death Block death signaling pathways Scavenge free radicals Downregulate death receptors or ligands Inactivate death sensors pathways	Inhibit apoptosis Activate death signaling pathways Alter apoptotic signaling pathways
10.	Interfere with TLRs	Block or hijack TLR signaling Prevent TLR recognition	Alter TLR ligands to decrease recognition Bind to TLR to dampen inflammation Inject effectors to inhibit downstream inflammation signaling

(Table 1) cont.....

S. No.	Strategy	Viral Examples	Bacterial Examples
11.	Block antimicrobial small molecules	Prevent iNOS induction Inhibit antiviral RNA silencing	Secrete proteases to degrade Alter cell surface to avoid peptide insertion Use pumps to transport peptide Directly sense small molecules to trigger defense mechanisms
12.	Block intrinsic cellular pathways	Inhibit RNA editing Regulate ubiquitin/ISgylation pathways	Alter ubiquitin pathway Alter transcriptional programs

Avoiding Immune Detection

The main feature of bacterial and viral pathogenic microorganisms is the ability to avoid detection by either the innate or acquired immune system of host cells. There are two ways by which they can avoid detection; one is the concealment of the surface of their cells and another is to lessen immune response. To provide machinery for the transport of protein onto the surface of a cell, and secretion of virus-encoded immunomodulators, viruses rely on the infected host cell, unlike bacteria.

Proteins secreted by viruses interact directly with the immune system through virion surface or extracellular. These viral immunomodulator proteins have been used as biopharmaceuticals to treat diseases of hyperacute inflammation due to their potent -anti-inflammatory properties [47]. Viral proteins that show immunomodulatory properties include CD homologs, superantigens, complement inhibitors, ligands, receptor mimics, regulators of leukocyte activation (NK cells, T cells, dendritic cells, and Macrophages), and binding proteins [48]. The major problem associated with a bacterial surface is hiding or disguising the presence of surfaces by capsules and thus preventing opsonization. However, some molecules can be used as immunomodulators like TLR agonists such as LPS (Lipid A), peptidoglycan, and flagella [49].

Alternatively, pathogens once internalized, can adopt different patterns of infection within the host cell-like, they can thrive inside macrophages or dendritic cells which show antimicrobial defense or endosomal compartments of host cells like neutrophiles or fibroblasts, or epithelial cells [50]. By acquiring this, the pathogen does not encounter any competition with other microbes, gains nutrients sources for survival, and is protected from antibody attack. Also, it can replicate without disturbing host cell function and integrity and therefore, evolving strategies of bypassing the killing mechanism of the host immune system [51]. These strategies have led to the improvement of our knowledge of the biology of infection and for the development of vaccines and appropriate therapeutics.

Existing and Potential Innate Immune Targets for The Development of Anti-infectives

The abundance of potential targets is available for therapeutic intervention that takes advantage of the convolutions of innate immunity. Cytokine-based immunomodulators are used because of their role in showing antimicrobial responses against infections. Examples include recombinant or modified forms of IFN-a and IFN-b for the treatment of viral diseases like HCV, HBV, and herpes virus-associated diseases in immunocompromised patients. CSF (Colony Stimulating factors) is used for the treatment of neutropenia (depletion of neutrophils) in patients with damaged bone marrow. For example, GM-CSF restores and stimulates neutrophil functions to fight bacterial and fungal functions.

Other examples are also there that can act on innate immunity targets. In the treatment of papillomavirus-associated genital warts Imiquimod, a synthetic TLR-7 agonist can be used which works through receptor-mediated cytokine secretion and Macrophage or NK cell activation [52]. For the treatment of HSV, EBV, and Viral hepatitis, Isoprinosine can be used as an immunostimulant that enhances T cell proliferation. Products like Bronchomunal1 (lek) and Luviac1 (Daiichi Sankyo Co.) are used as treatments for RTI and human immunoglobulin is used for pediatric HIV, sepsis, and C.

ANTIMICROBIAL PEPTIDES AS ANTI-INFECTIVES

Antimicrobial peptides are gene-encoded multifunctional effector molecules, having a direct antimicrobial activity and/or immunomodulatory properties [53]. AMPs are folded into amphipathic structures and can destabilize the plasma membranes of target cells. Antimicrobial peptides (AMPs) are active to various degrees against a variety of organisms including bacteria, enveloped viruses, protozoa, and fungi [54]. Although AMPs are a good alternative to conventional antibiotics, they are not devoid of drawbacks. They are proteinaceous, rarely available, and are unstable; these two features have severely hampered clinical progress to date. Therefore, to overcome these disadvantages, various modifications have been introduced to develop synthetic analogs that mimic the properties of AMPs [55]. Among the most promising AMPs, multimeric peptides *i.e.* peptidic dendrimers have been reported with antimicrobial properties. These peptides modulate host immunity by modulating inflammation and activating immunocytes.

Naturally occurring AMPs are often referred to as 'host defense peptides' (HDP), or innate defense regulatory (IDR) peptides, [56]. AMPs in prokaryotes are produced by both Gram-negative and Gram-positive bacteria, with one abundant class being the bacteriocins [57]. Dendrimeric AMPs containing multiple Arginine and tryptophan dipeptides, named as (RW)4D, can be used to kill gram-negative bacteria through the membranolytic mechanism. Peptide binding to cell walls and membranes of bacterial targets is governed by Arginine which provides cationic charges and Tryptophan anchored peptides to the outer leaflet of the membrane perturbing its integrity.

Novel antimicrobial peptide dendrimer G3KL, against *Acinetobacter baumannii* and *Pseudomonas aeruginosa* strain with natural lysine and leucine residues alternating in the branches, act as a membrane-disrupting compound, is a peptide dendrimer of a third generation [58]. Other dendrimeric peptides identified as SB041, a tetra branched peptide against Escherichia coli cells also found effective against Gram-negative microorganisms, with intensity comparable to that of colistin and polymyxin B [59]. Another example is 2D-24, a dendrimeric peptide with antibiofilm activity, a new synthetic compound containing RWR Arg-Tr--Arg) and RTtbR(2) tripeptide branches [60]. This molecule was able to kill biofilm cells of two strains of *Pseudomonas aeruginosa*, namely the wild-type PAO1 and its mucoid mutant PDO300, in a dose-dependent manner.

Peptide-derivatized dendrimers like SB105 and its derivative SB105-A10 also can act as an antiviral agent and inhibit the replication process of several strains of human cytomegalovirus (HCMV) in both primary fibroblasts and endothelia cells [61]. HCMV is a challenging pathogen of organ transplant patients, bone marrow recipients, and patients with immunocompromised acquired immune deficiency syndrome (AIDS). More recently, SB105 and SB105-A10 directly inhibit herpes simplex virus 1 (HSV-1) and HSV-2 *in vitro* replication process by blocking virion attachment to target cells [62]. Based on its membranotropic nature, gH625–644 domain acts as an antiviral agent against HSV-1 and HSV-2 at the time of entry process, by interacting with the glycoproteins that form the viral envelope [63].

Mode of Action

There are two modes of mechanisms by which AMP functions, which include artificial membranes and nonlytic methods. Some AMPs act using both mechanisms [64] and some by switching from one to another based on the characteristics of specific microorganisms.

The functions of AMP include:

1. **Disruption of Membrane Integrity -** AMP often disrupts the membrane of infectious microorganisms, making it permeable so considered as the primary inactivation mechanism. AMP is amphipathic, and possesses interfacial activity, resulting in functional diversity. This allows AMP to remain active against a narrow or broad spectrum of microbial species [65]. AMPs result in membrane disruption by the initial attraction of AMP to the membrane, causing conformational change and insertion. For example, maculatin, isolated from the skin glands of a green-eyed tree frog Litoria genimaculata, acts by pore formation [66] and by the successive addition of peptide molecules to an already existing transmembrane to form a growing oligomer.
2. **Non-Lytic Action -** Some AMPs do not act on membrane but act on intracellular and extracellular targets, resulting in the inactivation of specific metabolically essential components and cell wall biogenesis. For example, Trp-rich AMPs enter into bacteria by direct translocation, but without resulting in cell lysis [67]. The proline-rich AMPs enter bacterial cells using specific membrane transport proteins.
3. **Nucleic Acid Biosynthesis and Metabolism Inhibitors -** This group includes helical buforin II and Trp-rich indolicidin which are homologous to DNA-binding protein histone H_2A and act by disrupting the bacterial membrane and inhibiting DNA synthesis, or, more specifically, inactivating DNA topoisomerase [68].
4. **Inhibitors of Protein Biosynthesis and Folding -** AMPs like bovine cathelicidin Bac7, a long peptide isolated from bovine neutrophils, proline-rich peptides with PR-39, CP10A, interferes by disrupting protein synthesis, and protein-folding. Pyrrhocoricin, apidaecin, drosocin, and Bac71-35 all inhibit DnaK, and ATPase activity and prevent DnaK from refolding misfolded proteins [69].
5. **Inhibitors of Bacterial Proteases -** Some AMPs, like histatin-5, inhibit/dysregulate proteases [70] which in turn act as a therapeutic agent to reduce extracellular matrix degradation caused by host proteases. These AMPs reduce virulence and are antimicrobial.
6. **Cell Division Inhibitors -** CRAMP, an antimicrobial peptide orthologous to human LL-37, is a potent membranolytic, which interferes with the septation process, inhibiting bacterial cytokinesis. C18G inhibits cell division by strongly stimulating the PhoQ/PhoP signaling system. This, in turn, results in increased synthesis of QueE, which is an enzyme that inhibits septation by interacting with the divisome [71].
7. **Lipopolysaccharide (LPS)-Binding Peptides-** These AMPs specifically act on the surface of Gram-negative bacteria, can bind to LPS, and disrupt the

outer membrane, affecting the cell's structural integrity and survival, for example, frog peptides temporins A and B from Rana temporaria [72].

Therapeutic Potential

AMPs have often been used as novel therapeutic agents for treating microbial infections as an alternative to classical antibiotics treatment due to several advantages like they are multimodal, multifunctional, fast-acting, and have healing activities [73]. Several AMPs, such as the membrane-active gH625 and its analog gH625-GCGKKKK, are found to be active against biofilm-forming bacteria. Even polymyxin B and gramicidin S [74] have recently been reported to be active against multidrug-resistant strains and biofilms of *Pseudomonas aeruginosa*.

Several AMPs *e.g.* bacitracin, polymyxin, and tyrothricin are produced by Bacillus sp and used as a topical agent due to hemolytic properties. Polymyxin is used for the treatment of gram-negative infections and MDR, and Bacitracin, a mixture of cyclic polypeptides, is used in combination with polymyxin and neomycin (Neosporin™) for topical treatment of eye and skin infections [75]. Nisin, a natural (34-residue) AMP produced by *Lactococcus lactis*, is effective against Gram-positive bacteria, in particular mastitis pathogens.

Finally, another cyclic lipopeptide, daptomycin, is utilized for the treatment of infections caused by MDR Gram-positive pathogens [76]. There are several antimicrobial peptides that are obtained from marine organisms such as bacteria, sponges, mud crabs, ascidian, spider crabs, jellyfish, and fish. Aurelin (1) exhibited activity against gram-positive and gram-negative bacteria (Listeria monocytogenes and Escherichia coli) [77]. Lee *et al.* reported that arenicin-1 (2), isolated from the marine polychaete Arenicola marina, exhibited significant antibacterial activity against *Pseudomonas aeruginosa* and *Staphylococcus aureus* [78].

Tauramamide (3), inhibits gram-positive human pathogen Enterococcus sp. and Methicillin-resistant S. aureus., produced from marine bacterial isolate Brevibacillus laterosporus PNG276, obtained from Papua New Guinea [79]. Scygonadin (5), an anionic antimicrobial peptide, from the seminal plasma of Scylla Serrata [80], inhibits Micrococcus luteus, *E. coli*, P. aeruginosa, S. aureus, and Streptococcus pyogenes. Halocidin (36), from hemocytes of a marine ascidian, and Cyclopeptide pedein A (39), from myxobacterium Chondromyces pediculatus, are antimicrobial peptides that show potent antifungal activity against *C. Albicans* [81].

Three cyclic depsipeptides, mirabamides A (85), C (86), and D (87), isolated from the sponge Siliquariaspongia mirabilis, papuamides, are a class of marine sponge-derived cyclic depsipeptides, asperterrestide A (98), a cyclic tetrapeptide isolated from the marine-derived fungus Aspergillus terreus, which are thought to have cytoprotective activity against HIV and influenza virus strains A/WSN/33 (H1N1) [82].

BACTERIOPHAGES AS ANTI-INFECTIVE AGENTS

Bacteriophages are organisms that kill bacterial cells. They are most abundant on earth and reduce the global bacterial population. Bacteriophage characteristics make it attractive for next-generation therapeutic agents, with several benefits over conventional antibiotics. Phages facilitate effective treatment by low phage dose delivery, get amplified at the infection site, and therefore, can be used as a therapeutic approach. The western scientific community started the assessment of various applications of phages and their products for the treatment of infectious diseases due to the increasing prevalence of antibiotic resistance among bacterial pathogens [83]. Bacteriophages can be used against pathogens including Pseudomonas spp [84], vancomycin-resistant Enterococci [85], antibiotic-resistant Staphylococci [86], multidrug-resistant Klebsiella pneumonia [87], imipenem-resistant [88], and multidrug-resistant *Pseudomonas aeruginosa* [89], antibiotic-resistant strains of Escherichia coli [90], and methicillin-resistant *Staphylococcus aureus* [91]. There are different strategies derived from phages to combat bacterial infections such as enzybiotics and whole-phage therapy [92].

Whole phage therapy may contain one or few phage strains or a mixture of several phages. The use of this therapy has advantages because of its specificity, self-destruction capability, with no side effects, wide administration routes, exponential reproduction, and a single dose efficiency to treat infection [93].

Nowadays, bacteriophages are used as a source of biochemical reagents for the treatment of human and animal diseases and as anti-infective agents for diagnostics and therapeutic delivery technologies. There are at least 20 lytic bacteriophages, which target clinically relevant, dominant ribotypes which are associated with hospital infection outbreaks. These bacteriophages are of significant therapeutic potential for anaerobic pathogens too. Ian Connerton (University of Nottingham, UK) highlighted the potential of bacteriophages as alternatives to conventional antimicrobial approaches for food-borne pathogens control, in particular Campylobacter jejuni [94].

Bacteriophages can reduce the high incidence of Campylobacter carriage in poultry (up to 80%) [95], and this reduces their entry into the human food chain.

Campylobacter bacteriophages prove themselves as potentially useful agents for therapy, bio-sanitation, food processing, and packaging reduce the number of food-borne pathogens in poultry products. Bacteriophages are also effective in controlling C. jejuni and biofilms *in vitro* [96].

The use of bacteriophages for decontamination of poultry products, treatment of *Pseudomonas aeruginosa* infections causing pulmonary infections, biofilm disruption, are the potential applications of bacteriophages as an anti-infective therapy. Isolation and identification of two novel enzymes namely polyγ-glutamate and a polysaccharide lyase of bacteriophage likely to be involved in the initial degradation of the host mucoid capsule may be useful in disruption of the exopolysaccharide biofilm matrix.

A novel class of protein– RNA toxin-antitoxin (TA) pair, ToxIN, represents the phage abortive infection system obtained from Erwinia carotovora subspecies atroseptica, which consists of a protein toxin and a specific RNA antitoxin [97]. Positive therapeutic results were obtained in patients with a wide range of bacterial infections caused by the pathogenic Staphylococci, Klebsiella, Escherichia, Proteus, and Pseudomonas bacteria [98]. Also, bacteriophages were used for treating chronic skin infections caused by Pseudomonas, Staphylococcus, Klebsiella, Proteus, and *E. coli* [99]. More recently in the same group, antibiotic-resistant septicemia was treated with phage therapy, and complete recovery was achieved in 85.1% of cases, whereas in 14.9% of cases, phage therapy was ineffective [100].

Phage Endolysins as Therapeutics

Bacteriophages encode enzymes called peptidoglycan-degrading enzymes, responsible for the lysis of the host bacterial cell at the end of the lytic cycle. These are known as Endolysins and they require a lysis factor called holin which helps in penetration in the cell membrane [101] by forming pores in the membrane and providing access to reach its target and causes cell lysis [102]. Lysins are of different types depending upon the acting cleavage site within the peptidoglycan named as N-acetyl-β-D-muramidase, lytic transglycosylase, N-acetyl-β-D-glucosaminidases, N- acetylmuramoyl-L-alanine amidases, L-alanoy--D-glutamate endopeptidases, and interpeptide bridge-specific endopeptidases [103]. Phage C1 produces endolysin known as streptococcal lysine which is specific for groups A, C, and E Streptococci [104], and lysin from phage γ of *B. anthracis* is effective against vegetative cells and germinating spores [105].

Staphylococcal phage MR11 was found to be active against Staphylococcus infections in mice, and lysin PlyV12 was active against *E. faecalis* and other

Gram-positive pathogens, such as Staphylococci and Streptococci [106]. Gram-negative endolysins have antibacterial applications, for example, *Pseudomonas aeruginosa* produces endolysins having a broad target range, but its application as an antibacterial is compromised due to the presence of the outer membrane. Thus, antibacterial activity is only possible after the treatment of the outer membrane of Gram-negative cells with EDTA [107] or by the fusion of hydrophobic amino acids to the endolysin, which enables the movement of the endolysin across the outer membrane.

Phage therapy as a Therapeutic Approach to Mycobacterial Infections

More than 4200 bacteriophages can infect Mycobacterium spp resulting in the application of bacteriophage as a candidate for alternative therapy in non-mycobacterial infection, and showing that bacteriophage has a high capacity to efficiently eradicate pathogenic bacteria. Bacteriophages cannot infect human cells and replicate only in the target bacterium and cause the lyses at the site of infection. Also, their administration is easier and the concentration of phages increases at the site of infection; therefore, very few doses are required, and they are highly virulent against MTB [108]. The use of nonvirulent mycobacterium, M. smegmatis as a delivery system, for the treatment of mycobacterial infection could deliver phage to the intracellular pathogen, and also high proliferation rate of bacteriophage also provide an appropriate environment for its activity within mononuclear cells [109].

The emergence of MDR and XDR in M. tuberculosis has attracted different research groups to investigate the bacteriophage roles as a suitable alternative to antibiotics in the treatment of TB. Bacteriophages can be used as an alternative to antibiotics to infect and kill mycobacteria. Different bacteriophages against TB as therapeutic options are available which include Phage DS-6A, Phage TM4, Phage D29, *etc.*

THERAPY BASED ON ANTIBODY

In the 1890s to treat human infections, antibody-based (serum) therapies were first used, including Haemophilus influenza, Corynebacterium diphtheriae, *Streptococcus pneumonia*, and *Neisseria meningitides*, group A streptococcus, and Clostridium tetani [110]. Major advances in the technology of antibody production have led to the use of antibodies as antimicrobial agents. Hybridoma technology provided the means to produce monoclonal antibodies (human antibodies and humanize murine MABs) in unlimited amounts [111]. Today antibody therapy is used in few situations, including toxin neutralization (diphtheria, tetanus, and botulism), replacement therapy in immunoglobulin-deficient patients, and post-exposure prophylaxis against several viruses (*e.g.*, rabies, measles, hepatitis A and B, varicella). Three recent developments in antibody-based therapies opened an option for serious consideration in treatment. First, difficulties involved in the treatment of immunocompromised patients can be resolved; Second, human antibody reagents can be synthesized and associated toxicities can be avoided; and Third, the emergence of new, old, and drug-resistant pathogens can be declined. Also, MABs recognize one epitope and have higher specific activity than polyclonal antibodies, resulting in greater therapeutic efficiency.

Due to its homogeneity, specific activity, safety, and constancy, MABs are superior over polyclonal antibodies. However, different therapeutic monoclonal antibodies can be combined to produce polyvalent antibodies with multiple specificities and isotypes. Antibodies can be produced within the human body against all existing pathogens from combinations of variable gene elements and also against an extraordinarily large number of antigens. During the production of an immune response, somatic mutations are introduced into genes for higher affinity and diversity [112]. Hence, antibody-based therapies can be used against any pathogen, although the level of antibody immunity differs among different pathogens. Natural antibodies can be generated against two fungi, *Candida albicans* and *Cryptococcus neoformans* [113] but the MABs enhance the therapeutic efficacy of chemical antibiotics against *C. neoformans* in models of cryptococcosis. Antibody therapy is not limited to extracellular pathogens, but intracellular pathogens can also be treated with MABs.

Some IgA MABs can neutralize intracellular viruses, and interfere with the intracellular replication of *Toxoplasma gondii* [114]. It has been proposed that intracellular virus neutralization by IgA occurs by antibodies binding to viral proteins and interfering with viral assembly. Additional evidence for intracellular antibody activity comes from the observation that IgG anti-DNA autoantibodies can enter the cytoplasm and nucleus of living cells. Antibody functions through different mechanisms, including neutralization, inhibition of microbial attachment, agglutination, antibody-directed cellular cytotoxicity, complement activation, and opsonization. MABs exhibit versatile activities: some are active directly against the pathogen, some neutralize the toxic products of infection, and others enhance the efficacy of host effector cells. The versatility of antibody-based therapies is illustrated by the ability of digoxin-binding antibodies to reverse digoxin toxicity and recent attempts to treat septic shock by employing MABs that bind cytokines [115]. Monoclonal antibodies could target a wide range of biological agents, including bacterial, viral pathogens, fungi, and associated toxins [116].

Monoclonal antibodies bind to the components of structural cell surface followed by bactericidal clearance or antibody-dependent cytotoxicity [117]. Monoclonal antibodies show potent activity against viral epitopes and can target receptors and coreceptors located on host cells and induce antibody-dependent cytotoxicity. For example, MABs (ibalizumab) are licensed for HIV therapy in adults and RSV infection in high-risk children [118]. Concerning RSV, palivizumab interferes with virus attachment and fusion by binding RSV F protein [119]. MABs are also used to treat influenza or neutralize MABs against Ebola and Middle East respiratory syndrome coronavirus (MERS-CoV) (Table **2**).

Table 2. Examples of Potential MABs.

Category	Target	Comments
Bioterrorism	Anthrax (*B. anthacis*) Small Pox Ebola virus	Need for immediate dispersal upon exposure Population of non-immune individuals Highly virulent
Emerging diseases	SARS COV Influenza virus	Also, potential bioterrorists agents Possibility of recurrence of 2003 pandemic, H1N1 and H5N1 are pandemic threats
Susceptible populations	Parainfluenza virus Candida Sp.	An important class of nosocomial infection
MDR bacteria	MRSA, VRSA *Pseudomonas aeruginosa*	Increasing prevalence in the community An important class of nosocomial infection

PROBIOTICS AS BIOTHERAPEUTIC AGENTS

Probiotics are live microorganisms that confer a health effect on the host when administered in adequate amounts by enhancing gut health and overall human well-being, resulting in their increased demand. The most common strains of probiotic bacteria are from the genera Lactobacillus (*i.e., L. rhamnosus, L. acidophilus, L. plantarum, L. casei, L. delbrueckii* subsp. Bulgaricus, *etc.*) and Bifidobacterium (*i.e., B. infantis, B. animalis* subsp. lactis, *B. longum, etc.*). The most common probiotics are certain strains from the genera *Lactococcus lactis* subsp. lactis, *Pediococcus acidilactici, Bacillus subtilis, Leuconostoc mesenteroides, Enterococcus faecium, Streptococcus thermophilus, Escherichia coli* Nissle 1917, *etc.* Certain yeasts such as Saccharomyces boulardii are also probiotics [120]. Probiotics not only improve gut health but also exert other health-promoting effects, including chronic diseases such as high serum cholesterol, cancer, allergy, and slow disease progression and symptoms of HIV

[121]. Probiotics modulate the gut microbiota, enhance the working of gut barrier functions, degrade carcinogens, and enhance the immune system [122].

A study conducted by Ma *et al.* [123] found that probiotic Bacillus polyfermenticus exerts an anticancer effect on human colon cancer cells stimulating IgG production and modulates the number of CD4þ, CD8þ, or NK cells. In another study, 54 women found that daily probiotic consumption for 6 months enhanced the clearance of human papillomavirus (HPV), causing cervical cancer [124]. The administration of probiotics causes an improvement of lipid profiles, including reduction of serum/plasma total cholesterol, LDL-cholesterol, and triglycerides [125].

For example, probiotic *Lactobacillus reuteri* NCIMB 30242 and a few other Lactobacillus and Bifidobacterium strains have the potential to reduce serum cholesterol levels, thereby reducing the risk of cardiovascular diseases, hypertension, hyperlipidemia, and build-up of atherosclerotic plaque in the arteries [126]. Also, probiotic intake reduces the prevalence of allergic diseases, including atopic dermatitis, rhinoconjunctivitis, and asthma as well as alleviate the common symptoms associated with HIV patients.

Nowadays, consortia of different probiotic species deliver a superior impact on human health as compared to the use of a single probiotic strain. For example, probiotic VSL#3 consists of 8 different mixtures of probiotics and was proven to be effective in treating several diseases, including ulcerative colitis, irritable bowel disease, diarrhea, improving hepatic insulin resistance in diabetic patients, enhancing the immune system of the consumer, and many more [127]. In addition, combinations of Bifidobacterium infantis with Lactobacillus acidophilus were found to be effective in reducing the incidence of necrotizing enterocolitis (NEC) and NEC-associated mortality in critically ill neonates [128].

Probiotics' important characteristics are their antimicrobial activity against pathogens, which makes them beneficial for maintaining the homeostasis of the intestinal flora. The antagonistic activity of probiotics against another includes competition, immune modulation, alleviating host defense systems, production of organic acids or hydrogen peroxide that lower pH, production of antimicrobials, such as bacteriocins, antioxidants, production of signaling molecules that trigger changes in gene expression [129].

Probiotics can produce antimicrobial substances such as lactic acid, acetic acid, formic acid, phenyl lactic acid, and benzoic acid, as well as other organic acids, short-chain fatty acids, hydrogen peroxide, carbon dioxide, acetaldehyde, acetoin, diacetyl, bacteriocins, and bacteriocins-like inhibitory substances and others [130]. Lactobacillus strains exert bacteriostatic activity against pathogenic bacteria by strain-specific production of bacteriocins and block the growth of enterovirulent bacteria, including *H. pylori*, EHEC, Shigella, Salmonella, and Campylobacter [131].

The most common bacteriocins include enterocin, enterolysin, lacticin, plantaricin, and nisin, which show bactericidal activity against various Gram-negative and Gram-positive gastric or enterovirulent bacteria like Shigella, *E. coli*, Vibrio cholerae, *etc*. Probiotics strains are also an alternative therapy for the disruption of the natural balance of skin microbiota, and they have a positive effect on host health and skin healing through the production of immune cells. Probiotics inhibit the growth of pathogen's by the release of bioactive molecules which interfere with the pathogen's quorum sensing system, facilitating removal from the skin *via* peristaltic elimination. Probiotics act on the epidermis and dermis by functioning as signaling receptors against pathogens, and they activate the production of beta-defensins and promote wound healing of the skin [132]. Several studies have indicated the positive effects of probiotics on wound healing, various skin problems, surgical site infections by mechanisms mainly included immune modulation including production of TNF –α and IL 10, systemic cellular immune response, modulation of the gene expression of SOCS3, and pathogen inhibition [133].

NANOTECHNOLOGY-BASED ANTI-INFECTIVES TO FIGHT MICROBIAL INTRUSIONS

Nowadays, nanotechnology is emerging as a new strategy to potentiate its therapeutic benefits and circumvent multiple disadvantages of antiviral drugs and antibiotics [134]. In this aspect, a variety of nanoparticles have been investigated to improve the efficacy of various therapeutics for the treatment of infectious diseases [135]. Nanomaterials sizes are of the same order as biomolecules and have a greater surface area to volume ratios, which results in enhanced chemical reactivities and bioactivities. Nanoparticles increase drug solubility/ stability, prolong the circulation time, overcome biological barriers, enhance bioavailability and modulate drug release profiles relevant to pathological changes [136]. Nanoparticle-based strategies reduce resistance development and reverse acquired resistance by changing the route of delivery, conferring antibiofilm effect, modulating the interaction between drug and pathogen, and promoting the uptake of nanoparticles [137].

Also, nanoparticles amplify the activity of adjuvants and antigens, and protect them from degradation by enzymes, and can achieve target delivery in immunity-related tissues, APCs, and subcellular compartments [138]. For achieving desirable immune responses, nanoparticles allow lower doses of vaccines and inhibit the nonspecific immune activation resulting from systemic delivery of soluble antigens [139]. Also, antigens can be delivered at the specific site, thereby generating expected immunity for protection against pathogens [140].

Nanoparticles made of metals act as a promising antimicrobial agent with a broad range of activity and with the ability to integrate into numerous materials such as foams, fibers, plastics, and coating materials [141]. Nanotechnology develops new products and also modifies old ones to enhance the efficacy by loading drugs on nanoparticles through chemical conjugation, physical adsorption, and encapsulation in the polymer. Drugs laded nanoparticles improve the efficiency of drugs through endocytosis for the treatment of microbial infections [142]. Recently, biomimetic strategies in combination with nanotechnology create nanoparticles with optimized surface physicochemical properties for drug delivery and vaccine development [143].

Advantages of using these biomimetic nanoparticles include diversity, tailorability, and reproducibility of synthetic nanomaterials as well as the functionality, complexity, and biocompatibility of biological materials [144]. These nature-inspired nanoparticles can function as effective nanotherapies against infectious diseases and serve as advanced nanocarriers for site-specific delivery of therapeutics.

Nanomaterials for the Infections Control

Nanomaterials can be used for various biomedical applications in managing various diseases. The application of nanoparticles (NPs) provides a potential strategy to manage infections caused by MDROs. Some of them are:

Carbon Nanotubes

Carbon nanotubes (CNTs) have drawn a lot of attention due to their outstanding physical properties and tuneable morphologies [25]. Functionalized carbon nanotubes (f-CNT) are emerging as a new family of nanovectors for therapeutic delivery, proving innovative and efficient for the transport and cellular translocation of therapeutic molecules [19, 26 - 38]. This f-CNT can be prepared with one or more bioactive substances from the group containing peptides, proteins, nucleic acids, and drugs, and can be delivered to cells or organs. CNTs are cylindrical nanostructures consists of hexagonal arrays of covalently bonded carbon atoms. These possess strong antimicrobial activity [145] but have poor solubility [146].

Solubility of CNTs can be enhanced after stabilization by surfactants [147]. Functionalized CNTs is fixed with drug either on the surface or inside. The conjugate obtained is then introduced into the body of the animal by different ways (oral, injection) or directly to the target site through the use of a magnetic conjugate, for example, lymphatic nodes. The cell ingests the drug CNT capsule, and finally, the nanotube spills its contents into the cell, and thus the drug is delivered.

Recently, Venkatesan *et al.* [148] reported chitosan conjugated CNT hydrogel with antimicrobial activity against *Staphylococcus aureus*, Escherichia coli, and Candida tropicalis. CNT can be used as a novel tool for vaccination against cancer and some infectious diseases [149]. According to Orecchioni *et al.* [150], various body cells, including cells of the immune system such as macrophages, monocytes, natural killer, dendritic cells, T and B cells, can uptake the CNTs, but nanotubes do not damage the functionality of these cells [151]. CNTs also have antiparasitic activity against parasitic infections like visceral leishmaniasis, for example, CNTs-Amphotericin B complex drug [152].

CNT functionalized within gelatin fluoroquinolones bioconjugates and dapsone functionalized carboxylated MWCNTs demonstrated the antibacterial activity against *Klebsiella pneumoniae* and *E. coli* [153]. Moreover, pegylated silver-coated SWCNTs were also found effective against food-borne Salmonella species [154].

b. **Fullerenes**: They are carbon engineered nanomaterials, a er-ball-shaped structure composed of 60 carbon atoms with both hydrophobic (C60) and hydrophilic derivatives which help them in better interaction with the cell wall of pathogens. Functionalization of fullerene by hydroxyl groups leads to the formation of polyhydroxy fullerenes (PHFs) and is found to possess antioxidant properties and inhibit allergic response [155]. A coating of polyhydroxyl fullerene and titanium oxide results in the rapid destruction of microbes [156] and can be efficiently used for the treatment of various diseases like cancer therapy, viral infection, *etc*.

Yu *et al.* [157] demonstrated the antibacterial activity of a sulfobutyl fullerene derivative on environmental bacteria, and Mizuno *et al.* [158] demonstrated cationic- substituted fullerene derivative effectivity against broad-spectrum pathogens, including Gram-positive (Staphlyococcus aureus), Gram-negative bacterium (*E. coli*) and fungus (*Candida albicans*). Deryabin *et al.* [159] prepared conjugated fullerene derivatives and compared their antibacterial activity against *E. coli*.

c. **Dendrimers:** Dendrimers are ordered structures with the functional group on the surface of the dendrimers. Substantial antimicrobial activity of the dendrimer is due to the type and size of a functional group [160]. Amino terminated PAMAM dendrimers were found to possess the strongest antibacterial activity as compared to PAMAM-OH and PAMAM-COOH because the amino group promotes the disruption of the bacterial membrane through electrostatic interaction [161]. The development of an coumarin-derived dendrimer for the detection of malaria by detecting the malarial antigen along with FLISA (Fluorescence-linked immunosorbent assay) makes this technique more sensitive and efficient than that of enzyme-linked immunosorbent assay (ELISA) [162]. Recently, biocompatible phloroglucinol succinic acid dendrimer was found to be potential against a Gram-positive bacterium *Staphylococcus aureus*, E. coli, and human pathogenic *C. Albicans* [163].

Nanocomposites

Nanocomposites are organic or inorganic with unique properties [164]. Silver bio-nanocomposites (Ag BNCs) were explored for their antibacterial activity against Gram-negative and Gram-positive bacteria [165]. Chitosan-silver nanocomposites were evaluated for their antimicrobial activity against *Staphylococcus aureus* (MTCC 1809), *Pseudomonas aeruginosa* (MTCC 424), and *Salmonella enterica* (MTCC 1253) [166]. Tobramycin-silver nanocomposite and chitosan–silver oxide encapsulated nanocomposite were demonstrated as novel antimicrobial agents [167] against different antibiotic-resistant microorganisms such as *Staphylococcus aureus*, *Klebsiella pneumoniae*, *Pseudomonas aeruginosa*, *Acinetobacter baumannii*, and *Proteus mirabilis*.

Nanocomposite like Polyacrylamide Ce(IV) silicophosphate (PAM–CSP) has efficient antimicrobial activity against *E. coli* and *Staphylococcus aureus*. Pinto *et al.* (2013) [168] prepared nanocomposites comprising copper nanofillers in cellulose matrices by *in situ* and *ex-situ* methods and studied antibacterial activity of these nanocomposites against *Staphylococcus aureus* and *Klebsiella pneumoniae*. Armentano *et al.* (2014) [169] studied polymeric nanocomposites and surface-engineered materials and antimicrobial modifications of polymers using a nanocomposite approach. It also signifies a promising alternative to classic antibiotic therapies or antimicrobial-coated or loaded biomaterials.

Recently, for the biological treatment of drinking water, chitosan-based nanocomposites have been developed to kill waterborne pathogens. Numerous waterborne pathogens are responsible for the diseases like cholera, hepatitis A, amoebiasis, *etc.* Chitosan-based nanocomposites were developed and incorporated in the membrane filters and used for the treatment of drinking water [170]. This approach of treating wastewater was very efficient in killing the pathogens present and ultimately useful for the management of infections caused due to waterborne pathogens.

e. Metal nanoparticles: Nanoparticles such as silver, copper, titanium, magnesium, gold, and alginate have strong antibacterial capabilities, and silver nanoparticles are used for antibacterial wound dressing. Magnetic nanoparticles, ZnO, and CuO nanomaterials can be used for wound healing and against *Staphylococcus aureus* biofilm Gram-positive, and Gram-negative bacteria [171]. Silver, titanium dioxide, and silica dioxide nanoparticles show efficacy against Streptococcus mutans and *E. coli, Pseudomonas aeruginosa*, and *Staphylococcus aureus* [172]. Nanomedicines are also effective against HIV eradication through nanomaterials-based targeted drug delivery.

PEG-based nanocarriers for delivery of antiretroviral in HIV patients were found to be effective [173]; for example, pentasaccharide conjugated with PEG for the delivery of enfuvirtide (antiviral drug)showed several-fold increases in half-life enabling weekly dosing of the drug and showed strong potency as a novel long-lasting anti-HIV-1 drug.

Polyvinyl alcohol-melamine formaldehyde films coated with silver nanoparticles were developed for foot ulcers in diabetic patients [174]. These dressings showed potential antibacterial activity against *Staphylococcus aureus*, Proteus Vulgaris, *Pseudomonas aeruginosa*, and *E. cloacae* species isolated from wound samples.

Antibiotic-resistant pathogens show sensitivity against silver nanoparticles making them stable and enhances their antimicrobial efficacy for a longer duration. Similarly, chitosan stabilized silver nanoparticles in conjugation with antibiotics fabricated the wound dressings [175]. To prevent biofilm formation over the surface of the dental materials silver nanoparticles are used frequently nowadays to reduce dental infections such as Streptococcus mutans and Lactobacillus spp [176].

Recently, modified antimicrobial restorative materials incorporated with silver nanoparticles have been developed for the reduction of infections from organisms causing a dental problem. Modification of metal nanoparticles enhances their bioactivity. For example, simple magnetic (Fe_3O_4) nanoparticles with PAMAM showed considerably good antimicrobial activity against Staph. aureus and *E. coli* [177].

Mechanism of Nanoparticles Against Bacteria

NPs, to achieve their antibacterial function, need to be in contact with bacterial cells through van der Waals forces, electrostatic attraction, receptor-ligand, and hydrophobic interactions. After contact, NPs can cross the bacterial membrane, influencing the shape and function of the cell membrane, interacting with the bacterial cell's basic components, and leading to oxidative stress, alterations, disorders, inhibition, deactivation, and changes in gene expression.

The following mechanisms are:

a. Oxidative stress: An important antibacterial mechanism of NPs is ROS-induced oxidative stress. ROS are reactive intermediates that have strong positive redox potential. The four types of ROS which exhibit different levels of dynamics and activity include superoxide radical, hydroxyl radical, hydrogen peroxide, and singlet oxygen. For example, O_2^- is generated by magnesium and calcium oxide NPs, whereas H_2O_2 and OH are generated by zinc oxide NPs. The produced O_2^- and H_2O_2 cause less acute stress reactions, whereas OH and O_2 can lead to acute microbial death [178].

Oxidative stress causes a change in the permeability of the cell membrane, which induces bacterial cell membrane damage. Nanosilver ions can activate the oxygen in air or water, leading to the production of hydroxyl radicals and reactive oxygen ions and preventing the proliferation of bacteria [179] Also, ROS can attack proteins and depress the activity of enzymes carried out some physiological processes in bacterial cells. ROS can be produced from NPs by different mechanisms like the photocatalytic method, resulting in the production of reactive reactants [180] that attack intracellular organic matter in bacteria. Another method of ROS production is ultrasonic activation, in which NPS can split water into ions and react with dissolved oxygen to generate H_2O_2 in an environment containing water and oxygen and penetrate the cell membrane to kill bacteria.

b. Dissolved Metal Ions: Metal oxide produces ions that slowly release and absorb through the cell membrane, followed by direct interaction with the functional groups of proteins and nucleic acids, leading to the damage to enzyme activity change in cell structure and ultimately inhibiting the microorganism [181].

c. Non-oxidative Mechanisms: MgO NPs have good antibacterial effects on *E. coli* under UV light, natural light, or complete darkness and are unrelated to the membrane lipid peroxidation caused by oxidative stress.

There are three approaches:

1) When the bacterial cell membrane is broken and surface pores are visible, MgO NPs are not observed in the cell, and no excessive Mg ions are visible in X-ray

spectroscopy spectra, resulting in damage to the cell membrane.

2) Only one type of MgO NP can detect small amounts of ROS, the other two cannot.

3) Lipopolysaccharide (LPS) and phosphatidylethanolamine (PE) in the cell wall are not significantly changed by MgO NP treatment, which indicates that MgO does not cause lipid peroxidation. In addition, the amount of ROS-associated protein in the cell is not increased, but many critical cellular metabolic processes related to proteins, including amino acid metabolism, carbohydrate metabolism, energy metabolism, and nucleotide metabolism, are significantly reduced [182]

Antiviral Mechanism of Nanoparticles

Virus infection mainly consists of attachment, penetration, replication, and budding, while antiviral nanoparticles inhibit viruses by blocking or suppressing some of these steps. The major way to suppress viruses is to inactivate them and change their capsid protein structure, which then dramatically reduce virulence. Viral infections proceed with attachment to host cells, by binding to the target receptor protein; however, nanoparticles can inhibit this attachment. For example, antiviral nanoparticles with heparan sulfate proteoglycans (Viral attachment ligands) can achieve efficient viral prevention through effective viral association with a binding simulated to be strong and multivalent to the VAL repeating units [183].

Another way to suppress viruses is to block their penetration and entry to host cells by changing the cell surface membrane and protein structures. For example, water-soluble fullerene- polyglycerol sulfates (FPS) with polyglycerol sulfate branches prevent interaction of vesicular stomatitis virus coat glycoprotein in baby hamster kidney cells.

On entry of the virus into the cell, destroying their replication machinery is the third effective strategy to inhibit the virus. This can be achieved by suppressing the expression of certain enzymes involved in the replication of virus DNA or RNA. The final strategy is to inhibit virus budding and excrete it from host cells. The offspring of a virus may be more virulent than its mother, and if functional nanoparticles prevent the virus from budding, it will be helpful in greatly reducing the number of offspring viruses.

CONCLUSION

Due to increasing MDR among microbes in this present era to many antibiotics, it is becoming very difficult to fight against diseases that cause mortality. Therefore, the exploration of novel approaches toward the improvement of human life should be focused on. It is evident that the search for alternatives for the treatment and control of microbial diseases is a complex path. According to the scientific reports presented in this chapter, it may be concluded that the application of nanotechnology in drug delivery systems has enormous potential and can be considered as an effective alternative for treatment in the near future.

CONSENT FOR PUBLICATION

Not Applicable.

CONFLICT OF INTEREST

The author declares no conflict of interest, financial or otherwise.

ACKNOWLEDGEMENTS

Declared none.

LIST OF ABBREVIATIONS

DALY	Disability-adjusted life years
DNA	Deoxyribonucleic Acid
WHO	World Health Organization
HIV	Human immunodeficiency virus
TB	Tuberculosis
MDR	Multi Drug Resistance
NP	Nanoparticle
DHFR	Dihydrofolate reductase
PDR	Pan Drug resistance
XDR	Extensively-drug resistant strains
AMR	Antimicrobial Resistance
ESBLs	Extended spectrum beta-lactamases
WWTPs	Wastewater treatment plants
ROI	Reactive Oxygen Intermediates
RNI	Reactive Nitrogen Intermediates
NADPH	Nicotinamide adenine dinucleotide phosphate
ROS	Reactive Oxygen Species
PACT	Photodynamic antimicrobial chemotherapy
PDT	Photodynamic therapy

NO	Nitric Oxide
TLR	Toll-like receptors
CD	Cluster of differentiation
NK	Natural Killer
LPS	Lipo Poly Saccharide
IFN	Interferon
HCV	hepatitis C virus
HBV	hepatitis B virus
CSF	Colony Stimulating factors
GMCSF	Granulocyte-macrophage Colony Stimulating factors
HSV	Herpes Simplex Virus
EBV	Epstein-Barr virus (EBV
RTI	Respiratory tract infections
AMP	Antimicrobial Peptides
HDP	Host defense peptides
IDR	Innate defense regulatory peptides
HCMV	Human cytomegalovirus
AIDS	Acquired immune deficiency syndrome
RNA	Ribonucleic acid
MAB	Monoclonal Antibody
HPV	Human papillomavirus
NEC	Necrotizing enterocolitis
EHEC	Enterohemorrhagic E.Coli
TNF	Tumor Necrosis Factor
CNT	Carbon Nanotubes
SWNTs	Single-walled nanotubes
MWNT	Multi-walled nanotubes
PHFs	polyhydroxy fullerenes
PAMAM	Polyamidoamine dendrimers
FLISA	Fluorescence-linked immunosorbent assay
ELISA	enzyme-linked immunosorbent assay
VAL	Viral attachment ligands
FPS	fullerene-polyglycerol sulfates

REFERENCES

[1] Mathers CD, Ezzati M, Lopez AD. Measuring the burden of neglected tropical diseases: the global burden of disease framework. PLoS Negl Trop Dis 2007; 1(2) e114
[http://dx.doi.org/10.1371/journal.pntd.0000114] [PMID: 18060077]

[2] Hsueh PR. New Delhi metallo-ß-lactamase-1 (NDM-1): an emerging threat among Enterobacteriaceae. J Formos Med Assoc 2010; 109(10): 685-7.
[http://dx.doi.org/10.1016/S0929-6646(10)60111-8] [PMID: 21033522]

[3] Poole K. Mechanisms of bacterial biocide and antibiotic resistance. J Appl Microbiol 2002; 92 (Suppl.): 55S-64S.
[http://dx.doi.org/10.1046/j.1365-2672.92.5s1.8.x] [PMID: 12000613]

[4] Jayaraman R. Antibiotic resistance: an overview of mechanisms and a paradigm shift. Curr Sci India 2009; 96(11): 1475-84.

[5] World Health Statistics on World Wide Web URL. www.who.int/whosis/whostat/2008/en/index.html

[6] Zhang L, Pfister M, Meibohm B. Concepts and challenges in quantitative pharmacology and model-based drug development. AAPS J 2008; 10(4): 552-9.
[http://dx.doi.org/10.1208/s12248-008-9062-3] [PMID: 19003542]

[7] Cui L, Su XZ. Discovery, mechanisms of action and combination therapy of artemisinin. Expert Rev Anti Infect Ther 2009; 7(8): 999-1013.
[http://dx.doi.org/10.1586/eri.09.68] [PMID: 19803708]

[8] Zaffiri L, Gardner J, Toledo-Pereyra LH. History of antibiotics. From salvarsan to cephalosporins. J Invest Surg 2012; 25(2): 67-77.
[http://dx.doi.org/10.3109/08941939.2012.664099] [PMID: 22439833]

[9] Nicolaou KC, Rigol S. A brief history of antibiotics and select advances in their synthesis. J Antibiot (Tokyo) 2018; 71(2): 153-84.
[http://dx.doi.org/10.1038/ja.2017.62] [PMID: 28676714]

[10] Kresge N, Simoni RD, Hill RL. Selman Waksman: The Father of Antibiotics. J Biol Chem 2004; 279 e7
[http://dx.doi.org/10.1016/S0021-9258(20)67861-9]

[11] Wong RW, Hägg U, Samaranayake L, Yuen MK, Seneviratne CJ, Kao R. Antimicrobial activity of Chinese medicine herbs against common bacteria in oral biofilm. A pilot study. Int J Oral Maxillofac Surg 2010; 39(6): 599-605.
[http://dx.doi.org/10.1016/j.ijom.2010.02.024] [PMID: 20418062]

[12] Aminov RI, Mackie RI. Evolution and ecology of antibiotic resistance genes. FEMS Microbiol Lett 2007; 271(2): 147-61.
[http://dx.doi.org/10.1111/j.1574-6968.2007.00757.x] [PMID: 17490428]

[13] Prestinaci F, Pezzotti P, Pantosti A. Antimicrobial resistance: a global multifaceted phenomenon. Pathog Glob Health 2015; 109(7): 309-18.
[http://dx.doi.org/10.1179/2047773215Y.0000000030] [PMID: 26343252]

[14] World Health Organization. WHO global strategy for containment of antimicrobial resistance. Geneva: WHO 2001.

[15] World Health Organization. The evolving threat of antimicrobial resistance Options for action. Geneva: WHO Library Cataloguing-in-Publication Data 2012.

[16] World Health Organization. Antimicrobial resistance: global report on surveillance 2014. Geneva, Switzerland: WHO 2014.

[17] Maciá MD, Blanquer D, Togores B, Sauleda J, Pérez JL, Oliver A. Hypermutation is a key factor *Role of antibiotics and antibiotic resistance* in development of multiple-antimicrobial resistance in *Pseudomonas aeruginosa* strains causing chronic lung infections. Antimicrob Agents Chemother

2005; 49: 3382-6.
[http://dx.doi.org/10.1128/AAC.49.8.3382-3386.2005] [PMID: 16048951]

[18]   Lee HH, Molla MN, Cantor CR, Collins JJ. Bacterial charity work leads to population-wide resistance. Nature 2010; 467(7311): 82-5.
[http://dx.doi.org/10.1038/nature09354] [PMID: 20811456]

[19]   Centres for Disease Control and Prevention, US Department of Health and Human Services. Antibiotic resistance threats in the United States. Atlanta: CDC 2013.

[20]   ECDC/EMEA. The bacterial challenge: time to react. Stockholm: European Center for Disease Prevention and Control 2009.

[21]   Ibrahim OM, Polk RE. Benchmarking antimicrobial drug use in hospitals. Expert Rev Anti Infect Ther 2012; 10(4): 445-57.
[http://dx.doi.org/10.1586/eri.12.18] [PMID: 22512754]

[22]   Marshall BM, Levy SB. Food animals and antimicrobials: impacts on human health. Clin Microbiol Rev 2011; 24(4): 718-33.
[http://dx.doi.org/10.1128/CMR.00002-11] [PMID: 21976606]

[23]   Stockwell VO, Duffy B. Use of antibiotics in plant agriculture. Rev Sci Tech 2012; 31(1): 199-210.
[http://dx.doi.org/10.20506/rst.31.1.2104] [PMID: 22849276]

[24]   Novo A, André S, Viana P, Nunes OC, Manaia CM. Antibiotic resistance, antimicrobial residues and bacterial community composition in urban wastewater. Water Res 2013; 47(5): 1875-87.
[http://dx.doi.org/10.1016/j.watres.2013.01.010] [PMID: 23375783]

[25]   Grigoryan L, Burgerhof JG, Degener JE, *et al.* Attitudes, beliefs and knowledge concerning antibiotic use and self-medication: a comparative European study. Pharmacoepidemiol Drug Saf 2007; 16(11): 1234-43.
[http://dx.doi.org/10.1002/pds.1479] [PMID: 17879325]

[26]   Gartin M, Brewis AA, Schwartz NA. Nonprescription antibiotic therapy: cultural models on both sides of the counter and both sides of the border. Med Anthropol Q 2010; 24(1): 85-107.
[http://dx.doi.org/10.1111/j.1548-1387.2010.01086.x] [PMID: 20420303]

[27]   Bengtsson B, Wierup M. Antimicrobial resistance in Scandina*via*after ban of antimicrobial growth promoters. Anim Biotechnol 2006; 17(2): 147-56.
[http://dx.doi.org/10.1080/10495390600956920] [PMID: 17127526]

[28]   Li Y, Zhang Y. PhoU is a persistence switch involved in persister formation and tolerance to multiple antibiotics and stresses in *Escherichia coli.* Antimicrob Agents Chemother 2007; 51(6): 2092-9.
[http://dx.doi.org/10.1128/AAC.00052-07] [PMID: 17420206]

[29]   Ejim L, Farha MA, Falconer SB, *et al.* Combinations of antibiotics and nonantibiotic drugs enhance antimicrobial efficacy. Nat Chem Biol 2011; 7(6): 348-50.
[http://dx.doi.org/10.1038/nchembio.559] [PMID: 21516114]

[30]   Francolini I, Donelli G. Prevention and control of biofilm-based medical-device-related infections 2010.
[http://dx.doi.org/10.1111/j.1574-695X.2010.00665.x]

[31]   Cai W, Wu J, Xi C, Ashe AJ III, Meyerhoff ME. Carboxyl-ebselen-based layer-by-layer films as potential antithrombotic and antimicrobial coatings. Biomaterials 2011; 32(31): 7774-84.
[http://dx.doi.org/10.1016/j.biomaterials.2011.06.075] [PMID: 21794909]

[32]   Silver LL. Challenges of antibacterial discovery. Clin Microbiol Rev 2011; 24(1): 71-109.
[http://dx.doi.org/10.1128/CMR.00030-10] [PMID: 21233508]

[33]   Nathan C, Shiloh MU. Reactive oxygen and nitrogen intermediates in the relationship between mammalian hosts and microbial pathogens. Proc Natl Acad Sci USA 2000; 97(16): 8841-8.
[http://dx.doi.org/10.1073/pnas.97.16.8841] [PMID: 10922044]

[34] Singh R, Manjunatha U, Boshoff HI, *et al.* PA-824 kills nonreplicating *Mycobacterium tuberculosis* by intracellular NO release. Science 2008; 322(5906): 1392-5.
[http://dx.doi.org/10.1126/science.1164571] [PMID: 19039139]

[35] Kalyanaraman B, Darley-Usmar V, Davies KJ, *et al.* Measuring reactive oxygen and nitrogen species with fluorescent probes: challenges and limitations. Free Radic Biol Med 2012; 52(1): 1-6.
[http://dx.doi.org/10.1016/j.freeradbiomed.2011.09.030] [PMID: 22027063]

[36] Winterbourn CC, Hampton MB, Livesey JH, Kettle AJ. Modeling the reactions of superoxide and myeloperoxidase in the neutrophil phagosome: implications for microbial killing. J Biol Chem 2006; 281(52): 39860-9.
[http://dx.doi.org/10.1074/jbc.M605898200] [PMID: 17074761]

[37] Singh H, Khurana H, Singh H, Singh M. Photodynamic therapy: truly a marriage between a drug and a light. Muller Journal of Medical Sciences and Research 2014; 5: 48-55.
[http://dx.doi.org/10.4103/0975-9727.128946]

[38] Diogo P, Goncalves Y, Palma P, Santos JM. Photodynamic antimicrobial chemotherapy for root canal system asepsis: a narrative literature review. 2015.

[39] Nathan C. Nitric oxide as a secretory product of mammalian cells. FASEB J 1992; 6(12): 3051-64.
[http://dx.doi.org/10.1096/fasebj.6.12.1381691] [PMID: 1381691]

[40] Long R, Light B, Talbot JA. Mycobacteriocidal action of exogenous nitric oxide. Antimicrob Agents Chemother 1999; 43(2): 403-5.
[http://dx.doi.org/10.1128/AAC.43.2.403] [PMID: 9925545]

[41] Creagh EM, O'Neill LA. TLRs, NLRs and RLRs: a trinity of pathogen sensors that co-operate in innate immunity. Trends Immunol 2006; 27(8): 352-7.
[http://dx.doi.org/10.1016/j.it.2006.06.003] [PMID: 16807108]

[42] Casadevall A, Pirofski LA. The damage-response framework of microbial pathogenesis. Nat Rev Microbiol 2003; 1(1): 17-24.
[http://dx.doi.org/10.1038/nrmicro732] [PMID: 15040176]

[43] Finlay BB, McFadden G. Anti-immunology: evasion of the host immune system by bacterial and viral pathogens. Cell 2006; 124(4): 767-82.
[http://dx.doi.org/10.1016/j.cell.2006.01.034] [PMID: 16497587]

[44] Cantin R, Méthot S, Tremblay MJ. Plunder and stowaways: incorporation of cellular proteins by enveloped viruses. J Virol 2005; 79(11): 6577-87.
[http://dx.doi.org/10.1128/JVI.79.11.6577-6587.2005] [PMID: 15890896]

[45] Perfettini JL, Castedo M, Roumier T, *et al.* Mechanisms of apoptosis induction by the HIV-1 envelope. Cell Death Differ 2005; 12 (Suppl. 1): 916-23.
[http://dx.doi.org/10.1038/sj.cdd.4401584] [PMID: 15719026]

[46] Madden JC, Ruiz N, Caparon M. Cytolysin-mediated translocation (CMT): a functional equivalent of type III secretion in gram-positive bacteria. Cell 2001; 104(1): 143-52.
[http://dx.doi.org/10.1016/S0092-8674(01)00198-2] [PMID: 11163247]

[47] Lucas A, McFadden G. Secreted immunomodulatory viral proteins as novel biotherapeutics. J Immunol 2004; 173(8): 4765-74.
[http://dx.doi.org/10.4049/jimmunol.173.8.4765] [PMID: 15470015]

[48] Lodoen MB, Lanier LL. Viral modulation of NK cell immunity. Nat Rev Microbiol 2005; 3(1): 59-69.
[http://dx.doi.org/10.1038/nrmicro1066] [PMID: 15608700]

[49] Portnoy DA. Manipulation of innate immunity by bacterial pathogens. Curr Opin Immunol 2005; 17(1): 25-8.
[http://dx.doi.org/10.1016/j.coi.2004.11.002] [PMID: 15653306]

[50] Cossart P, Helenius A. Endocytosis of viruses and bacteria. Cold Spring Harb Perspect Biol 2014; 6(8)

a016972
[http://dx.doi.org/10.1101/cshperspect.a016972] [PMID: 25085912]

[51] Foley J. Mini-review: strategies for variation and evolution of bacterial antigens. Comput Struct Biotechnol J 2015; 13: 407-16.
[http://dx.doi.org/10.1016/j.csbj.2015.07.002] [PMID: 26288700]

[52] Bilu D, Sauder DN. Imiquimod: modes of action. Br J Dermatol 2003; 149 (Suppl. 66): 5-8.
[http://dx.doi.org/10.1046/j.0366-077X.2003.05628.x] [PMID: 14616337]

[53] Cederlund A, Gudmundsson GH, Agerberth B. Antimicrobial peptides important in innate immunity. FEBS J 2011; 278(20): 3942-51.
[http://dx.doi.org/10.1111/j.1742-4658.2011.08302.x] [PMID: 21848912]

[54] Manzo G, Carboni M, Rinaldi AC, Casu M, Scorciapino MA. Characterization of sodium dodecylsulphate and dodecylphosphocholine mixed micelles through NMR and dynamic light scattering. Magn Reson Chem 2013; 51(3): 176-83.
[http://dx.doi.org/10.1002/mrc.3930] [PMID: 23364831]

[55] Scorciapino MA, Rinaldi AC. Antimicrobial peptidomimetics: reinterpreting nature to deliver innovative therapeutics. Front Immunol 2012; 3: 171.
[http://dx.doi.org/10.3389/fimmu.2012.00171] [PMID: 22798960]

[56] Hilchie AL, Wuerth K, Hancock REW. Immune modulation by multifaceted cationic host defense (antimicrobial) peptides. Nat Chem Biol 2013; 9(12): 761-8.
[http://dx.doi.org/10.1038/nchembio.1393] [PMID: 24231617]

[57] Hassan M, Kjos M, Nes IF, Diep DB, Lotfipour F. Natural antimicrobial peptides from bacteria: characteristics and potential applications to fight against antibiotic resistance. J Appl Microbiol 2012; 113(4): 723-36.
[http://dx.doi.org/10.1111/j.1365-2672.2012.05338.x] [PMID: 22583565]

[58] Stach M, Siriwardena TN, Köhler T, van Delden C, Darbre T, Reymond JL. Combining topology and sequence design for the discovery of potent antimicrobial peptide dendrimers against multidrug-resistant *Pseudomonas aeruginosa*. Angew Chem Int Ed Engl 2014; 53(47): 12827-31.
[http://dx.doi.org/10.1002/anie.201409270] [PMID: 25346278]

[59] Scorciapino MA, Pirri G, Vargiu AV, *et al.* A novel dendrimeric peptide with antimicrobial properties: structure-function analysis of SB056. Biophys J 2012; 102(5): 1039-48.
[http://dx.doi.org/10.1016/j.bpj.2012.01.048] [PMID: 22404926]

[60] Bahar AA, Liu Z, Totsingan F, Buitrago C, Kallenbach N, Ren D. Synthetic dendrimeric peptide active against biofilm and persister cells of *Pseudomonas aeruginosa*. Appl Microbiol Biotechnol 2015; 99(19): 8125-35.
[http://dx.doi.org/10.1007/s00253-015-6645-7] [PMID: 26012420]

[61] Luganini A, Giuliani A, Pirri G, Pizzuto L, Landolfo S, Gribaudo G. Peptide-derivatized dendrimers inhibit human cytomegalovirus infection by blocking virus binding to cell surface heparan sulfate. Antiviral Res 2010; 85(3): 532-40.
[http://dx.doi.org/10.1016/j.antiviral.2010.01.003] [PMID: 20083141]

[62] Luganini A, Nicoletto SF, Pizzuto L, *et al.* Inhibition of herpes simplex virus type 1 and type 2 infections by peptide-derivatized dendrimers. Antimicrob Agents Chemother 2011; 55(7): 3231-9.
[http://dx.doi.org/10.1128/AAC.00149-11] [PMID: 21576438]

[63] Zieli ´ nska, P.; Staniszewska, M.; Bondaryk, M.; Koronkiewicz, M.; Urba'nczyk-Lipkowska, Z. Design and studies of multiple mechanism of anti-Candida activity of a new potent Trp-rich peptide dendrimers. Eur J Med Chem 2015; 105: 106-19.
[http://dx.doi.org/10.1016/j.ejmech.2015.10.013]

[64] Lee TH, Hall KN, Aguilar MI. Antimicrobial Peptide Structure and Mechanism of Action: A Focus on the Role of Membrane Structure. Curr Top Med Chem 2016; 16(1): 25-39.

[http://dx.doi.org/10.2174/1568026615666150703121700] [PMID: 26139112]

[65] Guha S, Ghimire J, Wu E, Wimley WC. Mechanistic Landscape of Membrane-Permeabilizing Peptides. Chem Rev 2019; 119(9): 6040-85.
[http://dx.doi.org/10.1021/acs.chemrev.8b00520] [PMID: 30624911]

[66] Sani M-A, Whitwell TC, Gehman JD, *et al.* Maculatin 1.1 disrupts *Staphylococcus aureus* lipid membranes *via* a pore mechanism. Antimicrob Agents Chemother 2013; 57(8): 3593-600.
[http://dx.doi.org/10.1128/AAC.00195-13] [PMID: 23689707]

[67] Mishra AK, Choi J, Moon E, Baek K-H. Tryptophan-Rich and Proline-Rich Antimicrobial Peptides. Molecules 2018; 23(4): 815.
[http://dx.doi.org/10.3390/molecules23040815] [PMID: 29614844]

[68] Marchand C, Krajewski K, Lee H-F, *et al.* Covalent binding of the natural antimicrobial peptide indolicidin to DNA abasic sites. Nucleic Acids Res 2006; 34(18): 5157-65.
[http://dx.doi.org/10.1093/nar/gkl667] [PMID: 16998183]

[69] Le CF, Fang C-M, Sekaran SD. Intracellular Targeting Mechanisms by Antimicrobial Peptides. Antimicrob Agents Chemother 2017; 61(4): e02340-16.
[http://dx.doi.org/10.1128/AAC.02340-16] [PMID: 28167546]

[70] Gusman H, Travis J, Helmerhorst EJ, Potempa J, Troxler RF, Oppenheim FG. Salivary histatin 5 is an inhibitor of both host and bacterial enzymes implicated in periodontal disease. Infect Immun 2001; 69(3): 1402-8.
[http://dx.doi.org/10.1128/IAI.69.3.1402-1408.2001] [PMID: 11179305]

[71] Yadavalli SS, Carey JN, Leibman RS, *et al.* Antimicrobial peptides trigger a division block in *Escherichia coli* through stimulation of a signalling system. Nat Commun 2016; 7: 12340.
[http://dx.doi.org/10.1038/ncomms12340] [PMID: 27471053]

[72] Sun Y, Shang D. Inhibitory E_ects of Antimicrobial Peptides on Lipopolysaccharide-Induced Inflammation. Mediat. Inflamm 2015; p. 167572.

[73] Gordon YJ, Romanowski EG, McDermott AM. A review of antimicrobial peptides and their therapeutic potential as anti-infective drugs. Curr Eye Res 2005; 30(7): 505-15.
[http://dx.doi.org/10.1080/02713680590968637] [PMID: 16020284]

[74] Berditsch M, Jäger T, Strempel N, Schwartz T, Overhage J, Ulrich AS. Synergistic effect of membrane-active peptides polymyxin B and gramicidin S on multidrug-resistant strains and biofilms of *Pseudomonas aeruginosa*. Antimicrob Agents Chemother 2015; 59(9): 5288-96.
[http://dx.doi.org/10.1128/AAC.00682-15] [PMID: 26077259]

[75] Awais M, Shah AA, Hameed A, Hasan F. Isolation, identification and optimization of Bacitracin produced by *Bacillus* sp. Pak J Bot 2007; 39: 1303-12.

[76] Humphries RM, Pollett S, Sakoulas G. A current perspective on daptomycin for the clinical microbiologist. Clin Microbiol Rev 2013; 26(4): 759-80.
[http://dx.doi.org/10.1128/CMR.00030-13] [PMID: 24092854]

[77] Ovchinnikova TV, Balandin SV, Aleshina GM, *et al.* Aurelin, a novel antimicrobial peptide from jellyfish *Aurelia aurita* with structural features of defensins and channel-blocking toxins. Biochem Biophys Res Commun 2006; 348(2): 514-23.
[http://dx.doi.org/10.1016/j.bbrc.2006.07.078] [PMID: 16890198]

[78] Lee JU, Kang DI, Zhu WL, Shin SY, Hahm KS, Kim Y. Solution structures and biological functions of the antimicrobial peptide, arenicin-1, and its linear derivative. Biopolymers 2007; 88(2): 208-16.
[http://dx.doi.org/10.1002/bip.20700] [PMID: 17285588]

[79] Desjardine K, Pereira A, Wright H, Matainaho T, Kelly M, Andersen RJ. Tauramamide, a lipopeptide antibiotic produced in culture by *Brevibacillus laterosporus* isolated from a marine habitat: structure elucidation and synthesis. J Nat Prod 2007; 70(12): 1850-3.
[http://dx.doi.org/10.1021/np070209r] [PMID: 18044840]

[80] Wang KJ, Huang WS, Yang M, *et al.* A male-specific expression gene, encodes a novel anionic antimicrobial peptide, scygonadin, in *Scylla serrata.* Mol Immunol 2007; 44(8): 1961-8.
[http://dx.doi.org/10.1016/j.molimm.2006.09.036] [PMID: 17092560]

[81] D'Auria MV, Sepe V, D'Orsi R, Bellotta F, Debitus C, Zampella A. Isolation and structural elucidation of callipeltins J–M: Antifungal peptides from the marine sponge *Latrunculia* sp. Tetrahedron 2007; 63: 131-40.
[http://dx.doi.org/10.1016/j.tet.2006.10.032]

[82] Plaza A, Gustchina E, Baker HL, Kelly M, Bewley CA. Mirabamides A-D, depsipeptides from the sponge *Siliquariaspongia mirabilis* that inhibit HIV-1 fusion. J Nat Prod 2007; 70(11): 1753-60.
[http://dx.doi.org/10.1021/np070306k] [PMID: 17963357]

[83] Klein GO. [Bacteriophage therapy can be the rescue when antibiotics no longer work]. Lakartidningen 2009; 106(40): 2530-3.
[PMID: 19908622]

[84] Ahmad SI. Treatment of post-burns bacterial infections by bacteriophages, specifically ubiquitous *Pseudomonas* spp. notoriously resistant to antibiotics. Med Hypotheses 2002; 58(4): 327-31.
[http://dx.doi.org/10.1054/mehy.2001.1522] [PMID: 12027527]

[85] Biswas B, Adhya S, Washart P, *et al.* Bacteriophage therapy rescues mice bacteremic from a clinical isolate of vancomycin-resistant *Enterococcus faecium.* Infect Immun 2002; 70(1): 204-10.
[http://dx.doi.org/10.1128/IAI.70.1.204-210.2002] [PMID: 11748184]

[86] O'Flaherty S, Ross RP, Meaney W, Fitzgerald GF, Elbreki MF, Coffey A. Potential of the polyvalent anti-Staphylococcus bacteriophage K for control of antibiotic-resistant *staphylococci* from hospitals. Appl Environ Microbiol 2005; 71(4): 1836-42.
[http://dx.doi.org/10.1128/AEM.71.4.1836-1842.2005] [PMID: 15812009]

[87] Vinodkumar CS, Neelagund YF, Kalsurmath S. Bacteriophage in the treatment of experimental septicemic mice from a clinical isolate of multidrug resistant *Klebsiella pneumoniae.* J Commun Dis 2005; 37(1): 18-29.
[PMID: 16637396]

[88] Wang J, Hu B, Xu M, *et al.* Use of bacteriophage in the treatment of experimental animal bacteremia from imipenem-resistant *Pseudomonas aeruginosa.* Int J Mol Med 2006; 17(2): 309-17.
[http://dx.doi.org/10.3892/ijmm.17.2.309] [PMID: 16391831]

[89] Wright A, Hawkins C H, Anggard E E, Harper D R. D. R. A controlled clinical trial of a therapeutic bacteriophage preparation in chronic otitis due to antibiotic-resistant *Pseudomonas aeruginosa*; a preliminary report of efficacy. Clinical Otolaryngology, 2009, 34(4), 349□357, 2009..

[90] Viscardi M, Perugini AG, Auriemma C, *et al.* Isolation and characterisation of two novel coliphages with high potential to control antibiotic-resistant pathogenic *Escherichia coli* (EHEC and EPEC). Int J Antimicrob Agents 2008; 31(2): 152-7.
[http://dx.doi.org/10.1016/j.ijantimicag.2007.09.007] [PMID: 18082374]

[91] Mann NH. The potential of phages to prevent MRSA infections. Res Microbiol 2008; 159(5): 400-5.
[http://dx.doi.org/10.1016/j.resmic.2008.04.003] [PMID: 18541414]

[92] Hermoso JA, García JL, García P. Taking aim on bacterial pathogens: from phage therapy to enzybiotics. Curr Opin Microbiol 2007; 10(5): 461-72.
[http://dx.doi.org/10.1016/j.mib.2007.08.002] [PMID: 17904412]

[93] Skurnik M, Strauch E. Phage therapy: facts and fiction. Int J Med Microbiol 2006; 296(1): 5-14.
[http://dx.doi.org/10.1016/j.ijmm.2005.09.002] [PMID: 16423684]

[94] Connerton PL, Timms AR, Connerton IF. Campylobacter bacteriophages and bacteriophage therapy. J Appl Microbiol 2011; 111(2): 255-65.
[http://dx.doi.org/10.1111/j.1365-2672.2011.05012.x] [PMID: 21447013]

[95] Siringan P, Connerton PL, Payne RJ, Connerton IF. Bacteriophage-mediated dispersal of *Campylobacter jejuni* biofilms. Appl Environ Microbiol 2011; 77(10): 3320-6.
[http://dx.doi.org/10.1128/AEM.02704-10] [PMID: 21441325]

[96] Morello E, Saussereau E, Maura D, Huerre M, Touqui L, Debarbieux L. Pulmonary bacteriophage therapy on *Pseudomonas aeruginosa* cystic fibrosis strains: first steps towards treatment and prevention. PLoS One 2011; 6(2) e16963
[http://dx.doi.org/10.1371/journal.pone.0016963] [PMID: 21347240]

[97] Fineran PC, Blower TR, Foulds IJ, Humphreys DP, Lilley KS, Salmond GPC. The phage abortive infection system, ToxIN, functions as a protein-RNA toxin-antitoxin pair. Proc Natl Acad Sci USA 2009; 106(3): 894-9.
[http://dx.doi.org/10.1073/pnas.0808832106] [PMID: 19124776]

[98] Slopek S, Kucharewicz-Krukowska A, Weber-Dabrowska B, Dabrowski M. Results of bacteriophage treatment of suppurative bacterial infections. V. Evaluation of the results obtained in children. Arch Immunol Ther Exp (Warsz) 1985; 33(2): 241-59.
[PMID: 2935116]

[99] Weber-Dabrowska B, Mulczyk M, Górski A. Bacteriophage therapy of bacterial infections: an update of our institute's experience. Arch Immunol Ther Exp (Warsz) 2000; 48(6): 547-51.
[PMID: 11197610]

[100] Weber-Dabrowska B, Mulczyk M, Górski A. Bacteriophages as an efficient therapy for antibiotic-resistant septicemia in man. Transplant Proc 2003; 35(4): 1385-6.
[http://dx.doi.org/10.1016/S0041-1345(03)00525-6] [PMID: 12826166]

[101] Loessner MJ, Kramer K, Ebel F, Scherer S. C-terminal domains of *Listeria monocytogenes* bacteriophage murein hydrolases determine specific recognition and high-affinity binding to bacterial cell wall carbohydrates. Mol Microbiol 2002; 44(2): 335-49.
[http://dx.doi.org/10.1046/j.1365-2958.2002.02889.x] [PMID: 11972774]

[102] Wang IN, Smith DL, Young R. Holins: the protein clocks of bacteriophage infections. Annu Rev Microbiol 2000; 54: 799-825.
[http://dx.doi.org/10.1146/annurev.micro.54.1.799] [PMID: 11018145]

[103] Oliveira H, Melo LD, Santos SB, *et al.* Molecular aspects and comparative genomics of bacteriophage endolysins. J Virol 2013; 87(8): 4558-70.
[http://dx.doi.org/10.1128/JVI.03277-12] [PMID: 23408602]

[104] Nelson D, Loomis L, Fischetti VA. Prevention and elimination of upper respiratory colonization of mice by group A streptococci by using a bacteriophage lytic enzyme. Proc Natl Acad Sci USA 2001; 98(7): 4107-12.
[http://dx.doi.org/10.1073/pnas.061038398] [PMID: 11259652]

[105] Yoong P, Schuch R, Nelson D, Fischetti VA. PlyPH, a bacteriolytic enzyme with a broad pH range of activity and lytic action against *Bacillus anthracis*. J Bacteriol 2006; 188(7): 2711-4.
[http://dx.doi.org/10.1128/JB.188.7.2711-2714.2006] [PMID: 16547060]

[106] Yoong P, Schuch R, Nelson D, Fischetti VA. Identification of a broadly active phage lytic enzyme with lethal activity against antibiotic-resistant *Enterococcus faecalis* and *Enterococcus faecium*. J Bacteriol 2004; 186(14): 4808-12.
[http://dx.doi.org/10.1128/JB.186.14.4808-4812.2004] [PMID: 15231813]

[107] Walmagh M, Briers Y, dos Santos SB, Azeredo J, Lavigne R. Characterization of modular bacteriophage endolysins from Myoviridaephages OBP, 201□2-1 and PVP-SE1. PLoS One 2012; 7(5) e36991
[http://dx.doi.org/10.1371/journal.pone.0036991] [PMID: 22615864]

[108] Sulakvelidze A, Alavidze Z, Morris JG Jr. Bacteriophage therapy. Antimicrob Agents Chemother 2001; 45(3): 649-59.

[http://dx.doi.org/10.1128/AAC.45.3.649-659.2001] [PMID: 11181338]

[109] Nieth A, Verseux C, Barnert S, Süss R, Römer W. A first step toward liposome-mediated intracellular bacteriophage therapy. Expert Opin Drug Deliv 2015; 12(9): 1411-24.
[http://dx.doi.org/10.1517/17425247.2015.1043125] [PMID: 25937143]

[110] Casadevall A, Scharff MD. Return to the past: the case for antibody-based therapies in infectious diseases. Clin Infect Dis 1995; 21(1): 150-61.
[http://dx.doi.org/10.1093/clinids/21.1.150] [PMID: 7578724]

[111] Wright A, Shin SU, Morrison SL. Genetically engineered antibodies: progress and prospects. Crit Rev Immunol 1992; 12(3-4): 125-68.
[PMID: 1476621]

[112] French DL, Laskov R, Scharff MD. The role of somatic hypermutation in the generation of antibody diversity. Science 1989; 244(4909): 1152-7.
[http://dx.doi.org/10.1126/science.2658060] [PMID: 2658060]

[113] Casadevall A. Antibody immunity and invasive fungal infections. Infect Immun 1995; 63(11): 4211-8.
[http://dx.doi.org/10.1128/iai.63.11.4211-4218.1995] [PMID: 7591049]

[114] Mineo JR, Khan IA, Kasper LH. *Toxoplasma gondii*: a monoclonal antibody that inhibits intracellular replication. Exp Parasitol 1994; 79(3): 351-61.
[http://dx.doi.org/10.1006/expr.1994.1097] [PMID: 7525337]

[115] Bodmer M, Fournel MA, Hinshaw LB. Preclinical review of anti-tumor necrosis factor monoclonal antibodies. Crit Care Med 1993; 21(10) (Suppl.): S441-6.
[http://dx.doi.org/10.1097/00003246-199310001-00005] [PMID: 8403982]

[116] Wang-Lin SX, Balthasar JP. Pharmacokinetic and pharmacodynamic considerations for the use of monoclonal antibodies in the treatment of bacterial infections. Antibodies (Basel) 2018; 7(1): 5.
[http://dx.doi.org/10.3390/antib7010005] [PMID: 31544858]

[117] Soares MM, King SW, Thorpe PE. Targeting inside-out phosphatidylserine as a therapeutic strategy for viral diseases. Nat Med 2008; 14(12): 1357-62.
[http://dx.doi.org/10.1038/nm.1885] [PMID: 19029986]

[118] Klein F, Mouquet H, Dosenovic P, Scheid JF, Scharf L, Nussenzweig MC. Antibodies in HIV-1 vaccine development and therapy. Science 2013; 341(6151): 1199-204.
[http://dx.doi.org/10.1126/science.1241144] [PMID: 24031012]

[119] Zhu Q, McLellan JS, Kallewaard NL, Ulbrandt ND, Palaszynski S, Zhang J. A highly potent extended half-life antibody as a potential RSV vaccine surrogate for all infants 2017.
[http://dx.doi.org/10.1126/scitranslmed.aaj1928]

[120] Vanderhoof JA, Young RJ. Use of probiotics in childhood gastrointestinal disorders. J Pediatr Gastroenterol Nutr 1998; 27(3): 323-32.
[http://dx.doi.org/10.1097/00005176-199809000-00011] [PMID: 9740206]

[121] Fijan S. Influence of the growth of *Pseudomonas aeruginosa* in milk fermented by multispecies probiotics and Kefir microbiota. J Probiotics Health 2016; 3: 136.

[122] Park SY, Lim SD. Probiotic characteristics of *Lactobacillus plantarum* FH185 isolated from human feces. Han-gug Chugsan Sigpum Hag-hoeji 2015; 35(5): 615-21.
[http://dx.doi.org/10.5851/kosfa.2015.35.5.615] [PMID: 26761889]

[123] Ma EL, Choi YJ, Choi J, Pothoulakis C, Rhee SH, Im E. The anticancer effect of probiotic *Bacillus* polyfermenticus on human colon cancer cells is mediated through ErbB2 and ErbB3 inhibition. Int J Cancer 2010; 127(4): 780-90.
[PMID: 19876926]

[124] Verhoeven V, Renard N, Makar A, *et al.* Probiotics enhance the clearance of human papillomavirus-related cervical lesions: a prospective controlled pilot study. Eur J Cancer Prev 2013; 22(1): 46-51.

[http://dx.doi.org/10.1097/CEJ.0b013e328355ed23] [PMID: 22706167]

[125] Ettinger G, MacDonald K, Reid G, Burton JP. The influence of the human microbiome and probiotics on cardiovascular health. Gut Microbes 2014; 5(6): 719-28.
[http://dx.doi.org/10.4161/19490976.2014.983775] [PMID: 25529048]

[126] Sayin SI, Wahlström A, Felin J, *et al.* Gut microbiota regulates bile acid metabolism by reducing the levels of tauro-beta-muricholic acid, a naturally occurring FXR antagonist. Cell Metab 2013; 17(2): 225-35.
[http://dx.doi.org/10.1016/j.cmet.2013.01.003] [PMID: 23395169]

[127] Dong J, Teng G, Wei T, Gao W, Wang H, Green J. Methodological quality assessment of meta-analyses and systematic reviews of probiotics in inflammatory bowel disease and pouchitis. PLoS One 2016; 11(12) e0168785
[http://dx.doi.org/10.1371/journal.pone.0168785] [PMID: 28005973]

[128] Nair V, Soraisham AS. Probiotics and prebiotics: role in prevention of nosocomial sepsis in preterm infants. 2013.

[129] Ratsep M, Naaber P, Koljalg S, Smidt I, Shkut E, Sepp E. Effect of *Lactobacillus plantarum* strains on clinical isolates of *Clostridium difficile in vitro*. J Probiotics Health 2014; 2: 119.
[http://dx.doi.org/10.4172/2329-8901.1000119]

[130] Tharmaraj N, Shah NP. Antimicrobial effects of probiotics against selected pathogenic and spoilage bacteria in cheese-based dips. Int Food Res J 2009; 16: 261-76.

[131] Zamfir M, Callewaert R, Cornea PC, Savu L, Vatafu I, De Vuyst L. Purification and characterization of a bacteriocin produced by *Lactobacillus acidophilus* IBB 801. J Appl Microbiol 1999; 87(6): 923-31.
[http://dx.doi.org/10.1046/j.1365-2672.1999.00950.x] [PMID: 10664915]

[132] Reid G, Jass J, Sebulsky MT, McCormick JK. Potential uses of probiotics in clinical practice. Clin Microbiol Rev 2003; 16(4): 658-72.
[http://dx.doi.org/10.1128/CMR.16.4.658-672.2003] [PMID: 14557292]

[133] Pagnini C, Saeed R, Bamias G, Arseneau KO, Pizarro TT, Cominelli F. Probiotics promote gut health through stimulation of epithelial innate immunity. Proc Natl Acad Sci USA 2010; 107(1): 454-9.
[http://dx.doi.org/10.1073/pnas.0910307107] [PMID: 20018654]

[134] Singh L, Kruger HG, Maguire GEM, Govender T, Parboosing R. The role of nanotechnology in the treatment of viral infections. Ther Adv Infect Dis 2017; 4(4): 105-31.
[http://dx.doi.org/10.1177/2049936117713593] [PMID: 28748089]

[135] Xiong MH, Bao Y, Yang XZ, Zhu YH, Wang J. Delivery of antibiotics with polymeric particles. Adv Drug Deliv Rev 2014; 78: 63-76.
[http://dx.doi.org/10.1016/j.addr.2014.02.002] [PMID: 24548540]

[136] Zhou L, Qiu T, Lv F, Liu L, Ying J, Wang S. Self-assembled nanomedicines for anticancer and antibacterial applications. Adv Healthc Mater 2018; 7(20) e1800670
[http://dx.doi.org/10.1002/adhm.201800670] [PMID: 30080319]

[137] Kumar M, Curtis A, Hoskins C. Application of nanoparticle technologies in the combat against anti-microbial resistance. Pharmaceutics 2018; 10(1) E11
[http://dx.doi.org/10.3390/pharmaceutics10010011] [PMID: 29342903]

[138] Al-Halifa S, Gauthier L, Arpin D, Bourgault S, Archambault D. Nanoparticle-based vaccines against respiratory viruses. Front Immunol 2019; 10: 22.
[http://dx.doi.org/10.3389/fimmu.2019.00022] [PMID: 30733717]

[139] Lybaert L, Vermaelen K, De Geest BG, Nuhn L. Immunoengineering through cancer vaccines - A personalized and multi-step vaccine approach towards precise cancer immunity. J Control Release 2018; 289: 125-45.
[http://dx.doi.org/10.1016/j.jconrel.2018.09.009] [PMID: 30223044]

[140] Narasimhan B, Goodman JT, Vela Ramirez JE. Rational design of targeted next-generation carriers for drug and vaccine delivery. Annu Rev Biomed Eng 2016; 18: 25-49.
[http://dx.doi.org/10.1146/annurev-bioeng-082615-030519] [PMID: 26789697]

[141] Huh AJ, Kwon YJ. "Nanoantibiotics": a new paradigm for treating infectious diseases using nanomaterials in the antibiotics resistant era. J Control Release 2011; 156(2): 128-45.
[http://dx.doi.org/10.1016/j.jconrel.2011.07.002] [PMID: 21763369]

[142] Zhang L, Pornpattananangku D, Hu CM, Huang CM. Development of nanoparticles for antimicrobial drug delivery. Curr Med Chem 2010; 17(6): 585-94.
[http://dx.doi.org/10.2174/092986710790416290] [PMID: 20015030]

[143] Zhou X, Zhang X, Han S, *et al.* Yeast microcapsule-mediated targeted delivery of diverse nanoparticles for imaging and therapy *via* the oral route. Nano Lett 2017; 17(2): 1056-64.
[http://dx.doi.org/10.1021/acs.nanolett.6b04523] [PMID: 28075596]

[144] Meyer RA, Sunshine JC, Green JJ. Biomimetic particles as therapeutics. Trends Biotechnol 2015; 33(9): 514-24.
[http://dx.doi.org/10.1016/j.tibtech.2015.07.001] [PMID: 26277289]

[145] Yang C, Mamouni J, Tang Y, Yang L. Antimicrobial activity of single-walled carbon nanotubes: length effect. Langmuir 2010; 26(20): 16013-9.
[http://dx.doi.org/10.1021/la103110g] [PMID: 20849142]

[146] Brahmachari S, Mandal SK, Das PK. Fabrication of SWCNT-Ag nanoparticle hybrid included self-assemblies for antibacterial applications. PLoS One 2014; 9(9) e106775
[http://dx.doi.org/10.1371/journal.pone.0106775] [PMID: 25191756]

[147] Popp BV, Miles DH, Smith JA, Fong IM, Pasquali M, Ball ZT. Stabilization and functionalization of single-walled carbon nanotubes with polyvinylpyrrolidone copolymers for applications in aqueous media. J Polym Sci A Polym Chem 2015; 53: 337-43.
[http://dx.doi.org/10.1002/pola.27365]

[148] Venkatesan J, Jayakumar R, Mohandas A, Bhatnagar I, Kim SK. Antimicrobial activity of chitosancarbon nanotube hydrogels. Materials (Basel) 2014; 7(5): 3946-55.
[http://dx.doi.org/10.3390/ma7053946] [PMID: 28788658]

[149] Gottardi R, Douradinha B. Carbon nanotubes as a novel tool for vaccination against infectious diseases and cancer. J Nanobiotechnology 2013; 11: 30.
[http://dx.doi.org/10.1186/1477-3155-11-30] [PMID: 24025216]

[150] Orecchioni M, Bedognetti D, Sgarrella F, Marincola FM, Bianco A, Delogu LG. Impact of carbon nanotubes and graphene on immune cells. J Transl Med 2014; 12: 138.
[http://dx.doi.org/10.1186/1479-5876-12-138] [PMID: 24885781]

[151] Pescatori M, Bedognetti D, Venturelli E, *et al.* Functionalized carbon nanotubes as immunomodulator systems. Biomaterials 2013; 34(18): 4395-403.
[http://dx.doi.org/10.1016/j.biomaterials.2013.02.052] [PMID: 23507086]

[152] Prajapati VK, Awasthi K, Yadav TP, Rai M, Srivastava ON, Sundar S. An oral formulation of amphotericin B attached to functionalized carbon nanotubes is an effective treatment for experimental visceral leishmaniasis. J Infect Dis 2012; 205(2): 333-6.
[http://dx.doi.org/10.1093/infdis/jir735] [PMID: 22158723]

[153] Spizzirria UG, Hampel S, Cirilloab G, *et al.* Functional gelatin-carbon nanotubes nanohybrids with enhanced antibacterial activity. Int J Poly Mater Poly Biomater 2015; 64: 439-47.
[http://dx.doi.org/10.1080/00914037.2014.958833]

[154] Chaudhari AA, Jasper SL, Dosunmu E, *et al.* Novel pegylated silver coated carbon nanotubes kill Salmonella but they are non-toxic to eukaryotic cells. J Nanobiotechnology 2015; 13: 23.
[http://dx.doi.org/10.1186/s12951-015-0085-5] [PMID: 25888864]

[155] Yang X, Ebrahimi A, Li J, Cui Q. Fullerene-biomolecule conjugates and their biomedicinal applications. Int J Nanomedicine 2014; 9: 77-92.
[http://dx.doi.org/10.2147/IJN.S71700] [PMID: 24379667]

[156] Bai W, Krishna V, Wang J, Moudgil B, Koopman B. Enhancement of nano titanium dioxide photocatalysis in transparent coatings by polyhydroxy fullerene. Appl Catal B 2012; 125: 128-35.
[http://dx.doi.org/10.1016/j.apcatb.2012.05.026]

[157] Yu C, Canteenwala T, Chiang LY, Wilson B, Pritzker K. Photodynamic effect of hydrophilic C60-derived nanostructures for catalytic antitumoral antibacterial applications. Synth Met 2005; 153: 37-40.
[http://dx.doi.org/10.1016/j.synthmet.2005.07.247]

[158] Mizuno T, Masuda Y, Irie K. The Saccharomyces cerevisiae AMPK, Snf1, Negatively Regulates the Hog1 MAPK Pathway in ER Stress Response. PLoS Genet 2015; 11(9) e1005491
[http://dx.doi.org/10.1371/journal.pgen.1005491] [PMID: 26394309]

[159] Deryabin DG, Davydova OK, Yankina ZZ, *et al.* The activity of Fullerene derivatives bearing amine and carboxylic solubilizing groups against Escherichia coli: a comparative study. J Nanomater 2014; 2014: 1-9.
[http://dx.doi.org/10.1155/2014/907435]

[160] Lind TK, Polcyn P, Zielinska P, Cárdenas M, Urbanczyk-Lipkowska Z. On the antimicrobial activity of various peptide-based dendrimers of similar architecture. Molecules 2015; 20(1): 738-53.
[http://dx.doi.org/10.3390/molecules20010738] [PMID: 25574818]

[161] Xue XY, Mao XG, Li Z, *et al.* A potent and selective antimicrobial poly(amidoamine) dendrimer conjugate with LED209 targeting QseC receptor to inhibit the virulence genes of gram negative bacteria. Nanomedicine (Lond) 2015; 11(2): 329-39.
[http://dx.doi.org/10.1016/j.nano.2014.09.016] [PMID: 25461286]

[162] Yeo SJ, Huong DT, Han JH, *et al.* Performance of coumarin-derived dendrimer-based fluorescence-linked immunosorbent assay (FLISA) to detect malaria antigen. Malaria, 2014, J 13, 266..

[163] Kumar MS, Karthikeyan S, Ramprasad C, *et al.* Investigation of phloroglucinol succinic acid dendrimer as antimicrobial agent against *Staphylococcus aureus*, Escherichia coli and *Candida albicans*. Nano Biomed Eng 2015; 7: 62-74.
[http://dx.doi.org/10.5101/nbe.v7i2.p62-74]

[164] Alateyah AI, Dhakal HN, Zhang ZY. Processing, properties, and applications of polymer nanocomposites based on layer silicates: a review. Adv Polym Technol 2013; 32: 21368.
[http://dx.doi.org/10.1002/adv.21368]

[165] Ahmed F, Santos CM, Mangadlao J, Advincula R, Rodrigues DF. Antimicrobial PVK:SWNT nanocomposite coated membrane for water purification: performance and toxicity testing. Water Res 2013; 47(12): 3966-75.
[http://dx.doi.org/10.1016/j.watres.2012.10.055] [PMID: 23545165]

[166] Kaur P, Thakur A. Synthesis of chitosan-silver nanocomposites and their antibacterial activity. Int J Sci Eng Res 2013; 4: 879-82.

[167] Helal H, El-Din T, Ali A, Hamouda HH, Zedan H. Tobramycin-Silver nanocomposite: a new trend of antimicrobials against resistant strains. J Pharm Biol Sci 2014; 9: 54-61.
[http://dx.doi.org/10.9790/3008-09615461]

[168] Pinto R, Daina S, Sadocco P, Neto CP, Trindade T. Antibacterial activity of nanocomposites of copper and cellulose. BioMed Rese Int 2013; pp. 1-10.

[169] Armentano I, Arciola CR, Fortunati E, *et al.* The interaction of bacteria with engineered nanostructured polymeric materials: a review. ScientificWorldJournal 2014; 2014 410423
[http://dx.doi.org/10.1155/2014/410423] [PMID: 25025086]

[170] Rajendran R, Abirami M, Prabhavathi P, Premasudha P, Kanimozhi B, Manikandan A. Biological treatment of drinking water by chitosan based nanocomposites. Afr J Biotechnol 2015; 14: 930-6.

[171] Azam A, Ahmed AS, Oves M, Khan MS, Habib SS, Memic A. Antimicrobial activity of metal oxide nanoparticles against Gram-positive and Gram-negative bacteria: a comparative study. Int J Nanomedicine 2012; 7: 6003-9.
[http://dx.doi.org/10.2147/IJN.S35347] [PMID: 23233805]

[172] Guzman M, Dille J, Godet S. Synthesis and antibacterial activity of silver nanoparticles against gram-positive and gram-negative bacteria. Nanomedicine (Lond) 2012; 8(1): 37-45.
[http://dx.doi.org/10.1016/j.nano.2011.05.007] [PMID: 21703988]

[173] Huet T, Kerbarh O, Schols D, et al. Long-lasting enfuvirtide carrier pentasaccharide conjugates with potent anti-human immunodeficiency virus type 1 activity. Antimicrob Agents Chemother 2010; 54(1): 134-42.
[http://dx.doi.org/10.1128/AAC.00827-09] [PMID: 19805567]

[174] Kakkar T, Madgula K, Nehru YVS, Kakkar J. Polyvinyl alcohol-melamine formaldehyde films and coatings with silver nanoparticles as wound dressings in diabetic foot disease. Eur Chem Bull 2015; 4: 98-105.

[175] Namasivayam SKR, James J. Biocompatible polymer chitosan stabilized silver nanoparticlesAzithromycin (CS-AgNP-AZ) and levofloxacin (CS-AgNPLF) drug nano conjugate fabricated wound dressing for the improved antibacterial activity against human pyogenic bacteria. Der Pharmacia Lett 2015; 7: 100-11.

[176] Melo MA, Guedes SFF, Xu HHK, Rodrigues LK. Nanotechnology-based restorative materials for dental caries management. Trends Biotechnol 2013; 31(8): 459-67.
[http://dx.doi.org/10.1016/j.tibtech.2013.05.010] [PMID: 23810638]

[177] El-Sigeny SM, Abou-Taleb MF. Synthesis, characterization, and application of dendrimer modified magnetite nanoparticles as antimicrobial agent. Life Sci J 2015; 12: 161-70.

[178] Yang W, Shen C, Ji Q, et al. Food storage material silver nanoparticles interfere with DNA replication fidelity and bind with DNA. Nanotechnology 2009; 20(8) 085102
[http://dx.doi.org/10.1088/0957-4484/20/8/085102] [PMID: 19417438]

[179] Malka E, Perelshtein I, Lipovsky A, et al. Eradication of multi-drug resistant bacteria by a novel Zn-doped CuO nanocomposite. Small 2013; 9(23): 4069-76.
[http://dx.doi.org/10.1002/smll.201301081] [PMID: 23813908]

[180] Depan D, Misra RD. On the determining role of network structure titania in silicone against bacterial colonization: mechanism and disruption of biofilm. Mater Sci Eng C 2014; 34: 221-8.
[http://dx.doi.org/10.1016/j.msec.2013.09.025] [PMID: 24268253]

[181] Hussein-Al-Ali SH, El Zowalaty ME, Hussein MZ, Geilich BM, Webster TJ. Synthesis, characterization, and antimicrobial activity of an ampicillin-conjugated magnetic nanoantibiotic for medical applications. Int J Nanomedicine 2014; 9: 3801-14.
[http://dx.doi.org/10.2147/IJN.S61143] [PMID: 25143729]

[182] Leung YH, Ng AM, Xu X, et al. Mechanisms of antibacterial activity of MgO: non-ROS mediated toxicity of MgO nanoparticles towards Escherichia coli. Small 2014; 10(6): 1171-83.
[http://dx.doi.org/10.1002/smll.201302434] [PMID: 24344000]

[183] Cagno V, Andreozzi P, D'Alicarnasso M, *et al.* Broad-spectrum non-toxic antiviral nanoparticles with a virucidal inhibition mechanism. Nat Mater 2018; 17(2): 195-203.
[http://dx.doi.org/10.1038/nmat5053] [PMID: 29251725]

CHAPTER 5

Anti-infective Agents against Severe Acute Respiratory Syndrome Coronavirus 2 (SARS CoV-2)

Ramadevi Mohan[1] **and Subhashree Venugopal**[1,*]

[1] *Department of Integrative Biology, VIT University, Vellore-632014, Tamil Nadu, India*

Abstract: SARS-CoV-2, a newly identified coronavirus, causes the coronavirus disease of 2019 usually termed COVID-19 and is considered a pandemic and spreads by zoonotic transmission. The human coronavirus SARS CoV2 is similar to SARS CoV and MERS CoV both belonging to the β-coronavirus group but the mild differences between them influence the greater pathogenicity in SARS-CoV-2. The virus produces 4 clinically important proteins that are responsible for host-cell receptor attachment, suppression of host gene expression, and replication leading to multiple infections. It is much important to get insights into the essence of the virus and the virus-induced disease. Since the viruses have the ability to mutate quickly, the discovery of drugs against the virus is challenging. However, many scientists and researchers across the world are working hopefully to discover drugs or vaccines to slow down or stop the replication process of the virus. The repurposing of existing drugs has gained importance as it reduces time and cost-effectiveness during the drug-discovery process and development. In this chapter, we have highlighted the on-going researches on drugs against SARS-CoV-2 which are under various phases of a clinical trial. These include various FDA-approved (Food and Drug Administration) inhibitors such as protease inhibitors, polymerase inhibitors, antimalarial drugs, rheumatoid drugs, and lipid- lowering statins.

Keywords: Antimalarial drugs, Anti-infective agents, Coronavirus, COVID-19, Polymerase inhibitors, Protease inhibitors, Repurposing of drugs, SARS-CoV-2.

INTRODUCTION

Coronaviruses (also known as CoVs) constitute a crucial category of viruses predominantly infecting humans through the transmission of zoonoses. Over the past two decades, this novel coronavirus has emerged as the third instance, after SARS-CoV (severe acute respiratory syndrome) and MERS-CoV (Middle East

---

[*] **Corresponding author Subhashree Venugopal**: Department of Integrative Biology, School of Biosciences and Technology, VIT University, Vellore-632014, Tamil Nadu, India; Tel: +919486947377; E-mail: vsubhashree@vit.ac.in

Parvesh Singh, Vipan Kumar & Rajshekhar Karpoormath (Eds.)
All rights reserved-© 2021 Bentham Science Publishers

respiratory syndrome coronavirus) in the year 2003 and 2012, respectively [1, 2]. Genetic studies conducted by a group of researchers reveal that SARS-CoV-2 shares almost 80% sequence identity with SARS-CoV and 50% with MERS-CoV and therefore have been evaluated to be closely related to each other [3]. The genetic variations between SARS-CoV and SARS-CoV-2 are liable for differences in infectivity [4] and immune response [5].

Coronaviruses have the potential to affect a wide array of species including aves, domestic and wild mammals, especially humans [6, 7]. These viruses are familiar for their capacity to rapidly change the gene function, modify the ability of the host tissue to get infected, navigate the blockade of species, and are capable of adapting to various epidemiological conditions [6 - 8].

The coronavirus belongs to the Coronaviridae family and Nidovirales order and the subgroup of beta-coronaviruses. The World Health Organization (WHO) named '2019 novel coronavirus' to denote the coronavirus infecting pneumonia affected individuals in the lower respiratory tract in Wuhan, Hubei Province of China [9 - 11]. The International Committee on Taxonomy of Viruses (ICTV) gave the name SARS-CoV-2 and the disease COVID-19 [12, 13].

Structure of SARS-CoV-2

These viruses are categorized into a type of structurally enveloped viruses with non-segmented, positive-sense, single-stranded RNA genomes. Electron microscopic studies revealed its size of about 60 nm to 140 nm in diameter with unique spike-like projections that are extruded exterior giving it a shape a crown-like appearance; thus the virus got the name [2, 14]. The structure of the virus is shown in Fig. (**1**).

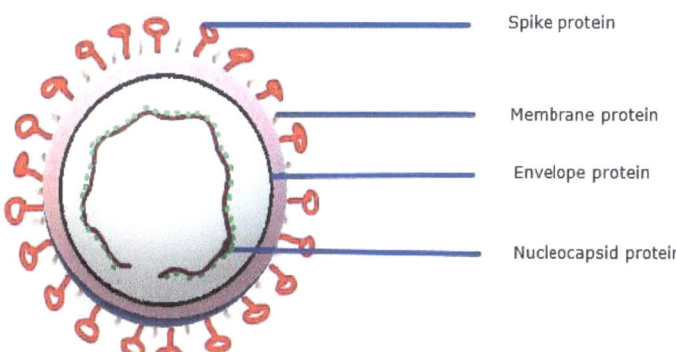

Fig. (1). Structure of SARS-CoV-2.

Structural Proteins

The RNA genome of the virus is 29,891 bp in length, and its G+C content is 38% [15]. The genome also consists of 7 genes that are preserved in the order of ORF1a, ORF1b, S, and OEF3, E, M and N in the 5' to 3' direction. Interestingly, the 2/3rd fraction part of its genome is occupied by the ORF1a/b that generates two replicase enzymes of poly-proteins type (PP1a and PP1ab). Also, 16 mature non-structural proteins (NSPs) emerge from additional refining of these two PPs. These NSPs are believed to involve in various roles including the development of the replicase-transcriptase complex. The excess part of the viral genome encodes an mRNA generating four important structural proteins namely spike (S) protein, nucleocapsid (N) protein, membrane (M) protein, and the envelope (E) protein necessary to form a structurally complete viral particle [16 - 18]. The RNA genome of CoV is stuffed with an envelope in the nucleocapsid protein [19].

S (Spike) Glycoprotein

The S protein has a crown-like shape; so named as 'Coronavirus' [14]. The size of the protein is between 9 and 12nm [20]. It mediates binding between the virus and the cell surface receptors in the host and following integration between them facilitates viral entry into the host cell [21, 22]. They are found exterior to the virion which gives the typical shape and has a receptor-binding domain (RBD). The protein consists of two active subunits which are S1 (bulb part) and S2 (stalk part) for receptor binding and membrane fusion respectively. The interaction of the S1 subunit with the associated cell surface receptor stimulates a radical structural alteration inducing endocytosis in the S2 part. This allows the virus envelope to combine with the cellular membrane and thereby liberating the nucleocapsid into the cytoplasm [16]. *In vitro* binding studies have also shown that the RBD is a pivotal role portion of the S1 part accountable for the attachment of ACE2 with SARS-CoV-2 [23]. The glycosylated spike (S) fusion protein and the ACE2 receptor control the host cell entry of the virus. The ability of S proteins to substantially rearrange the structure helps in the binding of the microbe and the host membranes [24]. The replication-transcription complex (RTC) is formed into double-membrane vesicles soon after the virus reaches the host cell, in order to initiate polyprotein 1a/1ab (pp1a/pp1ab) transcription. For the development of non-structural proteins, these proteins encode chymotrypsin-like protease (3CLpro), key protease (Mpro), and papain-like proteases (nsps) [25].

M (Membrane) Glycoprotein

The M protein refers to the structure of the viral envelope and is found in large amounts [26]. It is interpreted as the principal controller of CoV assembly which allows interaction with every other prime structural protein of the virus [16]. Homotypic interactions that occur between these membrane proteins are the major driving force for the development of virion envelopes [26]. The protein has three transmembrane regions and it is found to be glycosylated in Golgi apparatus [27] and this reformation is responsible for the antigenic property of the virion resulted from the fusion into the cell. One of the key features of the M protein is the stimulation of virions in the cell. M protein elicits the production and establishment of interchanging virions in the endoplasmic reticulum-Golgi apparatus intermediate compartment (ERGIC) with this complex [28, 29].

E (Envelope) Glycoprotein

The envelope protein is miniature among the extensive structural polypeptides of the virus consisting of 76 to 109 amino acids in which 30 aa belonging to the N-terminus are involved in attachment [30]. During replication, E protein is highly expressed in the damaged cell, but interestingly, only a little part is found to be integrated into the virion envelope [31]. Most of the proteins are confined to the intracellular region namely ER, Golgi, and ERGIC, where they are engaged in the formation of CoV assembly and budding [32]. E protein, together with M protein, forms the viral envelope whose interconnection is adequate for the generation and delivery of VLPs [17].

N (Nucleocapsid) Protein

It is the only structural protein that serves crucial to connect the CoV RNA genome thus creating a capsid around the enclosed nucleic acid to form nucleocapsid [33]. N protein is predominantly engaged in the processes linked to the viral genome by means of interaction with the viral membrane protein during viral assembly, assisting RNA synthesis and folding, virus budding, and affecting host cell reactions, comprising cell cycle and translation [18]. The interaction of M and N proteins equilibrate the nucleocapsid, and also the internal core of virions and eventually, assists the completion of the viral assembly [34, 35].

Clinical Outcomes

These deadly coronaviruses cause many clinical diseases in humans which extend from mild symptoms to severe diseases including the common cold, high temperature, croak, pharyngitis, headache, weariness, myalgia, watery stool, nausea and breathing difficulty, multi-organ dysfunction such as lung infection, arrhythmias, acute cardiac and kidney injury, shock, severe acute respiratory distress syndrome (ARDS), SARS and MERS [9, 36 - 39]. Also, the indications like pharyngeal pain, dizziness, dyspnea, abdominal pain, and malnutrition are more presumably seen in patients with severe illnesses [40]. These symptoms are interpreted to be more severe in cardiovascular disease patients and found to be related to rise in the production of ACE2 when compared with normal people. Further, individuals who have fundamental co-morbid conditions like high blood pressure and diabetes are highly probable to have worse results [41].

TRANSMISSION OF INFECTION

Intermediate Host Transmission

Most of the primary infected cases were connected to the wholesale market for Huanan seafood and wild animals, which was designated by the Chinese Health Authority as an epidemic center. Initial studies suggest that the virus may have originated in China from horseshoe bats and was then spread to other species that are normally consumed by humans [6]. The U.S.-based Center for Disease Control and Prevention (CDC) proposed that the Wuhan coronavirus possibly started from a 'spillover' that happens when the virus is transmitted from animal to human [42]. Research says there is evidence that COVID-19 originated from snakes sold on the market in Wuhan. They identified that the virus materializes to be a "recombination" of 2 coronaviruses. Homologous recombination within the newly recognized coronavirus' spike glycoprotein may increase the transmission of cross-species from the reptile to human [43]. Various studies prove the connection of COVID-19 with other known CoVs in bats, especially in the subspecies of Rhinolophus bat, which is found in huge amounts and predominantly seen in the regions of Southern China, Asia, the Middle East, Africa, and Europe [44, 45]. Several studies indicated that it was possible for snakes, minks, and pangolins to be intervening hosts, based on the preference for codon and patterns of viral infection [43, 46, 47].

Human-to-human Transmission

Infection caused by the virus is mainly transmitted through the large droplets that are produced during coughing and sneezing that are inhaled or contacted from patients and also subsequent touching of nose, mouth, and eyes [48, 49]. They could even proliferate from people with no symptoms and prior to the development of signs. The maturation period normally lies between 2 and 14 days. Moreover, the virus is seen in the stool and water contaminants and also by aerosolization/feco oral route [50]. In comparison with the throat, excess viral contents in the nasal cavity are found in both symptomatic and asymptomatic people [38, 51]. These viral-containing droplets can easily spread around 1–2 m and accumulate on various surfaces. The viruses are capable of living on surfaces for a period of time in good atmospheric conditions but are certainly demolished within a minute by ordinary disinfectants such as sodium hypochlorite, hydrogen peroxide, and so on [52].

Entry of COVID-19 and Interaction with a Host Cell Receptor

When the virus invades the host, it attaches to the extensive target cells namely enterocytes and pneumocytes and thus initiates infection and multiplication. Researchers have identified angiotensin receptor 2 (ACE2) as a significant functional cellular entry receptor through which both the viruses SARS-CoV-2 and SARS-CoV enter the respiratory mucosa [3, 53-56]. ACE2 is one of the members of the membrane-bound carboxy-dipeptidase family which is homology to ACE (an enzyme having a main role in the Renin-Angiotensin system) and is a selective protein for hypertension [57 - 59]. It is conventionally distributed in humans including the vascular endothelial cells, the renal tubular epithelium, and in Leydig cells in the testes [19, 60 - 62]. In addition to the kidneys, PCR results proved the presence of ACE-2 in the lungs and gastrointestinal tract, and the tissues are exhibited to possess SARS-CoV [63, 64]. In the lungs, ACE2 expression is strongly found in type II alveolar epithelial cells and macrophages and modestly in bronchial and tracheal epithelial cells [65]. *In vitro* results proclaim that the ciliated cells are primarily affected in the conducting airways [66].

Like SARS-CoV, SARS-CoV-2 also utilizes TMPRSS2 (transmembrane protease serine 2) enzyme to achieve the mechanism of entering into the target cells. The transmembrane S protein of the virus attaches to the target cells by interacting with the cell surface receptor, followed by the priming of S protein by means of TMPRSS2. This allows the integration of viral and hosts plasma membranes, thereby leading to SARS-CoV-2 entry and replication in the target cells [67]. Thus, SARS-CoV-2 illness is caused by the attachment of the spike protein to ACE2 [66].

Replication Process of SARS-CoV- 2

The mechanism of replication of the virus has been well-explained in a review [68]. The genomic RNA (gRNA) of the virus works as a template to translate the polyproteins and it is cut to form 16 non-structural proteins (NSPs) upon processing by the enzyme protease. The role of NSP1 and NSP2 is the termination of host gene expression and the development of a multidomain complex is performed by NSP3. NSP5 is an M protease with a specific role in replication [69] whereas NSP4 and NSP6 are transmembrane (TM) proteins [70].

The non-structural proteins NSP7 and NSP8 perform as primase [71] and NSP9, an RNA-binding protein, the dimeric form of which is essential for viral infection. NSP10 reacts as a cofactor to prompt the replicative enzyme [72]. NSP12 manifests RNA-dependent RNA polymerase activity, and NSP13 and NSP14 intimate helicase and exoribonuclease activity, respectively. NSP15 and NSP16 exhibit endoribonuclease and methyltransferase activity, respectively. Each NSP has a specific function in replication and transcription [70]. These nsps instigate the structural change in the plasma membrane to generate the double-membrane vesicles (DMVs) in the region where the viral replication transcription complexes (RTCs) are fixed [73]. Full-length gRNA is fairly multiplied through a negative-sense intermediate, and subgenomic RNA (sgRNA) species are incorporated by the process of discontinuous transcription. These sgRNAs encode structural and accessory proteins in the virus. Particle assembly takes place in the ER-Golgi intermediate complex (ERGIC), and grown virions are delivered in smooth-walled vesicles through the secretory pathway [73].

The disease progression by coronaviruses is associated with a substantial increase in inflammatory cytokines like IL2, IL7, IL10, IP10 (CXCL10), GCSF, MCP1, MIP1A, and TNFα [41]. CXCL10 is an interferon perceptive gene exhibiting an extraordinary signal/noise ratio in the alveolar type II cell response to both SARS-CoV and influenza [74, 75].

The properties of the virus such as indifferent properties of the disease, the infectivity surprisingly before the appearance of symptoms in the growing period, dissemination from persons without symptoms, elaborate developing period, tropism for mucosal surfaces such as the conjunctiva, prolonged duration of the illness, and transmission even after clinical recovery makes prevention difficult [11, 76].

TREATMENT

Uncertified medications should only be used under precise observations exclusively during the situations of morally sanctioned clinical trials or under the Monitored Emergency Use of Unregistered Interventions System (MEURI) [77].

However, many researchers around the world are conducting tests on various FDA-approved drugs against SARS-CoV-2 infection. Some of these approved drugs are in various phases of a clinical trial as they are shown to exert assured antiviral activity in cell culture as well as animal models [78].

The significant cost-effectiveness and the time that is taken for the process of modern drug discovery and development leads to the repurposing of 'old' drugs for the treatment of both common and rare diseases. Hence it is progressively turning out to be a captivating method that comprises the manipulation of de-risked compounds. A systematic approach in the identification of drugs is to check if the already available antiviral drugs are successful in curing the corresponding viral infections [79, 80].

Due to the increased and pandemic condition of nCoV 19, scientists and researchers are forced to recognize a variety of broad-spectrum antiviral agents (BSAAs) that might possibly act as powerful therapeutic drugs against various viral diseases [81]. BSAAs are usually small molecules that have the ability to suppress different infections by preventing viral replication [82 - 84]. These drugs have the ability to block the virus or host-related factors and stop the virus from proliferation and also lower the amount of the microorganism in the host to a degree that the immune system can obstruct their infection [85, 86]. BSAAs have mainly obtained peculiar attention with the rising of various new viral diseases. Repurposing of currently approved antiviral drugs can be used to cure current viral infections [15, 79, 87, 88].

Repurposing of Drugs for COVID-19 Treatment

It is well-known that drug re-purposing (also termed as repositioning, redirecting, reprofiling) is the process of examining already existing drugs to find therapeutic effects for new diseases [89, 90]. The major advantage of drug re-purposing over new drug discovery is that various information about drugs namely the phases of chemical synthesis, reliable safety, manufacturing methods, pharmacokinetic properties in several periods of clinical trials have been recognized earlier [91, 92].

Role of Artificial Intelligence (AI) in Drug Repositioning

Through the development of the learning-prediction model, AI is implemented in-field design and performs a simple virtual screening to show the output accurately. AI can easily identify drugs that can treat developing diseases like COVID-19 with a drug-repositioning technique [93]. Gysi and colleagues developed a framework found on the graph neural network and offered a SARS-CoV-2 model analysis with 81 identified possible repurposing candidates [94]. The knowledge graph of BenevolentAI is a broad store-house of organized clinical data with several links drawn out by machine learning from scientific publications [95]. By using an extensive scientific collection of 24 million PubMed reports, a group built a detailed COVID-19 information graph (called CoV-KGE) that contained 15 million edges over 39 kinds of associations linked to drugs, diseases, proteins, genes, pathways, and gene and protein expressions. To speculate if any remunerative antiviral drugs that are available will respond to SARS-CoV-2, Beck and colleagues invented a hybrid CNN and RNN model termed Molecule Transformer-Drug Target Interaction. Several recognized antiviral drugs namely atazanavir, remdesivir, efavirenz, ritonavir, and dolutegravir were estimated by the authors for the possible treatment of SARS-CoV-2 infection [96].

Various groups of researchers have shown the extensive use of antivirals that are productive against the prophylaxis of SARS-CoV-2 [97, 98]. Recently, the BSAAs are therapeutics or prophylaxis candidates against SARS CoV2 [99]. Anti-CoV drug progression is being confronted by the activity of a 3' to 5' proof-reading exo-ribonuclease that is unique to coronaviruses. The evolution of antiviral nucleoside and nucleotide analogues targeting viral RNA synthesis is found as powerful therapeutic drugs against CoV infections [100].

The drugs that are evaluated for the purpose of reusing in the treatment of COVID-19 likely to subject to two categories: Those that aim the viral replication cycle and those that challenges to regulate the indications of the disease [101]. Drugs belonging to different groups like nucleoside analogues, protease inhibitors, and host-targeted agents have been analyzed for if they possess antiviral property against SARS-CoV-2 infection. Due to its strong structural preservation of the binding site, the nucleoside analogue gives a less likelihood of resistance. In addition, amino acid sequence preservation of RdRp of coronavirus is comparatively more suggesting that nucleoside analogue could be possibly used in curing SARS-CoV-2 infections [102].

Polymerase Inhibitors

These are classified into nucleoside/nucleotide analogues and non-nucleoside inhibitors. They mimic natural nucleosides/nucleotides and inhibit the virus replication process by suppressing the function of the polymerase enzyme thereby resulting in an effective clinical therapy [103, 104]. Suppression of the specific enzyme is indispensable for viral proteolytic and additional necessary important activities [105].

The nucleoside analogues are converted into dNTPs and are integrated into the replication process by replacing cytosine, inhibiting, and targeting DNA methyl-transferases for degradation [106]. Adenine or guanine derivative nucleoside analogues are successful in targeting RNA-dependent RNA polymerases (RdRp) and blocking RNA synthesis in a wide variety of viruses, constituting human coronaviruses [107]. Some of the structures of polymerase inhibitors are shown in Fig. (**2**).

Favipiravir

Ribavirin

Galidesivir

Fig. (2). Chemical structures of polymerase inhibitors.

Remdesivir (GS-5734)

Remdesivir is a monophosphoramidate prodrug of an adenosine analogue that shows a wide antiviral spectrum including filoviruses, pneumoviruses, paramyxoviruses, and also coronaviruses. Remdesivir was invented by Gilead as a remedy for Ebola virus infections [108] but has shown antiviral and clinical effects against all types of human and animal coronaviruses in animal models [109 - 111].

It also inhibits SARS-CoV-2 multiplication in human nasal and bronchial airway epithelial cells. Remdesivir has been shown to be a potent antiviral agent that works by the mechanism of blocking RNA replication in which it incorporates with high-efficiency coronavirus RdRps resulting in slowing down the ending process of RNA synthesis thus escaping cut by the viral exonuclease [110, 112 - 114].

Research conducted by Wang *et al* showed CoVid19 (EC50 = 0.77 μM in Vero E6 cells) inhibition of remdesivir [111]. In a single-arm trial, the application of remdesivir in the individuals of the particular disease had promising preliminary results and the FDA granted remdesivir for critical situations limited to extremely infected COVID-19 cases [115]. In the month of February, 2 clinical trials of phase III were instigated to assess intravenous remdesivir (200 mg on day 1 and 100 mg once daily for 9 days) in 2019-nCoV cases.

Favipiravir (T-705)

Favipiravir (guanine nucleoside analogue), a apyrazinecarboxamide derivative, is a prodrug and is broken down to create ribofuranosyl-5′-triphosphate (favipiravir-RTP) to serve as purine mimetic binding to ATP- and GTP-binding sites on polymerase in a determined way [116, 117]. It works by the precise obstruction of viral RNA-dependent RNA polymerase [118]. It was originally developed by Toyama Chemical of Japan for the treatment of influenza [119]. Favipiravir can productively suppress RdRp of viruses such as influenza, Ebola, yellow fever, chikungunya, norovirus, and enterovirus [108]. Recently, favipiravir has been approved for use as a drug in clinical trials to treat nCoV 19 [120, 121]. In particular, favipiravir is precise to viral cells and so it does not block RNA or DNA synthesis in mammalian cells therefore it is harmless to them [122]. Also, an analysis revealed its action against 2019-nCoV (EC_{50} = 61.88 µM in Vero E6 cells) [123]. Patients with 2019-nCoV are evaluated for the efficacy in a combination of favipiravir with interferon-α (ChiCTR 2000029600) and favipiravir with baloxavir marboxil (a validated influenza inhibitor targeting the cap-dependent endonuclease) (ChiCTR2000029544). Further, research conducted on 80 cases found that it remarkably lessened viral removal time to 4 days and 91.43% of patients had improved CT scans with few side effects [124, 125].

Sofosbuvir/Velpatasvir (EPCLUSA)

Sofosbuvir is also known as a nucleotide analogue hepatitis C virus NS5B polymerase inhibitor. It is employed in the treatment of chronic hepatitis C as a constituent of a combined antiviral regimen. Additionally, the European Medicines Agency's Committee for Medicinal Products for Human Use has recommended the sanction of sofosbuvir for curing chronic hepatitis C [126]. The most notable drug target of the inhibitor is RdRp where it inhibits the RNA replication by the modifications at 2′ position. Furthermore, it could block RdRp of the hepatitis C virus by functioning as an RNA polymerase inhibitor by taking part with natural ribonucleotides. Since the hepatitis C virus and the coronavirus utilize a related viral genome replication process, the drug might inhibit COVID-19 [127]. When the activated triphosphate form of the drug is integrated with low-fidelity polymerases and SARS-CoV RNA-dependent RNA polymerases (RdRp), it leads to blockage of further incorporation by these polymerases.

β-D-N^4-hydroxycytidine (NHC)

NHC is a cytidine analogue with powerful, wide-spectrum antiviral activity against Venezuelan equine encephalitis virus (VEEV), influenza A virus (IAV), respiratory syncytial virus (RSV), chikungunya virus (CHIKV), influenza B virus (IBV), and CoVs. The drug exhibits antiviral activity mainly by RNA mutagenesis. Serial passaging with NHC resulted in low-level resistance for VEEV but not RSV, IAV, and bovine viral diarrhea virus which revealed a high resistance barrier [128 - 130]. The vigorous anti-CoV activity of NHC was observed for SARS-CoV and HCoV-NL63 [130, 131]. Similar to remdesivir, NHC also could interfere with CoV replication in a unique manner as evidence shown with the micromolar value of EC50; however, the inhibitory process is not well known. Its antiviral activity, either individually or in combination with other DAAs and immunomodulators, emphasizes more research in the treatment of CoV infections. As a matter of fact, it is another prodrug with broad-spectrum activity against coronaviruses by targeting its polymerase, even when it possesses complete proofreading operations [132, 133]. The isopropyl ester prodrug of the ribonucleotide analogue, NHC with enhanced bioavailability is shown to be a proven antiviral agent for the replication of human and bat SARS-Cov-2. It happens in the airway epithelial cells in mice and humans as well [134].

Ribavirin

Ribavirin is a guanosine analogue and was initially developed for curing HCV (hepatitis C virus) and RSV (respiratory syncytial virus). Its possible antiviral mechanism for RNA viruses is found to block mRNA capping and induce mutations in RNA-dependent viral replication. Coronaviruses produce exonuclease (nsp14-ExoN) in non-structural protein 14, which are seen commonly in the coronavirus family. The nsp14-ExoN is known to have an RNA proofing function [135]. In fact, it was clinically analyzed against MERS and SARS coronaviruses. But the drug is found to be linked with serious side effects like anaemia and hypoxia at large doses [136]. Additionally, following oral administration, the drug was expeditiously assimilated through sodium-dependent nucleoside transporters into the gastrointestinal tract. The oral bioavailability of the drug is 64 percent and it has a large distribution volume. Acetaminophen, acetazolamide, aspirin, acrivastine, and acyclovir are shown to lower the excretion value, resulting in an elevated ribavirin serum quantity. Thus ribavirin shows the little anti-CoV effect, *in vitro* but found to be effective against other RNA viruses [137].

Galidesivir (BCX4430)

It is an adenosine prodrug analogue originated by BioCryst Pharmaceuticals for HCV. It has the potent to suppress RNA polymerases from a wide spectrum of positive and negative-sense RNA viruses of 20 viruses in nine different families including Ebola, MERS-CoV and SARS-CoV, Marburg, Yellow Fever, and Zika viruses all of which are highly pathogenic as proven by the experimental studies in rodents and macaques [138-140]. *In vivo*, BCX4430 is functional following intramuscular, intra-peritoneal, and oral administration in different experimental infections. When BCX4430 moves into infected cells, it gets phosphorylated rapidly, and the generated nucleoside triphosphate works as an RNA chain terminator. As a broad-spectrum RNA virus inhibitor, BCX4430 has the potential to fight SARS-CoV-2.

Gemcitabine Hydrochloride

Gemcitabine, which is a NI deoxycytidine analogue, is a chemotherapy drug preventing SARS-CoV and MERS-CoV infections [130].

PROTEASES INHIBITORS

SARS-CoV-2 Main Protease Inhibitors

Inhibition of viral proteases is a proven strategy to fight against a number of viruses like human immunodeficiency virus (HIV) [141] and hepatitis C [142]. The suppression of coronavirus multiplication by employing protease inhibitors was established with the reusing of anti-HIV protease inhibitors to block the proteolytic activity [143]. The main protease (M^{pro}) of SARS-CoV-2 which is indispensable for viral proteolytic functions in the primary stages of its life cycle is regarded as an effective target for attacking the viral activity [144]. While the HIV protease uses an aspartate residue for the nucleophilic attack [145], coronavirus protease uses a cysteine residue [143]. The manipulation of drugs that inhibit M^{pro} of SARS-CoV as potential SARS-CoV-2 protease inhibitors are pragmatic [146]. Some of the structures of protease inhibitors are shown in Fig. (**3**).

Fig. (3). Chemical structures of protease inhibitors.

FDA-approved anti-HIV protease inhibitors namely lopinavir and ritonavir were proven as assured candidates for retarding the active site of SARS-CoV [147, 148]. Both the inhibitors were found to bind efficiently to the identical pocket in the active sites of M^{pro} of both SARS-CoV and SARS-CoV-2 [144].

A German Laboratory [146] designed a-ketoamide inhibitor based on a previously designed SARS-CoV protease inhibitor that successively inhibited the viral replication process in infected human Calu3 cells with an EC_{50} of 4–5 μM. These a-ketoamides form a bond on the Cys residue in the active site of the SARS-CoV series forming a thiohemiketal and this offers an advantage over HIV protease inhibitors used that lacks thiol reactivity [149, 150]. It also forms two hydrogen bonds at the catalytic active site of SARS-CoV-2 with Gly and Cys [151, 152].

Additionally, Scientists also tried to repurpose commercially available medicines to fit into the enzyme pocket of Mpro of SARS-CoV-2. Surprisingly, antibiotics and chemotherapeutic agents named colistin and valrubicin showed tight binding with 9 and 7 hydrogen bonds formed with essential amino acid residues in M^{pro} active site including THR^{24}, THR^{25}, and THR^{26} [145].

Serine Protease Inhibitors

Intriguingly, protease inhibitors are found to be potent anti-viral agents to fight against coronaviruses especially, for critical processes obstructing the proteolytic function needed for virus sustenance. Studies have revealed the application of serine protease inhibitors in interrupting the virus perforation into the host cell [67]. When the S1 part of spike protein enters the host cell, it binds to ACE 2, and thus the transmembrane serine protease (TMPRSS2) is accountable for S protein priming and enhances incision in both ACE 2 and S2 subunit generating irreversible alterations and allow viral integration with the host cell [153, 154]. Thus, the advantage of serine protease inhibitors is the prevention of entry of the virus into the host cell, and therefore suppressing its pathogenicity. Scientists are presently making an effort to reuse the already commercialized serine inhibitors for the possible treatment of COVID-19 caused by SARS-CoV-2.

In 2016, nafamostat, a blood thinner that functions by suppressing serine protease and was previously sanctioned in Japan to cure acute Pancreatitis, was repositioned to prevent MERS-CoV [155]. Recently, it is also being checked to examine if it can hinder SARS-CoV-2 entry from infecting human cells. Nafamostat may aid in the prevention of viral envelope integration with cell surface membranes in the host, which is the primary strategy in causing illness by SARS-CoV-2. Likewise, camostat, another inhibitor of TMPRSS2, prevents infection of human lung cells by minimizing the introduction of MERS-S, SARS-S, and SARS-2-S proteins into lung cell lines [67]. When compared to camostat, nafamostat inhibited viral membrane fusion at a 10 times lessened concentration [156]. In general, they both symbolize an intriguing category of compounds that could be effective in the modern COVID-19 endemic challenge.

Malaria Drugs in COVID-19

Chloroquine, hydroxychloroquine, and the structurally interconnected atovaquone and mefloquine are all drugs to treat malaria that have been employed for a long time. In animal studies, hydroxychloroquine, a hydroxyl analogue of chloroquine that was manufactured in the mid-twentieth century, was suggested to be a harmless derivative when compared to the parent chloroquine. They also have immunomodulatory effects and so they are employed in the treatment of rheumatoid arthritis or lupus erythematous diseases [157]. Some of the structures of malarial drugs are shown in Fig. (4).

An *in vivo* and *in vitro* antiviral activity of malaria drugs revealed that the use of antimalarial drugs to eradicate viral diseases could be productive particularly in the cases of viral resistance and emergencies [158]. The IC50 of chloroquine against SARS-CoV was 8.8 1.2 M in an *in vitro* study, which was lower when compared with the cytostatic activity possessing CC50 (261.3 14.5 M) with a selectivity index of 30. *In vitro*, the chloroquine's IC50 for SARS-CoV obstruction is similar to chloroquine plasma concentrations during malaria treatment. Chloroquine's antiviral activity was procrastinated for up to 5 hours after it was included in the sample cultures but there was no significant drop-in antiviral activity. Thus it facilitated the use of chloroquine for the suppression and remedy of SARS-CoV infections [159]. Also, *in vitro* study proved that chloroquine could prevent the viral multiplication and dispersion of CoV, and obstructs CoV infection in newly born mice, and thus it is recognized as an assuring powerful antiviral agent [160].

Chloroquine

Hydroxychloroquine

Fig. (4). Chemical structures of malarial drugs.

Another analysis revealed that, in comparison with chloroquine, hydroxychloroquine is thrice more effective in treating SARS-CoV-2 infected cells as inferred by EC50 = 5.47 and 0.72 M, respectively. This approach is based on the immunomodulatory properties of chloroquine and hydroxychloroquine, which could be advantageous in reducing cytokine stress in SARS-CoV-2 individuals [161]. Chloroquine is productive in blocking the dispersion of SARS-CoV in cell culture, according to Vincent and his colleagues [162]. This consequence was discovered in cells that had been treated with chloroquine before or after infection with SARS-CoV. The analysis found that chloroquine can raise endosomal pH or interrupt the cellular receptor's terminal glycosylation, angiotensin-converting enzyme-2 and hence, affecting virus receptor binding. In a modern study, hydroxychloroquine was recognized to be effective in obstructing SARS-CoV-2 *in vitro*. If the toxicity profile has been acclaimed by clinical research, it may diminish the inflammatory response connected with COVID-19 and thus fighting with the infection [163].

The N-cinnamoyl analogues of chloroquine 3a, b, have been shown to be productive *in vitro* in treating pneumocystis pneumonia caused by pulmonary viral, bacterial, mycobacterial, or parasitic diseases. Compounds 3a and 3b will be tested *in vivo* as powerful anti-pneumocystis pneumonia agents [151].

The framework of wide-ranging antiviral drugs of chloroquine and hydroxychloroquine is connected to a reduction in inflammatory mediators like TNF-α and IL6 production. It is also suggested that hydroxychloroquine and its analogues may be effective in the remedy of viral infections that are accompanied by inflammation or immune hyperactivity. Furthermore, a class of chloroquine analogues-4 has been shown to suppress the activity of tumor susceptibility gene (TSG101) expression as well as viral multiplication by obstructing delayed viral function, probably when viral protein synthesis gets completed [164]. Inhibition of this gene may prevent the virus from reaching the cell surface and, as a result, create an impact on budding [149].

Furthermore, the antimalarial drug atovaquone works by obstructing viral multiplication by delaying pyrimidine biosynthesis. Atovaquone could restrict Zika virus infection in an *in vitro* analysis using a human placental representation, implying that it could be used as a wide-ranging antiviral drug [165]. The antimalarial drugs mefloquine and HCl, as well as the antiparasitic drug selamectin, were recognized to be effective antiviral drugs for curing COVID-19 disease in a study conducted by Fan and colleagues [166].

The FDA sanctioned chloroquine as a remedy for COVID-19 disease with well-determined preventive measures in the mid of March 2020, which allowed to short-term use of the chloroquine and hydroxylchloroquine arm of the great, international Solidarity trial [167] from the May end to earlier June. The FDA invalidated the approval for these drugs in critical situations on June 15 following the re-evaluation of the generated data. Therefore, the drugs chloroquine and hydroxylchloroquine needed to be delivered with precaution when used for curing COVID-19 disease to counteract the probable cardiovascular complications [168].

Lipid Lowering Statins

Rosuvastatin (RSV), an FDA-approved statin, is utilized as a lipid-lowering agent. It works by inhibiting the HMG-CoA reductase enzyme, thereby decreasing or lowering the level of cholesterol, and is therefore inexpensive and safe [169]. It also enhances lung pathological changes by reducing cytokines mediated by T helper cells Th2 and Th17 in which the function is not correlated with its lipid-lowering mechanism [170].

In patients who were affected by severe SARS-CoV, Totura *et al.* proposed that toll-like receptor 3 (TLR3) signaling plays a defensive role in the innate immune response [171]. TLR-MYD88 agonists are FDA-approved statins that maintain TLR-MYD88 measures during hypoxia [172]. For the survival of MERS-CoV infection, timely statin administration may be crucial [173]. In a recent research review, it has been shown that ACE2 is upregulated by angiotensin receptor blockers and statins and thus offers prevention against acute respiratory disease syndrome and can minimize the death numbers [174]. Statins are considered to lessen the death rate of influenza-affected patients as a result of their anti-inflammatory and immuno-modulatory effect [175].

Furthermore, rosuvastatin reduces cytokines TNF-a, IFN-g, and Th-1 immune reaction during 72 h by employing rapid immunomodulatory effects [176]. Since the inhibitor does not produce any side effects, patients reported with viral respiratory infections, such as COVID-19, may benefit from continuing their statin therapy [174]. When statins, particularly rosuvastatin, are administered to COVID-19 individuals with severe infection, they decrease cardiovascular complications such as lethal myocardial infarction [177].

Rheumatoid Arthritis Drugs

Disease-Modifying Antirheumatic Drugs (DMARDs) are a different group of drugs, classified according to their utilization and protocol, for the remedy of inflammatory diseases like rheumatoid arthritis (RA). These are immunosuppressive and immunomodulatory agents having the potential to refine symptoms decrease joint damage and various sorts of aches and inflammations manifesting impact on heart and blood vessels [178]. They include:

Tocilizumab (TCZ)

It was established by Osaka University for curing inflammatory and autoimmune diseases [179]. Tocilizumab has ended with phase 2 clinical testing for the remedy of pulmonary arterial hypertension (PAH) [180]. China's National Health Commission recommends the drug for its safety and efficacy to employ 8 mg kg^{-1}/12 h in regulations to cure COVID-19 individuals either individually or in conjunction with favipiravir, a wide-ranging anti-viral drug. Out of twenty covid-19 patients involved in the Chinese clinical trial, within two weeks, 19 of them had shown good antiviral activity. Furthermore, Hong Zhao of Peking University First Hospital is leading a 150-patient trial evaluating tocilizumab, and Dongsheng Wang of The First Affiliated Hospital of University of Science and Technology of China (Anhui Provincial Hospital) is leading a 188-patient trial evaluating only tocilizumab [181].

Sarilumab

It is one of the two IL-6 receptor antagonists being analyzed to use as a powerful COVID-19 drug in the treatments. Similar to TCZ, sarilumab is sanctioned by the FDA in 2017 as a remedy for adults with average to extreme active rheumatoid arthritis [182]. In the mid of March 2020, in association with the FDA and the Biomedical Advanced Research and Development Authority (BARDA), the Phase II/III clinical program was carried out with 400 patients testing the antagonist in extreme COVID-19 patients. Long-term effects like lowering the requirement for hospitalization, and artificial oxygenation and lethality were assessed in the phase III trial [183].

Baricitinib

In June 2018, baricitinib was FDA-approved to treat average to seriously active rheumatoid arthritis (RA). It is used against Janus Kinase (JAK) and exerts its function by selective inhibition of the enzymes JAK1 and JAK2 [184]. Artificial intelligence (AI) software has been used by AI study groups and others to identify an already licensed drug to minimize infection [95]. Scientists revealed that the virus enters human cells by interacting with the cell-surface receptor, ACE2 [185]. The software aimed at the enzyme adaptor-associated protein kinase 1 (AAK1) as a probable target for the disease. AAK1 controls the mechanism of endocytosis which is known for its usual way of viral infection. AI selects the drug on the basis of its attraction for the kinase and its toxicity for more than 378 known AAK1 inhibitors. Janus-associated kinase (JAK) inhibitor baricitinib is indicted to lower the capacity of the virus to affect lung cells by the suppression of ACE2-mediated endocytosis [96].

Ruxolitinib, a potent anti-inflammatory and antiviral drug has been shown to function against the cytokine storm associated with COVID-19, where cytokine levels have been found to be substantially reduced and are therefore subjected to phase III clinical trials for COVID-19 [185].

Corticosteroids

Corticosteroid drugs are a group of synthetic steroid hormones that are originated in the adrenal cortex in healthy individuals. Corticosteroids, including glucocorticoids and mineralocorticoids, are used to treat a wide range of diseases and symptoms. In treating conditions such as chronic obstructive pulmonary disorder, extreme allergies, rheumatic problems, asthma, various skin conditions, swelling of the brain, and tuberculosis, one of the corticosteroid medications called dexamethasone, which is more specifically a glucocorticoid, is used [186]. As first reported in the RECOVERY study, the estimation of the experimental prospective studies, as well as the RCTs, confirmed the positive impact of corticosteroid treatment on the lethality in COVID-19 disease [187]. Dexamethasone decreases deaths by one-third in critically ill COVID-19 patients, according to a modern study large-scale RCT (the RECOVERY trial). Dexamethasone (6 mg/day for 10 days) was given to 2,100 individuals in the intervention category, while persons in the control group (n=4,300) obtained normal treatment for the disease [188].

Miscellaneous Drugs

In the treatment of COVID infections, certain other drug molecules or agents have possible beneficial effects. Study reports indicate that N-acetylcysteine in conjunction with antiviral agents would collaboratively minimize the mortal impact of influenza virus infection when antioxidants like ascorbic acid are used [189]. Another study revealed that integration of the influenza drug oseltamivir and N-acetylcysteine could boost the host protection process and reduce death rates by reducing oxidative stress related to viral disease [190, 191]. Cytoprotective effects on vital organs have been observed in dietary supplements like resveratrol, curcumin, and sulforaphane. It is possible to extrapolate this strategy to the affected lungs in coronavirus individuals. A current analysis found that the integration of thalidomide and celecoxib, the selective COX-2 inhibitor, could boost extreme COVID-19-related pneumonia by modulating activated NF-KB that promotes extreme pulmonary injury [192].

Ivermectin, an antiparasitic drug approved by the FDA, has been shown to have wide-ranging antiviral efficacy. Interestingly, modern studies have revealed that the particular treatment is a powerful SARS-CoV-2 inhibitor. Ivermectin induces a decrease in viral RNA of 5000 in two days; however, it needs potential human clinical investigation [193].

CONCLUDING REMARKS

The Covid-19 disease has created a world-wide health calamity. The capacity of the virus to mutate rapidly and modifications in tissue tropism has proposed formidable difficulties in finding drugs and vaccines. Repositioning of old drugs is indeed an attractive and useful technique for discovering drugs against various viruses, including SARS-CoV-2. Researchers and scientists around the world have come together for discovering drugs by repurposing the already available drugs for treating the disease. Plenty of drugs of various classes have been employed for reducing the risk of infection, and fortunately, many of the repurposed drugs possess antiviral activity against SARS-CoV-2 both in cell lines and animal studies.

CONSENT FOR PUBLICATION

Not Applicable.

CONFLICT OF INTEREST

The author declares no conflict of interest, financial or otherwise.

ACKNOWLEDGEMENTS

Declared none.

REFERENCES

[1] Ramadan N, Shaib H. Middle East respiratory syndrome coronavirus (MERS-CoV): A review. Germs 2019; 9(1): 35-42.
[http://dx.doi.org/10.18683/germs.2019.1155] [PMID: 31119115]

[2] Zhong NS, Zheng BJ, Li YM, *et al.* Epidemiology and cause of severe acute respiratory syndrome (SARS) in Guangdong, People's Republic of China, in February, 2003. Lancet 2003; 362(9393): 1353-8.
[http://dx.doi.org/10.1016/S0140-6736(03)14630-2] [PMID: 14585636]

[3] Zhou P, Yang XL, Wang XG, *et al.* A pneumonia outbreak associated with a new coronavirus of probable bat origin. Nature 2020; 579(7798): 270-3.
[http://dx.doi.org/10.1038/s41586-020-2012-7] [PMID: 32015507]

[4] Wrapp D, Wang N, Corbett KS, *et al.* Cryo-EM structure of the 2019-nCoV spike in the prefusion conformation. Science 2020; 367(6483): 1260-3.
[http://dx.doi.org/10.1126/science.abb2507] [PMID: 32075877]

[5] Phan T. Genetic diversity and evolution of SARS-CoV-2. Infect Genet Evol 2020; 81: 104260-2.
[http://dx.doi.org/10.1016/j.meegid.2020.104260] [PMID: 32092483]

[6] Cyranoski D. Did pangolins spread the China coronavirus to people? Nature 2020.
[http://dx.doi.org/10.1038/d41586-020-00364-2] [PMID: 33547428]

[7] Fan Y, Zhao K, Shi ZL, Zhou P. Bat Coronaviruses in China. Viruses 2019; 11(3): 210-23.
[http://dx.doi.org/10.3390/v11030210] [PMID: 30832341]

[8] Decaro N, Mari V, Elia G, *et al.* Recombinant canine coronaviruses in dogs, Europe. Emerg Infect Dis 2010; 16(1): 41-7.
[http://dx.doi.org/10.3201/eid1601.090726] [PMID: 20031041]

[9] Huang C, Wang Y, Li X, *et al.* Clinical features of patients infected with 2019 novel coronavirus in Wuhan, China. Lancet 2020; 395(10223): 497-506.
[http://dx.doi.org/10.1016/S0140-6736(20)30183-5] [PMID: 31986264]

[10] CDC 2019 Novel coronavirus, Wuhan, China. 2020. 2020.

[11] WHO. Novel coronavirus-china. 2020.

[12] Cui J, Li F, Shi ZL. Origin and evolution of pathogenic coronaviruses. Nat Rev Microbiol 2019; 17(3): 181-92.
[http://dx.doi.org/10.1038/s41579-018-0118-9] [PMID: 30531947]

[13] Gorbalenya AE, Baker SC, Baric RS, *et al.* Severe acute respiratory syndrome-related coronavirus: the species and its viruses-a statement of the Coronavirus Study Group BioRxiv 2020.
[http://dx.doi.org/10.1101/2020.02.07.937862]

[14] Richman DD, Whitley RJ, Hayden FG. Clinical Virology. 4th ed. Washington: ASM Press 2016; p. 9.
[http://dx.doi.org/10.1128/9781555819439]

[15] Chan JF, Kok KH, Zhu Z, *et al.* Genomic characterization of the 2019 novel human-pathogenic coronavirus isolated from a patient with atypical pneumonia after visiting Wuhan. Emerg Microbes Infect 2020; 9(1): 221-36.
[http://dx.doi.org/10.1080/22221751.2020.1719902] [PMID: 31987001]

[16] Masters PS. The molecular biology of coronaviruses. Adv Virus Res 2006; 66: 193-292.
[http://dx.doi.org/10.1016/S0065-3527(06)66005-3] [PMID: 16877062]

[17] Mortola E, Roy P. Efficient assembly and release of SARS coronavirus-like particles by a heterologous expression system. FEBS Lett 2004; 576(1-2): 174-8.
[http://dx.doi.org/10.1016/j.febslet.2004.09.009] [PMID: 15474033]

[18] McBride R, van Zyl M, Fielding BC. The coronavirus nucleocapsid is a multifunctional protein. Viruses 2014; 6(8): 2991-3018.
[http://dx.doi.org/10.3390/v6082991] [PMID: 25105276]

[19] Guo Y, Korteweg C, McNutt MA, Gu J. Pathogenetic mechanisms of severe acute respiratory syndrome. Virus Res 2008; 133(1): 4-12.
[http://dx.doi.org/10.1016/j.virusres.2007.01.022] [PMID: 17825937]

[20] Zhu N, Zhang D, Wang W, *et al.* A novel coronavirus from patients with pneumonia in China, 2019. N Engl J Med 2020; 382(8): 727-33.
[http://dx.doi.org/10.1056/NEJMoa2001017] [PMID: 31978945]

[21] Siu YL, Teoh KT, Lo J, *et al.* The M, E, and N structural proteins of the severe acute respiratory syndrome coronavirus are required for efficient assembly, trafficking, and release of virus-like particles. J Virol 2008; 82(22): 11318-30.
[http://dx.doi.org/10.1128/JVI.01052-08] [PMID: 18753196]

[22] Kirchdoerfer RN, Cottrell CA, Wang N, *et al.* Pre-fusion structure of a human coronavirus spike protein. Nature 2016; 531(7592): 118-21.
[http://dx.doi.org/10.1038/nature17200] [PMID: 26935699]

[23] Walls AC, Park YJ, Tortorici MA, Wall A, McGuire AT, Veesler D. Structure, Function, and Antigenicity of the SARS-CoV-2 Spike Glycoprotein. Cell 2020; 181(2): 281-292.e6.
[http://dx.doi.org/10.1016/j.cell.2020.02.058] [PMID: 32155444]

[24] Li F. Structure, function, and evolution of coronavirus spike proteins. Annu Rev Virol 2016; 3(1): 237-61.
[http://dx.doi.org/10.1146/annurev-virology-110615-042301] [PMID: 27578435]

[25] Cascella M, Rajnik M, Cuomo A, *et al.* Features, evaluation, and treatment of coronavirus (COVID-19).StatPearls. Treasure Island, FL: StatPearls Publishing 2021.

[26] Neuman BW, Kiss G, Kunding AH, *et al.* A structural analysis of M protein in coronavirus assembly and morphology. J Struct Biol 2011; 174(1): 11-22.
[http://dx.doi.org/10.1016/j.jsb.2010.11.021] [PMID: 21130884]

[27] Niemann H, Geyer R, Klenk HD, Linder D, Stirm S, Wirth M. The carbohydrates of mouse hepatitis virus (MHV) A59: structures of the *O*-glycosidically linked oligosaccharides of glycoprotein E1. EMBO J 1984; 3(3): 665-70.
[http://dx.doi.org/10.1002/j.1460-2075.1984.tb01864.x] [PMID: 6325180]

[28] Narayanan K, Maeda A, Maeda J, Makino S. Characterization of the coronavirus M protein and nucleocapsid interaction in infected cells. J Virol 2000; 74(17): 8127-34.
[http://dx.doi.org/10.1128/JVI.74.17.8127-8134.2000] [PMID: 10933723]

[29] Escors D, Ortego J, Laude H, Enjuanes L. The membrane M protein carboxy terminus binds to transmissible gastroenteritis coronavirus core and contributes to core stability. J Virol 2001; 75(3): 1312-24.
[http://dx.doi.org/10.1128/JVI.75.3.1312-1324.2001] [PMID: 11152504]

[30] Raamsman MJ, Locker JK, de Hooge A, *et al.* Characterization of the coronavirus mouse hepatitis virus strain A59 small membrane protein E. J Virol 2000; 74(5): 2333-42.
[http://dx.doi.org/10.1128/JVI.74.5.2333-2342.2000] [PMID: 10666264]

[31] Venkatagopalan P, Daskalova SM, Lopez LA, Dolezal KA, Hogue BG. Coronavirus envelope (E) protein remains at the site of assembly. Virology 2015; 478: 75-85.
[http://dx.doi.org/10.1016/j.virol.2015.02.005] [PMID: 25726972]

[32] Nieto-Torres JL, Dediego ML, Álvarez E, *et al.* Subcellular location and topology of severe acute respiratory syndrome coronavirus envelope protein. Virology 2011; 415(2): 69-82.
[http://dx.doi.org/10.1016/j.virol.2011.03.029] [PMID: 21524776]

[33] de Haan CA, Rottier PJ. Molecular interactions in the assembly of coronaviruses. Adv Virus Res 2005; 64: 165-230.
[http://dx.doi.org/10.1016/S0065-3527(05)64006-7] [PMID: 16139595]

[34] Fehr AR, Perlman S. Coronaviruses: An overview of their replication and pathogenesis Coronaviruses. Springer 2015; pp. 1-23.

[35] Escors D, Ortego J, Enjuanes L. The membrane M protein of the transmissible gastroenteritis coronavirus binds to the internal core through the carboxy-terminus. Adv Exp Med Biol 2001; 494: 589-93.
[http://dx.doi.org/10.1007/978-1-4615-1325-4_87] [PMID: 11774530]

[36] Duan YN, Qin J. Pre and post-treatment chest CT findings: 2019 novel coronavirus (2019-nCoV) pneumonia. Radiology 2020; 295(1): 21.
[http://dx.doi.org/10.1148/radiol.2020200323] [PMID: 32049602]

[37] Guan WJ, Ni ZY, Hu Y, *et al.* Clinical characteristics of 2019 novel coronavirus infection in China. medRxiv 2020.
[http://dx.doi.org/10.1101/2020.02.06.20020974]

[38] Lu R, Zhao X, Li J, *et al.* Genomic characterisation and epidemiology of 2019 novel coronavirus: implications for virus origins and receptor binding. Lancet 2020; 395(10224): 565-74.
[http://dx.doi.org/10.1016/S0140-6736(20)30251-8] [PMID: 32007145]

[39] Singhal T. A Review of Coronavirus Disease-2019 (COVID-19). Indian J Pediatr 2020; 87(4): 281-6.
[http://dx.doi.org/10.1007/s12098-020-03263-6] [PMID: 32166607]

[40] WMHC. Wuhan municipal health and health commission's briefing on the current pneumonia epidemic situation in our city. 2020.

[41] Chen N, Zhou M, Dong X, *et al.* Epidemiological and clinical characteristics of 99 cases of 2019 novel coronavirus pneumonia in Wuhan, China: a descriptive study. Lancet 2020; 395(10223): 507-13.

[http://dx.doi.org/10.1016/S0140-6736(20)30211-7] [PMID: 32007143]

[42] Li Q, Guan X, Wu P, *et al.* Early transmission dynamics in Wuhan, China, of novel coronavirus-infected pneumonia. N Engl J Med 2020; 382(13): 1199-207.
[http://dx.doi.org/10.1056/NEJMoa2001316] [PMID: 31995857]

[43] Ji W, Wang W, Zhao X, Zai J, Li X. Cross-species transmission of the newly identified coronavirus 2019-nCoV. J Med Virol 2020; 92(4): 433-40.
[http://dx.doi.org/10.1002/jmv.25682] [PMID: 31967321]

[44] Novel Coronavirus (2019-nCoV) (Situation Report – 22). Available at: https://apps.who.int/iris/handle/10665/330991

[45] Wang N, Li SY, Yang XL, *et al.* Serological evidence of bat SARS-related coronavirus infection in humans. Virol Sin 2018; 33(1): 104-7.
[http://dx.doi.org/10.1007/s12250-018-0012-7] [PMID: 29500691]

[46] Guo Q, Li M, Wang C, *et al.* Host and infectivity prediction of Wuhan 2019 novel coronavirus using deep learning algorithm. bioRxiv 2020.
[http://dx.doi.org/10.1101/2020.01.21.914044]

[47] Lam TT, Jia N, Zhang YW, *et al.* Identifying SARS-CoV-2-related coronaviruses in Malayan pangolins. Nature 2020; 583(7815): 282-5.
[http://dx.doi.org/10.1038/s41586-020-2169-0] [PMID: 32218527]

[48] Guan WJ, Liang WH, Zhao Y, *et al.* Comorbidity and its impact on 1590 patients with COVID-19 in China: a nationwide analysis. Eur Respir J 2020; 55(5): 2000547-60.
[http://dx.doi.org/10.1183/13993003.00547-2020] [PMID: 32217650]

[49] Rothan HA, Byrareddy SN. The epidemiology and pathogenesis of coronavirus disease (COVID-19) outbreak. J Autoimmun 2020; 109: 102433-6.
[http://dx.doi.org/10.1016/j.jaut.2020.102433] [PMID: 32113704]

[50] Han Y, Yang H. The transmission and diagnosis of 2019 novel coronavirus infection disease (COVID-19): A Chinese perspective. J Med Virol 2020; 92(6): 639-44.
[http://dx.doi.org/10.1002/jmv.25749] [PMID: 32141619]

[51] World Health Organization. Clinical management of severe acute respiratory infection when novel coronavirus (2019-nCoV) infection is suspected. Geneva: WHO 2020.

[52] Zou L, Ruan F, Huang M, *et al.* SARS-CoV-2 viral load in upper respiratory specimens of infected patients. N Engl J Med 2020; 382(12): 1177-9.
[http://dx.doi.org/10.1056/NEJMc2001737] [PMID: 32074444]

[53] Kampf G, Todt D, Pfaender S, Steinmann E. Persistence of coronaviruses on inanimate surfaces and their inactivation with biocidal agents. J Hosp Infect 2020; 104(3): 246-51.
[http://dx.doi.org/10.1016/j.jhin.2020.01.022] [PMID: 32035997]

[54] Li W, Moore MJ, Vasilieva N, *et al.* Angiotensin-converting enzyme 2 is a functional receptor for the SARS coronavirus. Nature 2003; 426(6965): 450-4.
[http://dx.doi.org/10.1038/nature02145] [PMID: 14647384]

[55] Turner AJ, Hiscox JA, Hooper NM. ACE2: from vasopeptidase to SARS virus receptor. Trends Pharmacol Sci 2004; 25(6): 291-4.
[http://dx.doi.org/10.1016/j.tips.2004.04.001] [PMID: 15165741]

[56] Wu Z, McGoogan JM. Characteristics of and important lessons from the coronavirus disease 2019 (COVID-19) outbreak in China: summary of a report of 72314 cases from the Chinese Center for Disease Control and Prevention. JAMA 2020; 323(13): 1239-42.
[http://dx.doi.org/10.1001/jama.2020.2648] [PMID: 32091533]

[57] Wan Y, Shang J, Graham R, Baric RS, Li F. Receptor recognition by novel coronavirus from Wuhan: An analysis based on decade-long structural studies of SARS. J Virol 2020; 94(7): e00127-20.

[http://dx.doi.org/10.1128/JVI.00127-20] [PMID: 31996437]

[58] Riordan JF. Angiotensin-I-converting enzyme and its relatives. Genome Biol 2003; 4(8): 225-9.
[http://dx.doi.org/10.1186/gb-2003-4-8-225] [PMID: 12914653]

[59] Cheng ZJ, Shan J. 2019 Novel coronavirus: where we are and what we know. Infection 2020; 48(2): 155-63.
[http://dx.doi.org/10.1007/s15010-020-01401-y] [PMID: 32072569]

[60] Kuba K, Imai Y, Ohto-Nakanishi T, Penninger JM. Trilogy of ACE2: a peptidase in the renin-angiotensin system, a SARS receptor, and a partner for amino acid transporters. Pharmacol Ther 2010; 128(1): 119-28.
[http://dx.doi.org/10.1016/j.pharmthera.2010.06.003] [PMID: 20599443]

[61] Jiang F, Yang J, Zhang Y, *et al.* Angiotensin-converting enzyme 2 and angiotensin 1-7: novel therapeutic targets. Nat Rev Cardiol 2014; 11(7): 413-26.
[http://dx.doi.org/10.1038/nrcardio.2014.59] [PMID: 24776703]

[62] Gu J, Korteweg C. Pathology and pathogenesis of severe acute respiratory syndrome. Am J Pathol 2007; 170(4): 1136-47.
[http://dx.doi.org/10.2353/ajpath.2007.061088] [PMID: 17392154]

[63] Harmer D, Gilbert M, Borman R, Clark KL. Quantitative mRNA expression profiling of ACE 2, a novel homologue of angiotensin converting enzyme. FEBS Lett 2002; 532(1-2): 107-10.
[http://dx.doi.org/10.1016/S0014-5793(02)03640-2] [PMID: 12459472]

[64] Leung WK, To KF, Chan PK, *et al.* Enteric involvement of severe acute respiratory syndrome-associated coronavirus infection. Gastroenterology 2003; 125(4): 1011-7.
[http://dx.doi.org/10.1016/j.gastro.2003.08.001] [PMID: 14517783]

[65] Hamming I, Timens W, Bulthuis ML, Lely AT, Navis G, van Goor H. Tissue distribution of ACE2 protein, the functional receptor for SARS coronavirus. A first step in understanding SARS pathogenesis. J Pathol 2004; 203(2): 631-7.
[http://dx.doi.org/10.1002/path.1570] [PMID: 15141377]

[66] Sims AC, Baric RS, Yount B, Burkett SE, Collins PL, Pickles RJ. Severe acute respiratory syndrome coronavirus infection of human ciliated airway epithelia: role of ciliated cells in viral spread in the conducting airways of the lungs. J Virol 2005; 79(24): 15511-24.
[http://dx.doi.org/10.1128/JVI.79.24.15511-15524.2005] [PMID: 16306622]

[67] Hoffmann M, Kleine-Weber H, Schroeder S, *et al.* SARS-CoV-2 cell entry depends on ACE2 and TMPRSS2 and is blocked by a clinically proven protease inhibitor. Cell 2020; 181(2): 271-280.e8.
[http://dx.doi.org/10.1016/j.cell.2020.02.052] [PMID: 32142651]

[68] Boopathi S, Poma AB, Kolandaivel P. Novel 2019 Coronavirus structure, mechanism of action, antiviral drug promises and rule out against its treatment. J Biomol Struct Dyn 2020; 1: 1-10.
[http://dx.doi.org/10.1080/07391102.2020.1758788] [PMID: 32306836]

[69] Stobart CC, Sexton NR, Munjal H, *et al.* Chimeric exchange of coronavirus nsp5 proteases (3CLpro) identifies common and divergent regulatory determinants of protease activity. J Virol 2013; 87(23): 12611-8.
[http://dx.doi.org/10.1128/JVI.02050-13] [PMID: 24027335]

[70] Wang H, Xue S, Yang H, Chen C. Recent progress in the discovery of inhibitors targeting coronavirus proteases. Virol Sin 2016; 31(1): 24-30.
[http://dx.doi.org/10.1007/s12250-015-3711-3] [PMID: 26920707]

[71] te Velthuis AJ, van den Worm SH, Snijder EJ. The SARS-coronavirus nsp7+nsp8 complex is a unique multimeric RNA polymerase capable of both *de novo* initiation and primer extension. Nucleic Acids Res 2012; 40(4): 1737-47.
[http://dx.doi.org/10.1093/nar/gkr893] [PMID: 22039154]

[72] Bouvet M, Lugari A, Posthuma CC, *et al.* Coronavirus Nsp10, a critical co-factor for activation of

multiple replicative enzymes. J Biol Chem 2014; 289(37): 25783-96.
[http://dx.doi.org/10.1074/jbc.M114.577353] [PMID: 25074927]

[73] Zhao X, Sehgal M, Hou Z, *et al.* Identification of residues controlling restriction versus enhancing activities of IFITM proteins on entry of human coronaviruses. J Virol 2018; 92(6): e01535-17.
[http://dx.doi.org/10.1128/JVI.01535-17] [PMID: 29263263]

[74] Qian Z, Travanty EA, Oko L, *et al.* Innate immune response of human alveolar type II cells infected with severe acute respiratory syndrome-coronavirus. Am J Respir Cell Mol Biol 2013; 48(6): 742-8.
[http://dx.doi.org/10.1165/rcmb.2012-0339OC] [PMID: 23418343]

[75] Wang J, Nikrad MP, Phang T, *et al.* Innate immune response to influenza A virus in differentiated human alveolar type II cells. Am J Respir Cell Mol Biol 2011; 45(3): 582-91.
[http://dx.doi.org/10.1165/rcmb.2010-0108OC] [PMID: 21239608]

[76] World Health Organization. Situation reports. Available at: https://www.who.int/emergencies/diseases/novel-coronavirus-2019/situation-reports/

[77] World Health Organization. Novel Coronavirus (2019-nCoV) situation report-14. 2020a. Available at: https://www.who.int/docs/default-source/coronaviruse/situationreports/20200203-sitrep-14-ncov.pdf

[78] Li G, De Clercq E. Therapeutic options for the 2019 novel coronavirus (2019-nCoV). Nat Rev Drug Discov 2020; 19(3): 149-50.
[http://dx.doi.org/10.1038/d41573-020-00016-0] [PMID: 32127666]

[79] Mercorelli B, Palù G, Loregian A. Drug repurposing for viral infectious diseases: How far are we? Trends Microbiol 2018; 26(10): 865-76.
[http://dx.doi.org/10.1016/j.tim.2018.04.004] [PMID: 29759926]

[80] Pizzorno A, Padey B, Terrier O, Rosa-Calatrava M. Drug repurposing approaches for the treatment of influenza viral infection: reviving old drugs to fight against a long-lived enemy. Front Immunol 2019; 10: 531-42.
[http://dx.doi.org/10.3389/fimmu.2019.00531] [PMID: 30941148]

[81] Andersen PI, Ianevski A, Lysvand H, *et al.* Discovery and development of safe-in-man broad-spectrum antiviral agents. International Journal of Infectious Diseases: IJID: Official Publication of the International Society for Infectious Diseases 2020; 93: 268-76.
[http://dx.doi.org/10.1016/j.ijid.2020.02.018] [PMID: 32081774]

[82] Ianevski A, Zusinaite E, Kuivanen S, *et al.* Novel activities of safe-in-human broad-spectrum antiviral agents. Antiviral Res 2018; 154: 174-82.
[http://dx.doi.org/10.1016/j.antiviral.2018.04.016] [PMID: 29698664]

[83] Pant S, Singh M, Ravichandiran V, *et al.* Peptide-like and small-molecule inhibitors against Covid-19. J Biomol Struct Dyn 2020; 1-10.
[PMID: 32306822]

[84] Xiong R, Zhang L, Li S, *et al.* Novel and potent inhibitors targeting DHODH, a rate-limiting enzyme in de novo pyrimidine biosynthesis, are broad-spectrum antiviral against RNA viruses including newly emerged coronavirus SARS-CoV-2. Protein Cell 2020; 11: 723-39.
[http://dx.doi.org/10.1007/s13238-020-00768-w] [PMID: 32754890]

[85] Xu J, Shi PY, Li H, Zhou J. Broad spectrum antiviral agent niclosamide and its therapeutic potential. ACS Infect Dis 2020; 6(5): 909-15.
[http://dx.doi.org/10.1021/acsinfecdis.0c00052] [PMID: 32125140]

[86] Cui H, Zhang C, Zhao Z, *et al.* Identification of cellular microRNA miR-188-3p with broad-spectrum anti-influenza A virus activity. Virol J 2020; 17(1): 12-23.
[http://dx.doi.org/10.1186/s12985-020-1283-9] [PMID: 32000791]

[87] Ji X, Li Z. Medicinal chemistry strategies toward host targeting antiviral agents. Med Res Rev 2020; 40(5): 1519-57.
[http://dx.doi.org/10.1002/med.21664] [PMID: 32060956]

[88] Kouznetsova J, Sun W, Martínez-Romero C, *et al.* Identification of 53 compounds that block Ebola virus-like particle entry *via* a repurposing screen of approved drugs. Emerg Microbes Infect 2014; 3(12): e84.
[http://dx.doi.org/10.1038/emi.2014.88] [PMID: 26038505]

[89] Xu M, Lee EM, Wen Z, *et al.* Identification of small-molecule inhibitors of Zika virus infection and induced neural cell death *via* a drug repurposing screen. Nat Med 2016; 22(10): 1101-7.
[http://dx.doi.org/10.1038/nm.4184] [PMID: 27571349]

[90] Aggarwal M, Leser GP, Lamb RA. Repurposing papaverine as an antiviral agent against influenza viruses and paramyxoviruses. J Virol 2020; 94(6): 1-14.
[http://dx.doi.org/10.1128/JVI.01888-19] [PMID: 31896588]

[91] Senathilake K, Samarakoon S, Tennekoon K. Virtual screening of inhibitors against spike glycoprotein of 2019 novel corona virus: A drug repurposing approach. Preprints 2020.

[92] Aanouz I, Belhassan A, ElKhatabi K, *et al.* Moroccan medicinal plants as inhibitors of COVID-19: Computational investigations. J Biomol Struct Dyn 2020; 6: 1-12.

[93] Mohanty S, Harun Ai Rashid M, Mridul M, Mohanty C, Swayamsiddha S. Application of Artificial Intelligence in COVID-19 drug repurposing. Diabetes Metab Syndr 2020; 14(5): 1027-31.
[http://dx.doi.org/10.1016/j.dsx.2020.06.068] [PMID: 32634717]

[94] Gysi DM, Do Valle I, Zitnik M, *et al.* Network medicine framework for identifying drug repurposing opportunities for COVID-19. arXiv 2020.

[95] Richardson P, Griffin I, Tucker C, *et al.* Baricitinib as potential treatment for 2019-nCoV acute respiratory disease. Lancet 2020; 395(10223): e30-1.
[http://dx.doi.org/10.1016/S0140-6736(20)30304-4] [PMID: 32032529]

[96] Beck BR, Shin B, Choi Y, Park S, Kang K. Predicting commercially available antiviral drugs that may act on the novel coronavirus (SARS-CoV-2) through a drug-target interaction deep learning model. Comput Struct Biotechnol J 2020; 18: 784-90.
[http://dx.doi.org/10.1016/j.csbj.2020.03.025] [PMID: 32280433]

[97] Gupta MK, Vemula S, Donde R, *et al.* In-silico approaches to detect inhibitors of the human severe acute respiratory syndrome coronavirus envelope protein ion channel. J Biomol Struct Dyn 2020; 15: 1-17.
[http://dx.doi.org/10.1080/07391102.2020.1751300] [PMID: 32238078]

[98] Jomah S, Asdaq SMB, Al-Yamani MJ. Clinical efficacy of antivirals against novel coronavirus (COVID-19): A review. J Infect Public Health 2020; 13(9): 1187-95.
[http://dx.doi.org/10.1016/j.jiph.2020.07.013] [PMID: 32773212]

[99] Elmezayen AD, Al-Obaidi A, Şahin AT, *et al.* Drug repurposing for coronavirus (COVID-19): In silico screening of known drugs against coronavirus 3CL hydrolase and protease enzymes. J Biomol Struct Dyn 2020; 26: 1-13.
[http://dx.doi.org/10.1080/07391102.2020.1798812] [PMID: 32306862]

[100] Senanayake SL. Drug repurposing strategies for COVID-19. Future Science 2020; 2: 1-3.

[101] D'Andrea G, Brisdelli F, Bozzi A. AZT: an old drug with new perspectives. Curr Clin Pharmacol 2008; 3(1): 20-37.
[http://dx.doi.org/10.2174/157488408783329913] [PMID: 18690875]

[102] https://www.nature.com/articles/d41591-020-00019-9

[103] https://sars-cov-2.creative-biolabs.com/nucleoside-analogue-for-the-treatment-of-sars-cov2.htm

[104] Chhikara BS, Rathi B, Singh J, *et al.* Corona virus SARS-CoV-2 disease COVID-19: Infection, prevention and clinical advances of the prospective chemical drug therapeutics. Chemical Biology Letters 2020; 7: 63-72.

[105] Abuo-Rahma GEA, Mohamed MFA, Ibrahim TS, *et al.* Potential repurposed SARS-CoV-2 (COVID-19) infection drugs. RSC Advances 2020; 10: 26895-916.
[http://dx.doi.org/10.1039/D0RA05821A]

[106] Pruijssers AJ, Denison MR. Nucleoside analogues for the treatment of coronavirus infections. Curr Opin Virol 2019; 35: 57-62.
[http://dx.doi.org/10.1016/j.coviro.2019.04.002] [PMID: 31125806]

[107] De Clercq E. New Nucleoside Analogues for the Treatment of Hemorrhagic Fever Virus Infections. Chem Asian J 2019; 14(22): 3962-8.
[http://dx.doi.org/10.1002/asia.201900841] [PMID: 31389664]

[108] Tchesnokov EP, Feng JY, Porter DP, Götte M. Mechanism of inhibition of Ebola virus RNA-dependent RNA polymerase by remdesivir. Viruses 2019; 11(4): 326-41.
[http://dx.doi.org/10.3390/v11040326] [PMID: 30987343]

[109] Ju J, Li X, Kumar S, *et al.* Nucleotide analogues as inhibitors of SARS-CoV Polymerase. Pharmacol Res Perspect 2020; 8(6): e00674-82.
[http://dx.doi.org/10.1002/prp2.674] [PMID: 33124786]

[110] Gordon CJ, Tchesnokov EP, Woolner E, *et al.* Remdesivir is a direct-acting antiviral that inhibits RNA-dependent RNA polymerase from severe acute respiratory syndrome coronavirus 2 with high potency. J Biol Chem 2020; 295(20): 6785-97.
[http://dx.doi.org/10.1074/jbc.RA120.013679] [PMID: 32284326]

[111] Wang Y, Wang Y, Chen Y, Qin Q. Unique epidemiological and clinical features of the emerging 2019 novel coronavirus pneumonia (COVID-19) implicate special control measures. J Med Virol 2020; 92(6): 568-76.
[http://dx.doi.org/10.1002/jmv.25748] [PMID: 32134116]

[112] Jordan PC, Liu C, Raynaud P, *et al.* Initiation, extension, and termination of RNA synthesis by a paramyxovirus polymerase. PLoS Pathog 2018; 14(2): e1006889-.
[http://dx.doi.org/10.1371/journal.ppat.1006889] [PMID: 29425244]

[113] Sarma P, Sekhar N, Prajapat M, *et al.* In-silico homology assisted identification of inhibitor of RNA binding against 2019-nCoV N-protein (N terminal domain). J Biomol Struct Dyn 2020; 18: 1-9.
[http://dx.doi.org/10.1080/07391102.2020.1753580] [PMID: 32266867]

[114] Warren TK, Jordan R, Lo MK, *et al.* Therapeutic efficacy of the small molecule GS-5734 against Ebola virus in rhesus monkeys. Nature 2016; 531(7594): 381-5.
[http://dx.doi.org/10.1038/nature17180] [PMID: 26934220]

[115] Ciliberto G, Mancini R, Paggi MG. Drug repurposing against COVID-19: focus on anticancer agents. J Exp Clin Cancer Res 2020; 39(1): 86-94.
[http://dx.doi.org/10.1186/s13046-020-01590-2] [PMID: 32398164]

[116] Julander JG, Smee DF, Morrey JD, Furuta Y. Effect of T-705 treatment on western equine encephalitis in a mouse model. Antiviral Res 2009; 82(3): 169-71.
[http://dx.doi.org/10.1016/j.antiviral.2009.02.201] [PMID: 19428608]

[117] Delang L, Segura Guerrero N, Tas A, *et al.* Mutations in the chikungunya virus non-structural proteins cause resistance to favipiravir (T-705), a broad-spectrum antiviral. J Antimicrob Chemother 2014; 69(10): 2770-84.
[http://dx.doi.org/10.1093/jac/dku209] [PMID: 24951535]

[118] Jin Z, Smith LK, Rajwanshi VK, Kim B, Deval J. The ambiguous base-pairing and high substrate efficiency of T-705 (Favipiravir) Ribofuranosyl 5′-triphosphate towards influenza A virus polymerase. PLoS One 2013; 8(7): e68347-56.
[http://dx.doi.org/10.1371/journal.pone.0068347] [PMID: 23874596]

[119] Mifsud EJ, Hayden FG, Hurt AC. Antivirals targeting the polymerase complex of influenza viruses. Antiviral Res 2019; 169: 104545-53.

[http://dx.doi.org/10.1016/j.antiviral.2019.104545] [PMID: 31247246]

[120] Sissoko D, Laouenan C, Folkesson E, *et al.* Experimental Treatment with Favipiravir for Ebola Virus Disease (the JIKI Trial): A Historically Controlled, Single-Arm Proof-of-Concept Trial in Guinea. PLoS Med 2016; 13(3): e1001967-.
[http://dx.doi.org/10.1371/journal.pmed.1001967] [PMID: 26930627]

[121] Maxmen A. More than 80 clinical trials launch to test coronavirus treatments. Nature 2020; 578(7795): 347-8.
[http://dx.doi.org/10.1038/d41586-020-00444-3] [PMID: 32071447]

[122] Furuta Y, Takahashi K, Shiraki K, *et al.* T-705 (favipiravir) and related compounds: Novel broad-spectrum inhibitors of RNA viral infections. Antiviral Res 2009; 82(3): 95-102.
[http://dx.doi.org/10.1016/j.antiviral.2009.02.198] [PMID: 19428599]

[123] Wang M, Cao R, Zhang L, *et al.* Remdesivir and chloroquine effectively inhibit the recently emerged novel coronavirus (2019-nCoV) *in vitro*. Cell Res 2020; 30(3): 269-71.
[http://dx.doi.org/10.1038/s41422-020-0282-0] [PMID: 32020029]

[124] Cai Q, Yang M, Liu D, *et al.* Experimental Treatment with Favipiravir for COVID-19: An Open-Label Control Study. Engineering (Beijing) 2020; 6(10): 1192-8.
[http://dx.doi.org/10.1016/j.eng.2020.03.007] [PMID: 32346491]

[125] Dong L, Hu S, Gao J. Discovering drugs to treat coronavirus disease 2019 (COVID-19). Drug Discov Ther 2020; 14(1): 58-60.
[http://dx.doi.org/10.5582/ddt.2020.01012] [PMID: 32147628]

[126] Keating GM, Vaidya A. Sofosbuvir: first global approval. Drugs 2014; 74(2): 273-82.
[http://dx.doi.org/10.1007/s40265-014-0179-7] [PMID: 24442794]

[127] Mani D, Wadhwani A, Krishnamurthy PT. Drug Repurposing in Antiviral Research: A Current Scenario. J Young Pharm 2019; 11: 117.
[http://dx.doi.org/10.5530/jyp.2019.11.26]

[128] Urakova N, Kuznetsova V, Crossman DK, *et al.* β-d-N^4-Hydroxycytidine Is a Potent Anti-alphavirus Compound That Induces a High Level of Mutations in the Viral Genome. J Virol 2018; 92(3): e01965-17.
[http://dx.doi.org/10.1128/JVI.01965-17] [PMID: 29167335]

[129] Yoon JJ, Toots M, Lee S, *et al.* Orally Efficacious Broad-Spectrum Ribonucleoside Analog Inhibitor of Influenza and Respiratory Syncytial Viruses. Antimicrob Agents Chemother 2018; 62(8): e00766-18.
[http://dx.doi.org/10.1128/AAC.00766-18] [PMID: 29891600]

[130] Pyrc K, Bosch BJ, Berkhout B, *et al.* Inhibition of human coronavirus NL63 infection at early stages of the replication cycle. Antimicrob Agents Chemother 2006; 50(6): 2000-8.
[http://dx.doi.org/10.1128/AAC.01598-05] [PMID: 16723558]

[131] Barnard DL, Hubbard VD, Burton J, *et al.* Inhibition of severe acute respiratory syndrome-associated coronavirus (SARSCoV) by calpain inhibitors and beta-D-N4-hydroxycytidine. Antivir Chem Chemother 2004; 15(1): 15-22.
[http://dx.doi.org/10.1177/095632020401500102] [PMID: 15074711]

[132] Agostini ML, Pruijssers AJ, Chappell JD, *et al.* Small-molecule antiviral β-d-N^4-hydroxycytidine inhibits a proofreading-intact coronavirus with a high genetic barrier to resistance. J Virol 2019; 93(24): e01348-19.
[http://dx.doi.org/10.1128/JVI.01348-19] [PMID: 31578288]

[133] Sheahan TP. An orally bioavailable broad-spectrum antiviral inhibits SARS-CoV-2 in human airway epithelial cell cultures and multiple coronaviruses in mice. Sci Transl Med 2020; 12: eabb5883-.

[134] Hannah B. Drug target review. 2020. Avaiable at: https://www.drugtargetreview.com/news/59567/eidd-2801-shows-efficacy-against-covid-19-in-human-cells-and-mice/

[135] Minskaia E, Hertzig T, Gorbalenya AE, *et al.* Discovery of an RNA virus 3'->5' exoribonuclease that is critically involved in coronavirus RNA synthesis. Proc Natl Acad Sci USA 2006; 103(13): 5108-13.
[http://dx.doi.org/10.1073/pnas.0508200103] [PMID: 16549795]

[136] Arabi YM, Shalhoub S, Mandourah Y, *et al.* Ribavirin and Interferon Therapy for Critically Ill Patients With Middle East Respiratory Syndrome: A Multicenter Observational Study. Clin Infect Dis 2020; 70(9): 1837-44.
[http://dx.doi.org/10.1093/cid/ciz544] [PMID: 31925415]

[137] Smith EC, Blanc H, Surdel MC, Vignuzzi M, Denison MR. Coronaviruses lacking exoribonuclease activity are susceptible to lethal mutagenesis: evidence for proofreading and potential therapeutics. PLoS Pathog 2013; 9(8): e1003565-.
[http://dx.doi.org/10.1371/journal.ppat.1003565] [PMID: 23966862]

[138] Zumla A, Chan JF, Azhar EI, Hui DS, Yuen KY. Coronaviruses - drug discovery and therapeutic options. Nat Rev Drug Discov 2016; 15(5): 327-47.
[http://dx.doi.org/10.1038/nrd.2015.37] [PMID: 26868298]

[139] Taylor R, Kotian P, Warren T, *et al.* BCX4430 - A broad-spectrum antiviral adenosine nucleoside analog under development for the treatment of Ebola virus disease. J Infect Public Health 2016; 9(3): 220-6.
[http://dx.doi.org/10.1016/j.jiph.2016.04.002] [PMID: 27095300]

[140] Warren TK, Wells J, Panchal RG, *et al.* Protection against filovirus diseases by a novel broad-spectrum nucleoside analogue BCX4430. Nature 2014; 508(7496): 402-5.
[http://dx.doi.org/10.1038/nature13027] [PMID: 24590073]

[141] Ghosh AK, Osswald HL, Prato G. Recent Progress in the Development of HIV-1 Protease Inhibitors for the Treatment of HIV/AIDS. J Med Chem 2016; 59(11): 5172-208.
[http://dx.doi.org/10.1021/acs.jmedchem.5b01697] [PMID: 26799988]

[142] de Leuw P, Stephan C. Protease inhibitors for the treatment of hepatitis C virus infection. GMS Infect Dis 2017; 5: Doc08.
[PMID: 30671330]

[143] Cinatl J Jr, Michaelis M, Hoever G, Preiser W, Doerr HW. Development of antiviral therapy for severe acute respiratory syndrome. Antiviral Res 2005; 66(2-3): 81-97.
[http://dx.doi.org/10.1016/j.antiviral.2005.03.002] [PMID: 15878786]

[144] Liu X, Wang XJ. Potential inhibitors against 2019-nCoV coronavirus M protease from clinically approved medicines. J Genet Genomics 2020; 47(2): 119-21.
[http://dx.doi.org/10.1016/j.jgg.2020.02.001] [PMID: 32173287]

[145] Todd S, Anderson C, Jolly DJ, Craik CS. HIV protease as a target for retrovirus vector-mediated gene therapy. Biochim Biophys Acta 2000; 1477(1-2): 168-88.
[http://dx.doi.org/10.1016/S0167-4838(99)00272-1] [PMID: 10708857]

[146] Zhang L, Lin D, Sun X, *et al.* Crystal structure of SARS-CoV-2 main protease provides a basis for design of improved α-ketoamide inhibitors. Science 2020; 368(6489): 409-12. a
[http://dx.doi.org/10.1126/science.abb3405] [PMID: 32198291]

[147] Chu CM, Cheng VC, Hung IF, *et al.* Role of lopinavir/ritonavir in the treatment of SARS: initial virological and clinical findings. Thorax 2004; 59(3): 252-6.
[http://dx.doi.org/10.1136/thorax.2003.012658] [PMID: 14985565]

[148] Cao B, Wang Y, Wen D, *et al.* A Trial of Lopinavir-Ritonavir in Adults Hospitalized with Severe Covid-19. N Engl J Med 2020; 382(19): 1787-99.
[http://dx.doi.org/10.1056/NEJMoa2001282] [PMID: 32187464]

[149] OBI and Justice E. Compositions and methods for treating warts associated with viral infections. Google Patents WO 2014/008248 A2 2014.

[150] Zhang H, Saravanan KM, Yang Y, *et al.* Deep learning based drug screening for novel Coronavirus 2019-nCov. Interdiscip Sci 2020; 12(3): 368-76.
[http://dx.doi.org/10.1007/s12539-020-00376-6] [PMID: 32488835]

[151] Gomes A, Ferraz R, Ficker L, *et al.* Chloroquine Analogues as Leads against Pneumocystis Lung Pathogens. Antimicrob Agents Chemother 2018; 62(11): e00983-18.
[http://dx.doi.org/10.1128/AAC.00983-18] [PMID: 30201816]

[152] Zhang L, Lin D, Kusov Y, *et al.* α-Ketoamides as Broad-Spectrum Inhibitors of Coronavirus and Enterovirus Replication: Structure-Based Design, Synthesis, and Activity Assessment. J Med Chem 2020; 63(9): 4562-78.
[http://dx.doi.org/10.1021/acs.jmedchem.9b01828] [PMID: 32045235]

[153] Patel AB, Verma A. Nasal ACE2 Levels and COVID-19 in Children. JAMA 2020; 323(23): 2386-7.
[http://dx.doi.org/10.1001/jama.2020.8946] [PMID: 32432681]

[154] Shulla A, Heald-Sargent T, Subramanya G, Zhao J, Perlman S, Gallagher T. A transmembrane serine protease is linked to the severe acute respiratory syndrome coronavirus receptor and activates virus entry. J Virol 2011; 85(2): 873-82.
[http://dx.doi.org/10.1128/JVI.02062-10] [PMID: 21068237]

[155] Yamamoto M, Matsuyama S, Li X, *et al.* Identification of Nafamostat as a Potent Inhibitor of Middle East Respiratory Syndrome Coronavirus S Protein-Mediated Membrane Fusion Using the Split-Protein-Based Cell-Cell Fusion Assay. Antimicrob Agents Chemother 2016; 60(11): 6532-9.
[http://dx.doi.org/10.1128/AAC.01043-16] [PMID: 27550352]

[156] Yamamoto M, Kiso M, Sakai-Tagawa Y, *et al.* The Anticoagulant Nafamostat Potently Inhibits SARS-CoV-2 S Protein-Mediated Fusion in a Cell Fusion Assay System and Viral Infection *In Vitro* in a Cell-Type-Dependent Manner. Viruses 2020; 12(6): 629.
[http://dx.doi.org/10.3390/v12060629] [PMID: 32532094]

[157] Al-Bari MAA. Chloroquine analogues in drug discovery: new directions of uses, mechanisms of actions and toxic manifestations from malaria to multifarious diseases. J Antimicrob Chemother 2015; 70(6): 1608-21.
[http://dx.doi.org/10.1093/jac/dkv018] [PMID: 25693996]

[158] D'Alessandro S, Scaccabarozzi D, Signorini L, *et al.* The Use of Antimalarial Drugs against Viral Infection. Microorganisms 2020; 8(1): 85-110.
[http://dx.doi.org/10.3390/microorganisms8010085] [PMID: 31936284]

[159] Keyaerts E, Vijgen L, Maes P, Neyts J, Van Ranst M. *In vitro* inhibition of severe acute respiratory syndrome coronavirus by chloroquine. Biochem Biophys Res Commun 2004; 323(1): 264-8.
[http://dx.doi.org/10.1016/j.bbrc.2004.08.085] [PMID: 15351731]

[160] Keyaerts E, Li S, Vijgen L, *et al.* Antiviral activity of chloroquine against human coronavirus OC43 infection in newborn mice. Antimicrob Agents Chemother 2009; 53(8): 3416-21.
[http://dx.doi.org/10.1128/AAC.01509-08] [PMID: 19506054]

[161] Yao X, Ye F, Zhang M, *et al. In Vitro* Antiviral Activity and Projection of Optimized Dosing Design of Hydroxychloroquine for the Treatment of Severe Acute Respiratory Syndrome Coronavirus 2 (SARS-CoV-2). Clin Infect Dis 2020; 71(15): 732-9.
[http://dx.doi.org/10.1093/cid/ciaa237] [PMID: 32150618]

[162] Vincent MJ, Bergeron E, Benjannet S, *et al.* Chloroquine is a potent inhibitor of SARS coronavirus infection and spread. Virol J 2005; 2: 69-78.
[http://dx.doi.org/10.1186/1743-422X-2-69] [PMID: 16115318]

[163] Liu Z, Xiao X, Wei X, *et al.* Composition and divergence of coronavirus spike proteins and host ACE2 receptors predict potential intermediate hosts of SARS-CoV-2. J Med Virol 2020; 92(6): 595-601.
[http://dx.doi.org/10.1002/jmv.25726] [PMID: 32100877]

[164] Njaria PM, Okombo J, Njuguna NM, Chibale K. Chloroquine-containing compounds: a patent review (2010 - 2014). Expert Opin Ther Pat 2015; 25(9): 1003-24.
[http://dx.doi.org/10.1517/13543776.2015.1050791] [PMID: 26013494]

[165] Cifuentes Kottkamp A, De Jesus E, Grande R, *et al.* Atovaquone inhibits arbovirus replication through the depletion of intracellular nucleotides. J Virol 2019; 93(11): e00389-19.
[http://dx.doi.org/10.1128/JVI.00389-19] [PMID: 30894466]

[166] Fan HH, Wang LQ, Liu WL, *et al.* Repurposing of clinically approved drugs for treatment of coronavirus disease 2019 in a 2019-novel coronavirus-related coronavirus model. Chin Med J (Engl) 2020; 133(9): 1051-6.
[http://dx.doi.org/10.1097/CM9.0000000000000797] [PMID: 32149769]

[167] Mehra MR, Ruschitzka F, Patel AN. Retraction-Hydroxychloroquine or chloroquine with or without a macrolide for treatment of COVID-19: a multinational registry analysis. Lancet 2020; 395(10240): 1820.
[http://dx.doi.org/10.1016/S0140-6736(20)31324-6] [PMID: 32511943]

[168] Zhang J, Xie B, Hashimoto K. Current status of potential therapeutic candidates for the COVID-19 crisis. Brain Behav Immun 2020; 87: 59-73.
[http://dx.doi.org/10.1016/j.bbi.2020.04.046] [PMID: 32334062]

[169] Jones PH, Davidson MH, Stein EA, *et al.* Comparison of the efficacy and safety of rosuvastatin versus atorvastatin, simvastatin, and pravastatin across doses (STELLAR* Trial). Am J Cardiol 2003; 92(2): 152-60.
[http://dx.doi.org/10.1016/S0002-9149(03)00530-7] [PMID: 12860216]

[170] Saadat S, Mohamadian Roshan N, Aslani MR, Boskabady MH. Rosuvastatin suppresses cytokine production and lung inflammation in asthmatic, hyperlipidemic and asthmatic-hyperlipidemic rat models. Cytokine 2020; 128: 154993.
[http://dx.doi.org/10.1016/j.cyto.2020.154993] [PMID: 32007867]

[171] Totura AL, Whitmore A, Agnihothram S, *et al.* Toll-Like Receptor 3 Signaling *via* TRIF Contributes to a Protective Innate Immune Response to Severe Acute Respiratory Syndrome Coronavirus Infection. MBio 2015; 6(3): e00638-15.
[http://dx.doi.org/10.1128/mBio.00638-15] [PMID: 26015500]

[172] Yuan X, Deng Y, Guo X, Shang J, Zhu D, Liu H. Atorvastatin attenuates myocardial remodeling induced by chronic intermittent hypoxia in rats: partly involvement of TLR-4/MYD88 pathway. Biochem Biophys Res Commun 2014; 446(1): 292-7.
[http://dx.doi.org/10.1016/j.bbrc.2014.02.091] [PMID: 24582748]

[173] Yuan S. Statins May Decrease the Fatality Rate of Middle East Respiratory Syndrome Infection. MBio 2015; 6(4): e01120-15.
[http://dx.doi.org/10.1128/mBio.01120-15] [PMID: 26265720]

[174] Fedson DS, Opal SM, Rordam OM. Hiding in Plain Sight: an Approach to Treating Patients with Severe COVID-19 Infection. MBio 2020; 11(2): e00398-20.
[http://dx.doi.org/10.1128/mBio.00398-20] [PMID: 32198163]

[175] Vandermeer ML, Thomas AR, Kamimoto L, *et al.* Association between use of statins and mortality among patients hospitalized with laboratory-confirmed influenza virus infections: a multistate study. J Infect Dis 2012; 205(1): 13-9.
[http://dx.doi.org/10.1093/infdis/jir695] [PMID: 22170954]

[176] Link A, Ayadhi T, Böhm M, Nickenig G. Rapid immunomodulation by rosuvastatin in patients with acute coronary syndrome. Eur Heart J 2006; 27(24): 2945-55.
[http://dx.doi.org/10.1093/eurheartj/ehl277] [PMID: 17012299]

[177] Kow CS, Hasan SS. Use of statins in patients with COVID-19. Int J Med (Dubai) 2020; 1-2.

[178] Saravanan V, Hamilton J. Advances in the treatment of rheumatoid arthritis: old versus new therapies.

Expert Opin Pharmacother 2002; 3(7): 845-56.
[http://dx.doi.org/10.1517/14656566.3.7.845] [PMID: 12083985]

[179] Ding C, Jones G. Anti-interleukin-6 receptor antibody treatment in inflammatory autoimmune diseases. Rev Recent Clin Trials 2006; 1(3): 193-200.
[http://dx.doi.org/10.2174/157488706778250168] [PMID: 18473972]

[180] Prins KW, Thenappan T, Weir EK, Kalra R, Pritzker M, Archer SL. Repurposing Medications for Treatment of Pulmonary Arterial Hypertension: What's Old Is New Again. J Am Heart Assoc 2019; 8(1): e011343-74.
[http://dx.doi.org/10.1161/JAHA.118.011343] [PMID: 30590974]

[181] Xu X, Han M, Li T, *et al.* Effective treatment of severe COVID-19 patients with tocilizumab. Proc Natl Acad Sci USA 2020; 117(20): 10970-5.
[http://dx.doi.org/10.1073/pnas.2005615117] [PMID: 32350134]

[182] Boyce EG, Rogan EL, Vyas D, Prasad N, Mai Y. Sarilumab: Review of a Second IL-6 Receptor Antagonist Indicated for the Treatment of Rheumatoid Arthritis. Ann Pharmacother 2018; 52(8): 780-91.
[http://dx.doi.org/10.1177/1060028018761599] [PMID: 29482351]

[183] Cennimo DJ. 2020. Avaiable at: https://www.medscape.com/answers/2500114-197456/what-is--he-role-of-the-il-6-inhibitor-sarilumab-kevzara-in-the-treatment-of-coronavirus-disease-2019-covid-19

[184] Mogul A, Corsi K, McAuliffe L. Baricitinib: The Second FDA-Approved JAK Inhibitor for the Treatment of Rheumatoid Arthritis. Ann Pharmacother 2019; 53(9): 947-53.
[http://dx.doi.org/10.1177/1060028019839650] [PMID: 30907116]

[185] Zhao Y, Zhao Z, Wang Y, Zhou Y, Ma Y, Zuo W. Single-cell RNA expression profiling of ACE2, the receptor of SARS-CoV-2. Am J Respir Crit Care Med 2020; 202(5): 756-9.
[http://dx.doi.org/10.1164/rccm.202001-0179LE] [PMID: 32663409]

[186] Ramamoorthy S, Cidlowski JA. Corticosteroids: Mechanisms of Action in Health and Disease. Rheum Dis Clin North Am 2016; 42(1): 15-31, vii.
[http://dx.doi.org/10.1016/j.rdc.2015.08.002] [PMID: 26611548]

[187] Horby P, Lim WS, Emberson JR, *et al.* Dexamethasone in hospitalized patients with covid-19: preliminary report. N Engl J Med 2021; 384(8): 693-704.
[http://dx.doi.org/10.1056/NEJMoa2021436] [PMID: 32678530]

[188] Ledford H. Coronavirus breakthrough: dexamethasone is first drug shown to save lives. Nature 2020; 582(7813): 469.
[http://dx.doi.org/10.1038/d41586-020-01824-5] [PMID: 32546811]

[189] Yeleswaram S, Smith P, Burn T, *et al.* Inhibition of cytokine signaling by ruxolitinib and implications for COVID-19 treatment. Clin Immunol 2020; 218: 108517-23.
[http://dx.doi.org/10.1016/j.clim.2020.108517] [PMID: 32585295]

[190] Uchide N, Toyoda H. Antioxidant therapy as a potential approach to severe influenza-associated complications. Molecules 2011; 16(3): 2032-52.
[http://dx.doi.org/10.3390/molecules16032032] [PMID: 21358592]

[191] Garozzo A, Tempera G, Ungheri D, Timpanaro R, Castro A. N-acetylcysteine synergizes with oseltamivir in protecting mice from lethal influenza infection. Int J Immunopathol Pharmacol 2007; 20(2): 349-54.
[http://dx.doi.org/10.1177/039463200702000215] [PMID: 17624247]

[192] Hada M. Chemotherapeutic strategy with synbiotics, thalidomide and celecoxib for severe COVID-19 pneumonia. Association between microbiota, chronic inflammation and pneumonia 2020; 10: 13140.

[193] Caly L, Druce JD, Catton MG, Jans DA, Wagstaff KM. The FDA-approved drug ivermectin inhibits the replication of SARS-CoV-2 *in vitro*. Antiviral Res 2020; 178: 104787-90.
[http://dx.doi.org/10.1016/j.antiviral.2020.104787] [PMID: 32251768]

CHAPTER 6

Bilayer Tablet - Approach for the Treatment of Sexually Transmitted Diseases with Fixed Dose Combination

Swati S. Gaikwad[1,*] **and Mansi L. Patil**[2]

[1] *Nagpur College of Pharmacy, Wanadongri, Hingna Road, Nagpur, India*

[2] *Department of Pharmaceutical Sciences, R. T. M. Nagpur University, Nagpur 440033, Maharashtra, India*

Abstract: The purpose of this study is to develop an efficient therapy of combination antibiotics for the treatment of sexually transmitted infections. The best-preferred combination of drugs Cefixime trihydrate and Ofloxacin was selected to prepare bilayer tablets. This combination work against several genito-urinary tract infections. The Bilayer tablet was prepared in order to tailor the release of the drug to maintain the peak plasma level of the drug. It contains Cefixime trihydrate as a quick release layer and Ofloxacin as an extended-release layer. In this tablet, super disintegrant was used for the rapid release of the Cefixime layer, whereas HPMC was used to prolong the release of the ofloxacin layer. Drug release study suggests that there is a complete release of Cefixime within 30 minutes followed by the simultaneous release of ofloxacin, which was extended up to 24 hours. Current research reveals that Cefixime trihydrate and ofloxacin bilayer have been successfully developed for use in combating sexually transmitted infections.

Keywords: Bilayer tablets, Cefixime trihydrate, Ofloxacin, Sexually transmitted diseases.

INTRODUCTION

(STDs) are also known as venereal diseases. STDs are a serious health problem for women, and these diseases are alarming worldwide. Bacteria that cause the development of STDS live above the skin or body fluids such as semen, vaginal fluid or blood. The mode of transmission of the disease from an infected person to a healthy one is usually through sexual contact with the skin, blood, or body fluids [1]. Common sexually transmitted diseases (STIs) are gonorrhea, trichomoniasis, chancroid, syphilis, bacterial vaginosis, and genital candidiasis [2].

---

* **Corresponding author Swati S. Gaikwad:** Nagpur College of Pharmacy, Wanadongri, Hingna Road, 441110 Nagpur, India; Tel: +91-7709493400; E-mail: swati.gaikwad05@gmail.com

Currently, in the treatment of simple pharyngeal, urogenital and anorectal gonorrhea, the CDC official recommended combined treatment [3].

Benefits of Antimicrobial Combination [4]

- Achieve collaboration
- Preventing the emergence of resistance
- Reducing the severity or incidence of side effects
- Expanding the spectrum of antimicrobial action

It has been observed that the conventional form of drug produces a wide range of variations in plasma drug concentration which leads to unwanted toxicity. Various factors like repeated drug dosing and unpredictable absorption develop the need for controlled drug delivery systems. Therefore, the main objective of this study is to develop drug delivery in order to improve drug efficacy and ensure patient safety and adherence.

BI-LAYER TABLET TECHNOLOGY

Bi-layer tablet technology is the most suitable form for the continuous release of two drugs, preferably when it is necessary to separate two incompatible drugs. In the Bilayer tablet, there is one immediate release layer needed to be released quickly as the first dose and the second layer as a maintenance dose. The bi-layered tablet is a novel technology prominently applied days for the formulation of a controlled drug release system for providing effective drug delivery. There is a wide range of applications for two-layer tablet technology in the form of integrated layers or various matrices [5].

ADVANTAGES OF BILAYER TABLET [6 - 8]

1. In combination therapy, bi-layered tablet technology is usually used to formulate the two layers of the tablet containing two different drugs
2. Dose frequency of the drug can be minimized, which may improve patient compliance.
3. Two incompatible substances can be formulated in order to deliver.
4. If the drugs have a low half-life, each layer consists of a loading dose and maintenance dose of the same, which increases the bioavailability of the drug.
5. The constant plasma drug concentration can be achieved for better efficacy of the drug.
6. Amongst all oral dosage forms, it has the greatest chemical and microbial stability.

7. If the drugs formulated in an extended release form, the control on drug absorption can be achieved.
8. Systemic adverse effects of high potency drugs can be reduced in the patient.

GENERAL PROPERTIES OF BI-LAYER TABLETS

1. It must be able to sustain the jerks of the machine during its packaging, production, transportation, and distribution.
2. There should be no defects such as chips, cracks, discoloration, and contamination.
3. It must have physicochemical stability to maintain its properties over time.
4. It should be able to dispense the drug in a predictable and reproductive way [6, 8, 9].

NEED

There are many difficulties associated with the current treatment of STIs (STDs), such as resistance from a single drug. There are limited drugs available to pregnant or allergic patients. The higher dose is required for treatment, and there is no single drug available for a wide range of sexually transmitted infections. Hence, it is required to formulate such a product that will help to subdue the above problems linked with the treatment of STDs.

OBJECTIVE

The present research is carried out with the idea of developing a Bilayer tablet for Cefixime trihydrate and Ofloxacin for improved therapeutically effective treatment of sexually transmitted infections. The primary aim of immediate-release layer is to provide the instant effect as well as the sustained release of drug to improve the efficacy of drugs by maintaining plasma concentration.

- To formulate the bilayered tablets of antibiotics acting synergistically for STDs in which one would be immediate release and another sustained release.
- To evaluate the formulated dosage units for physical parameters, *in-vitro* drug release study and comparison of optimized formulations with marketed reference product.

PLAN OF WORK

- Cefixime trihydrate and Ofloxacin two drugs selected for the development of bilayered tablet formulation
- Preformulation studies for Cefixime trihydrate and Ofloxacin
  - Confirmation of drug by

- UV spectroscopy
- Infra-red spectroscopy
  ○ Drug-excipients interaction study by
    - Infra-red spectroscopy's
- Standard calibration curve of cefixime trihydrate and ofloxacin in different dissolution media.
- Preparation of blend or granules for IR and SR tablet
- Precompression parameters study for cefixime trihydrate immediate release blend
- Post compression parameters study for cefixime trihydrate immediate release tablets
- Comparative study with marketed formulation of cefixime trihydrate
- Precompression parameters study for prepared ofloxacin sustained release granules
- Post compression parameters study for prepared ofloxacin sustained release tablets
- Comparative study with marketed formulation of Ofloxacin.
- Preparation of bilayer tablets by using best immediate release of cefixime trihydrate and sustained release layer of ofloxacin.
- Tablets evaluation study of bilayer tablets
- Accelerated stability study of optimized bilayer tablets.

MATERIAL AND METHODS

Drug Profile

Cefixime Trihydrate

Chemical Formula: $C_{16}H_{15}N_5O_7S_2, 3H_2O$

Molecular Weight: 507.5

Melting point: 218-225 °c

logP: 0.4

pKa: 3.26

Appearance: White coloured powder which is slightly hygroscopic in nature.

Pharmacodynamics: Cefixime is categorized as a third-generation cephalosporin. Its sability is high which is effective in the presence of beta-lactamase enzymes. Therefore, it is effective against many organisms resistant to penicillins. Its antibacterial activity is due to inhibition of bacterial cell wall synthesis.

Absorption: Cefixime is absorbed 40 to 50% on oral administration with or without food, maximum absorption achieved at 0.8 hours with food.

Protein binding: There is 65% protein binding.

Hepatic Metabolism: About 50% of the drug absorbed and excreted in the urine in 24 hours unchanged.

Half life: Cefixime t1/2 - 3-4 hours. The creatinine clearance at rate of 5 to 20 ml/min results in prolongation of t1/2 to an average of 11.5 hours in severe renal impairment.

Toxicity: Overdose of drug leads to symptoms like blood in the urine, nausea, diarrhoea, vomiting and upper abdominal pain.

Ofloxacin

Chemical Formula: $C_{18}H_{20}FN_3O_4$

Molecular Weight: 361.36

Melting point: 250-257 °C

Log P: 2.1

Solubility: Ofloxacin is slightly soluble in water, ethanol, and methanol but it is sparingly soluble in chloroform

Appearance: Drug is a pale yellow or bright yellow colour crystalline powder.

Pharmacodynamics: Ofloxacin belongs to quinolone/fluoroquinolone class of antibiotics. Ofloxacin works by blocking the DNA gyrase enzyme responsible for duplication or transcription and thus prevents normal cell division.

Absorption: Ofloxacin have 98% bioavailability in the tablet formulation

Protein binding: Ofloxacin have 32% protein binding.

Metabolism: It undergoes hepatic metabolism.

Half life: t ½ - 9 hours.

POLYMER/ EXCIPIENTS PROFILE

Hydroxy Propyl Methylcellulose

Chemical Name: Cellulose hydroxyl propyl methyl ether.

Category: HPMC is used as coating agent in tablets, rate-controlling polymer for achieving sustained release and film forming agent. It is also used as stabilizer, suspending agent, binder and viscosity enhancing agent.

Description: Hyproxypropyl methylcellulose is odorless and tasteless, a white to off white color granular powder.

Typical Properties: pH - 5.5–8.0 for a 1% w/w aqueous solution.

Microcrystalline Cellulose

Chemical Name: Cellulose

Category: Used as adsorbent, suspending agent, diluents and disintegrant.

Description: Microcrystalline cellulose exists as a white crystalline powder composed of porous particles, odourless and tasteless. It is available in market in based on different moisture grades and particle sizes which has varying properties and applications.

Solubility: MCC is slightly soluble in 5% w/v NaOH alkaline solution; and practically insoluble in polar solvent like H_2O, weak acid, and other organic solvents.

Crosscarmellose Sodium

Synonyms: Cross carmellose sodium is also known as Solutab/Ac-Di-Sol/ Primellose/ Vivasol/ Explocel.

Chemical Name: Chemically it is also known as Cellulose and carboxymethyl ether sodium salt.

Category: Disintegrant.

Description: It is odorless, white or grayish white powder.

Solubility: It is insoluble in polar solvent like water but it swells rapidly in contact with water. Also it is practically insoluble in organic solvents like toluene, acetone, and ethanol.

Sodium Starch Glycolate

Synonyms: Sodium starch glycolate is also known as Primojel /Explosol/ Glycolys/ Tablo/ Explotab/ Vivastar P.

Chemical Name: It's chemical name is Sodium carboxymethyl starch

Category: Disintegrant

Description: SSG odourless, tasteless, free-flowing white to off-white color powder.

Solubility: Sodium Starch glycolate is sparingly soluble in 95% ethanol and insoluble in H_2O.

Crospovidone

Synonyms: Crospovidone is also known as Polyplasdone /cross linked povidone/Kollidon / polyvinyl polypyrrolidone/ PVPP.

Chemical Name: Chemically it is 1-Ethenyl-2-pyrrolidinone homopolymer

Category: Disintegrant.

Description: It exist as white to off white color, odourless and tasteless, freely flowing fine hygroscopic powder.

Solubility: Crospovidone is insoluble in water and other organic solvents.

Lactose, Monohydrate

Chemical Name: Chemically it is known as O-b-D-Galactopyranosyl-(1,-)-a-D-glucopyranose monohydrate

Category: Functionally used as Binder and diluent.

Description: Lactose is white to off-white crystalline particles or powder odourless and slightly sweet in taste.

Solubility: It is slightly soluble in water but practically insoluble in chloroform, ethanol, and ether.

EXPERIMENTAL METHODS

Confirmation of Drugs

Drug Confirmation of was done by using infrared spectroscopy and UV spectroscopy

Fourier Transformed Infrared Spectroscopy (FT-IR)

Pure drug and drug with excipients that is to be used in core tablet were analysed by FT-IR spectrophotometer by using KBr disc method. Sample powder to be analyzed was triturated with KBr powder and disc is formed by hydrostatic press. The formed disc was analysed from 4600 to 400 cm-1 range at a resolution of 1 cm-1 at zero time and spectrum was recorded.

Spectrophotometric Analysis of Drug

a) Spectrophotometric determination of λ_{max} of drug (Cefixime trihydrate)

Stock solution of 1mg/ml drug concentration was prepared in pH 7.2 phosphate buffer. Further this solution was diluted to prepare 10 µg/ml concentration. Filtered and analyzed spectrophotometrically to determine λ_{max}.

b) Spectrophotometric determination of λ_{max} of drug (Ofloxacin)

Stock solution of 1mg/ml drug concentration was prepared in acid buffer (pH 1.2). Solution was further diluted to 10µg/ml concentration. Filtered and analyzed spectrophotometrically to determine λ_{max}.

Preformulation Studies

Drug-excipients Compatibility Study

To study compatibility between drug cefixime trihydrate and ofloxacin and excipients that to be used in formulation were placed in humidity control chamber at accelerated stability condition *i.e* 40°C ± 2°C temperature and 75 ± 5% relative humidity for duration of 6 months. After completion of 6 month storage the samples were withdrawn evaluated using FTIR spectroscopy and compared with the reference FTIR spectra obtained before exposing accelerated conditions.

Method of Preparation of Blend or Granules

Preparation of Powder Blend for Immediate Release Layer

Cefixime trihydrate and all other ingredients were mixed together properly using mortar pestle in appropriate compositions given in batches (Table 1). Finally powder mixture was passed through 40 mesh sieve. This blend was directly compressed for the formulation of Cefixime trihydrate (IR) tablets.

Preparation of Granules for Sustained Release (SR) Layer

The powder granules of Ofloxacin SR tablets were prepared with the approach of wet granulation technology. All the excipients along with drug were properly mixed together and sifted through 40 mesh sieve and granulation was carried out using water as a binder. The granules prepared were placed in oven at 40°C temperature for drying. They were then sifted through sieve (40#). Finally, glidant and lubricant were added with proper mixing.

Evaluation study of Physical Properties of Blend/granules

Prepared blend of drug and excipients for Cefixime trihydrate IR layer and granule of ofloxacin SR layer were lubricated and then evaluation study for various physical pre compression properties like bulk and tapped densities, angle of repose and % compressibility was evaluated [10, 11]. The prepared compressed tablets were studied for post compression properties such as thickness, hardness, friability, weight variation, and disintegration time. The drug content of Cefixime trihydrate in tablets was estimated as per the specified USP procedure. But, drug content of ofloxacin in tablets was estimated using UV-spectroscopy technique at 293 nm.

Formulation of Cefixime Trihydrate Immediate Release Tablets [12]

Cefixime trihydrate and Microcrystalline cellulose (MCC) was mixed properly with different superdisintegrant in varying concentration. In every batch trituration was carried out using mortar pestle as per the compositions given in (Table 1). The superdisintegrants like polyplasdone, cross carmellose sodium and sodium starch glycolate were tried at various concentrations. Exactly weighed amount of lubricated mix was filled manually to a compression machine die and directly compressed using nine millimeter size flat round formed punches at a fill volume of 350 mg. Force for compression was kept constant for all the formulation batches.

Table 1. Compositions of Immediate Release Tablet.

S. No.	Ingredients	C_1	C_2	C_3	C_4	C_5	C_6	C_7	C_8	C_9
		(Weight in mg)								
1.	Cefixime Trihydrate	200	200	200	200	200	200	200	200	200
2.	MCC PH 102	136	129	122	136	129	122	136	129	122

(Table 1) cont.....

S. No.	Ingredients	C_1	C_2	C_3	C_4	C_5	C_6	C_7	C_8	C_9
		(Weight in mg)								
3.	Sodium starch glycolate	10.5	17.5	24.5	-	-	-	-	-	-
4.	Cross carmelslose sodium	-	-	-	10.5	17.5	24.5	-	-	-
5.	Polyplasdone	-	-	-	-	-	-	10.5	17.5	24.5
6.	Magnesium stearate	1.75	1.75	1.75	1.75	1.75	1.75	1.75	1.75	1.75
7.	Aerosil (Colloidal silicon dioxide)	1.75	1.75	1.75	1.75	1.75	1.75	1.75	1.75	1.75

Evaluation Study of Cefixime Trihydrate Tablets

All the batches of cefixime trihydrate IR tablets were analysed for post compression parameters *i.e.* hardness of tablets, uniformity of weight, thickness, friability, disintegration time, uniformity in drug content and drug dissolution study [13].

Formulation of Ofloxacin SR Tablets

Accurately weighed amount of lubricated SR granules were weighed and filled manually to a die of compression machine and compressed using eleven millimeter flat featured round punches at a fill volume of 550 mg (Table **2**).

Table 2. Compositions of sustained release tablets.

S. No.	Ingredients	F1	F2	F3	F4	F5	F6	F7	F8
		(Weight in mg)							
1.	Ofloxacin	400	400	400	400	400	400	400	400
2.	MCC PH 101	50.25	44.75	39.25	58.5	62.65	53.70	35.80	26.85
3.	Lactose monohydrate	50.25	44.75	39.25	58.5	26.85	35.80	53.70	62.65
4.	HPMC K100M	44	55	66	82.5	55	55	55	55
5.	Magnesium stearate	2.75	2.75	2.75	2.75	2.75	2.75	2.75	2.75
6.	Aerosil	2.75	2.75	2.75	2.75	2.75	2.75	2.75	2.75

Evaluation Study of Sustained Release Tablets

All the prepared sustained release tablets were evaluated for post compression parameters such as hardness, friability, weight variation, thickness of tablets, ofloxacin drug content and percent drug dissolution [14].

Bilayer Tablets Preparation

Bilayer tablets were developed by using optimized batch of immediate release layer (C8) and sustained release layer (F8) (Table 3). Appropriate quantity of powder weighing about 350 mg of cefixime trihydrate immediate release blend and 550 mg of ofloxacin sustained release granules were taken. Bilayer tablets were produced by direct compression method according to formula given . Initially, powder blend of immediate release was fed into the die cavity of tablet compression machine manually and compressed at low force of compression in order to form uniform layer. Subsequently, granules of ofloxacin blend were added over the precompressed immediate release layer and compressed by using flat faced punch 19×10 mm capsule shaped punches [15, 16] (Fig. 1).

Table 3. Composition of optimized bilayered tablets.

S. No.	Ingredients	C8F8
1	Cefixime trihydrate	200
2	MCC PH 102	129
3	Polyplasdone	17.5
4	Magnesium stearate	1.75
5	Aerosil	1.75
6	Ofloxacin	400
7	MCC PH 101	26.85
8	Lactose	62.65
9	HPMC k-100m	55
10	Talc	2.75
11	Magnesium stearate	2.75

Evaluation Study of Bilayer Tablets

Bilayer tablets were evaluated for post compression parameters like hardness, uniformity of weight, and percent drug dissolution.

In-vitro Drug Release Study of Bilayer Tablets

In-vitro drug release study was done using type I (basket) apparatus at 100 rpm in phosphate buffer of 7.2 pH for immediate release layer of cefixime trihydrate and in pH 1.2 acid buffer, for first two hours, followed by pH 4.5 acetate buffer for next two hours, and pH 7.4 phosphate buffer for remaining hours for sustained release layer of ofloxacin. The 1 mL sample was withdrawn at predetermined time intervals for immediate release and 5ml for sustained release and in order to maintain sink condition replaced with same dissolution media respectively. Before analysis the samples solutions were diluted 20 times for immediate release and 2 times for sustained release samples and analyzed simultaneously by using HPTLC at λ_{max} 290 nm [17]. The test was performed on 3 tablets and mean ± SD was calculated (Fig. **2**).

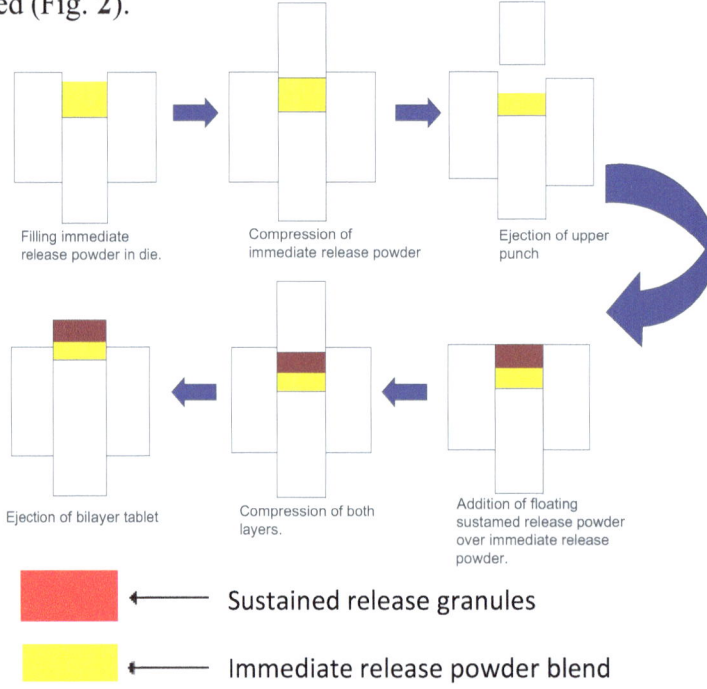

Fig. (1). Compression cycle for bilayer tablets preparation.

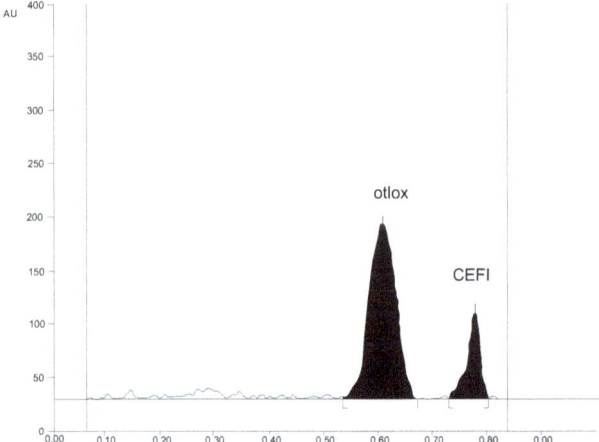

Fig. (2). Densitogram of mixture of standard solution of OFLOX (200 ng/band, Rf = 0.61 ± 0.10) and CEFI (200 ng/band, Rf = 0.78 ± 0.12).

Stability Studies and Storage Condition

The stability studies were carried out of the optimized batches of Bilayer tablets. Two optimized batch C8F2 and C8F8 was placed in stability chamber for accelerated stability condition at 40°C ± 2°C temperature and 75 ± 5% relative humidity for duration of 6 months [18, 19].

RESULTS AND DISCUSSION

Confirmation of Drug

Identification of drug was carried out by following methods

Fourier Transform Infrared Spectroscopy (FT-IR) Study

The FT-IR spectra analysis of cefixime trihydrate and ofloxacin showed the peaks which are characteristics of the drugs structures. This identified the supplied drugs (Figs. **3** and **4**).

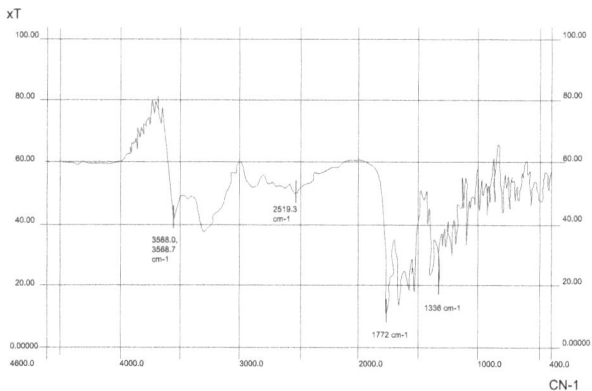

Fig. (3). Fourier Transform-Infra red (FT-IR) spectrum of Cefixime trihydrate.

Preformulation Studies

Drug-excipient Compatibility Study

The FT-IR spectra study of physical mixture of excipients which are proposed to be used in the development of tablets along with drug are shown in Figs. (**5** and **6**) respectively. When compared with Figs. (**3** and **4**), it was observed that the characteristic peaks of both drugs were present in FT-IR spectra of the physical mixture. No sign of interaction between the drug and excipients were observed, this indicates that the drug was compatible with the excipients.

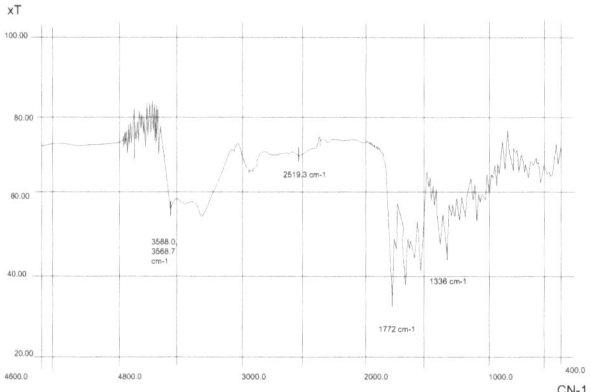

Fig. (4). Fourier Transform-Infra red (FT-IR) spectrum of ofloxacin.

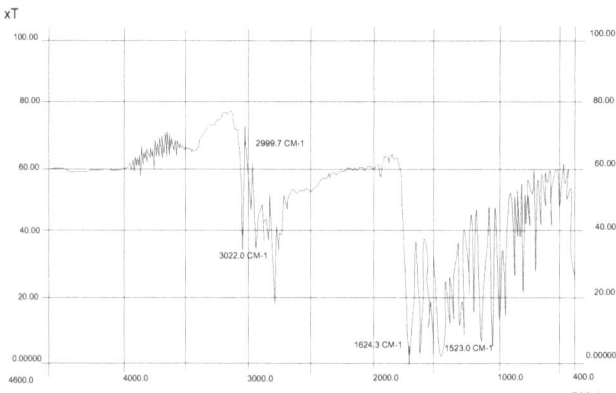

Fig. (5). Fourier Transform-Infra red (FT-IR) spectrum physical mixture of cefixime trihydrate with MCC PH-102 and polyplasdone.

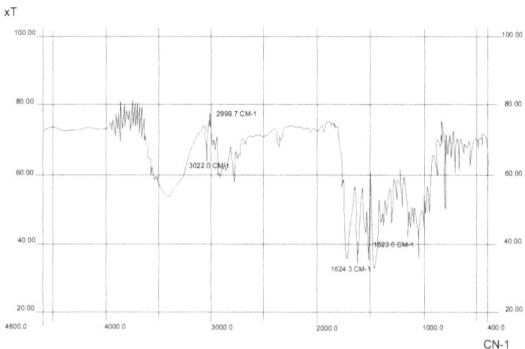

Fig. (6). Fourier Transform-Infra red (FT-IR) spectrum physical mixture of ofloxacin with MCC PH-101, Lactose monohydrate and HPMC k100M.

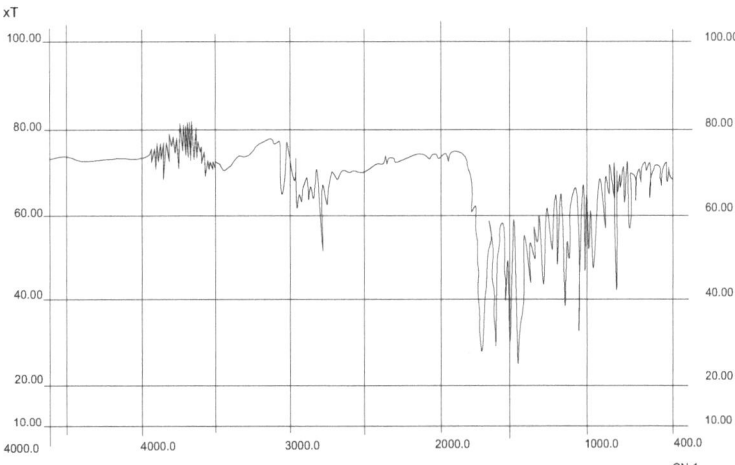

Fig. (7). Fourier Transform-Infra red (FT-IR) spectrum physical mixture of cefixime trihydrate and ofloxacin.

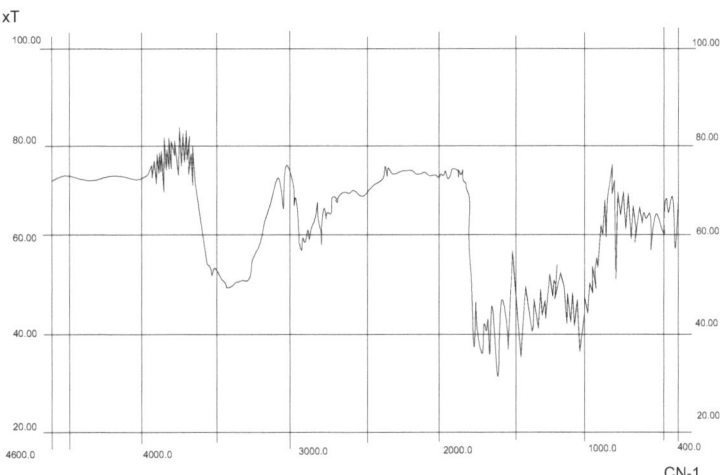

Fig. (8). Fourier Transform-Infra red (FT-IR) spectrum physical mixture of cefixime trihydrate blend+ ofloxacin granules.

Similarly, when Figs. (**7** and **8**) compared with Figs. (**3** and **4**), it was observed that all the characteristic peaks of both drugs were found in the FT-IR spectra of physical mixture. This indicates that there is no interaction between two drugs or drug-excipient. So the drugs and excipients can be used for further study.

Evaluation of Precompression Parameters for Cefixime Trihydrate Immediate Release Tablets (Table 4)

Physical Properties of Blend of Cefixime Trihydrate Tablets

Table 4. Physical properties of blend (Mean ± SD).

Test	C1	C2	C3	C4	C5	C6	C7	C8	C9
Angle of repose(°)	29.87 ±0.23	28.38 ±0.61	29.42 ±0.41	28.63 ±0.61	27.42 ±0.53	26.51 ±0.28	28.81 ±0.46	28.84 ±0.62	29.61 ±0.52
Bulk density (g/ml)	0.39 ±0.025	0.38 ±0.052	0.38 ±0.024	0.38 ±0.035	0.38 ±0.062	0.38 ±0.058	0.38 ±0.035	0.39 ±0.024	0.39 ±0.041
Tapped Density (g/ml)	0.44 ±0.084	0.44 ±0.012	0.44 ±0.032	0.44 ±0.021	0.44 ±0.039	0.44 ±0.085	0.44 ±0.053	0.44 ±0.074	0.45 ±0.023
Carr's index	11.11	11.15	11.10	11.13	11.15	11.11	11.14	11.15	11.12
Hausner's ratio	1.125	1.210	1.120	1.126	1.212	1.112	1.115	1.130	1.130

It is evident from above table that all the batches have bulk density in the range 0.3-0.5 g/cm3. All granules have shown good compression properties.

Evaluation of Post Compression Parameters of Cefixime Trihydrate (IR) Tablets (Table 5)

Table 5. Different evaluation parameters of Cefixime Trihydrate tablets.

Test	C1	C2	C3	C4	C5	C6	C7	C8	C9
Hardness (Kg/cm^2)	4-5	4-5	4-5	5-6	4-5	4-5	5-6	**4-5**	4-5
Friability (%)	0.22	0.13	0.14	0.13	0.22	0.21	0.13	**0.12**	0.12
Thickness (mm)	5.6	5.3	5.4	5.7	5.6	5.4	5.2	**5.3**	5.4
Drug content (%)	97.24±0.24	97.36±0.81	98.20±0.53	97.52±0.82	99.20±0.79	98.62±0.61	98.56±0.94	**98.42±0.63**	98.50±0.83
Weight variation (%)	3.75	3.26	3.49	4.56	3.48	4.64	3.34	**4.62**	3.45
Disintegration (in sec)	35 ±1.5	30 ±1.4	25 ±1.3	38 ±1.6	25 ±1.9	25 ±1.6	35 ±1.2	**20 ±1.1**	23 ±1.6

Weight variation of tablets was within ±5% deviation range and passed the weight variation test according to USP. The hardness of the tablets was in range of 4.0 – 6.0 kg/cm^2.

The friability of the tablets was found 0.1-0.3% which is within the desirable range and hence the tablets passed the friability. DT stands satisfactory with the time limit of <1 min for all the batches, as shown in table no. 23. However disintegration time (DT) of batch no. C8 found to be 20 sec which was lowest as compared to other batches. The batches C8 was selected to carry out further evaluation.

In-vitro Drug Release Studies of Cefixime Trihydrate (IR) Tablets

In vitro drug release profiles from cefixime trihydrate immediate release tablets are shown in Table **6** and Fig. (**9**).

Table 6. *In-vitro* drug release studies of Cefixime trihydrate tablets.

Time (Min)	Cumulative % Drug Released								
	C1	C2	C3	C4	C5	C6	C7	C8	C9
10	80.21±1.2	81.02±1.5	81.44±1.4	80.2±1.1	82.1±1.7	85.1±1.5	85.05±1.1	**86.21±1.3**	86.32±1.5
20	88.6±1.6	89.71±1.2	89.71±1.3	85.67±1.6	91.22±1.1	92.32±1.2	90.2±1.2	**97.9±1.5**	95.33±1.4
30	93.27±1.1	93.52±1.5	97.04±1.4	89.81±1.3	95.44±1.5	97.31±1.2	96.31±1.3	**100.01±1.4**	98.26±1.1
40	99.88±1.4	101.57±1.6	100.5±1.5	96.04±1.4	99.52±1.4	99.06±1.2	98.42±0.9	**101.53±0.7**	100.01±1.1
50	99.95±1.2	101.68±1.3	101.08±1.2	98.1±1.4	99.82±0.9	100.32±0.7	98.52±0.8	**101.64±0.6**	100.2±1.2

When drug release of C2, C5 and C8 batch is compared, it was found that C8 batch with Polyplasdone XL releases drug more readily and completely within 30 min. Hence, C8 batch is selected as optimized batch for cefixime trihydrate immediate release tablets.

Tablet disintegration and study of tablet all batches were performed in pH 7.2 phosphate buffer.

Precompression evaluation parameters for ofloxacin SR tablets (Table 7)

Table 7. Physical properties of granules.

Test	F1	F2	F3	F4	F5	F6	F7	F8
Angle of repose (°)	30.45 ±0.41	29.77 ±0.32	28.31 ±0.61	29.86 ±0.75	28.86 ±0.23	30.86 ±0.23	28.91 ±0.54	29.05 ±0.66
Bulk density (g/ml)	0.44 ±0.023	0.58 ±0.021	0.51 ±0.074	0.48 ±0.032	0.50 ±0.039	0.47 ±0.058	0.54 ±0.052	0.53 ±0.074
Tapped density (g/ml)	0.81 ±0.044	0.78 ±0.053	0.79 ±0.084	0.75 ±0.012	0.81 ±0.028	0.73 ±0.083	0.83 ±0.044	0.79 ±0.028
Carr's index	45.12	25.03	35.56	35.27	37.59	35.14	34.57	32.61
Hausner's ratio	1.822	1.333	1.552	1.545	1.602	1.542	1.528	1.484

Table depicts less than 30° the angle of repose depicts that granules have good flowability. Also, bulk density less than 1.25g/cm3 indicate good flowability. Granules of all the batches have bulk density in the range 0.4-0.6 g/cm3. All batches have good compression properties.

Evaluation of Post Compression Parameters of Ofloxacin (SR) Tablets (Table 8)

Table 8. Physical properties of SR Ofloxacin tablets.

Test	F1	F2	F3	F4	F5	F6	F7	F8
Hardness (Kg/cm^2)	5-6	6-7	6-7	6-7	5-6	6-7	5-6	6-7
Friability (%)	0.138	0.187	0.156	0.150	0.171	0.159	0.182	0.154
Thickness (mm)	6.1	6.2	6.2	6.4	6.3	6.4	6.3	6.2
Drug content %	98.10±1.54	98.31±1.58	98.64±1.64	97.87±1.54	98.50±1.66	97.64±1.72	97.53±1.64	98.05±1.59
Weight variation (%)	3.45	3.72	4.26	3.48	4.56	4.67	2.76	3.49

Weight variation test according to USP were within ±5% deviation range.
The hardness was found to be about 5.0 – 6.0 kg/cm^2.
The friability within the limit range 0.1-0.2% and hence the tablets passed the friability.

In-vitro Drug Release Studies of Ofloxacin (SR) Tablets

In vitro drug release profiles from ofloxacin SR tablets are shown in Table 9.

Table 9. *In- vitro* drug release studies of ofloxacin SR tablets.

Time (hrs)	Percentage Drug Release of Sustained Release Ofloxacin Tablets							
	F1	F2	F3	F4	F5	F6	F7	F8
1	25.19±0.23	16.45±0.34	15.92±0.52	12.72±0.41	16.01±0.53	17.21±0.36	17.56±0.43	18.74±0.51
2	39.94±0.47	22.94±0.42	21.62±0.51	20.24±0.55	25.24±0.75	25.62±0.82	25.52±0.85	26.26±0.73
3	43.39±0.81	32.89±0.65	30.7±0.88	27.31±0.95	34.68±0.84	35.12±0.76	34.21±0.69	35.72±0.85
4	45.77±0.68	34.76±0.75	32.64±0.66	30.02±0.75	35.56±0.88	36.04±0.74	35.62±0.64	40.13±0.61
5	47.11±0.52	39.37±0.64	35.16±0.72	32.62±0.81	39.04±0.91	37.34±0.83	38.47±0.76	42.72±0.68
6	53.13±0.66	41.97±0.61	38.22±0.70	35.11±0.73	42.62±0.81	43.52±0.89	43.62±0.94	45.84±0.87
7	68.75	50.07	42.16	37.33	55.72	56.12	56.46	50.73
8	80.18±0.57	55.42±0.68	45.01±0.80	41.08±0.79	58.61±0.81	59.49±0.75	58.12±0.76	56.35±0.74

(Table 9) cont.....

Time (hrs)	Percentage Drug Release of Sustained Release Ofloxacin Tablets							
	F1	F2	F3	F4	F5	F6	F7	F8
9	96.21±0.81	62.38±0.72	50.62±0.76	42.53±0.79	65.38±0.86	67.82±0.90	65.72±0.75	58.56±0.82
10	96.21±0.81	64.68±0.81	55.33±0.84	50.04±0.83	69.72±0.82	68.64±0.91	69.61±0.87	66.52±0.79
23	96.21±0.81	96.21±0.63	81.98±0.59	78.51±0.55	98.76±0.78	95.42±0.81	96.24±0.69	96.57±0.86
24	96.21±0.81	98.72±0.76	84.68±0.87	79.68±0.59	99.63±0.82	97.76±0.65	98.02±0.53	101.24±0.66

Release Kinetics Study

It was observed from results that the kinetics of *in-vitro* drug release of sustained release tablet was fitted with zero order, and plots showed the linearity (R^2 = 0.9792) for Crowell's (R^2 = 0.9786, Hixson- for Korsmeyer Peppas (R^2 = 0.9826), (n= 0.7912) and Higuchi's equation (R^2 = 0.9189), of optimized batch F8.

Mechanism of Drug Release

The plot for the Korsmeyer- Peppas indicated linearity (R^2 = 0.9826) and release exponent n was (n = 0.7912) for batch F8. It follows quasi Fickian diffusion drug release mechanism [20].

Bilayer Tablets

Development of bilayer tablets

Bilayer tablets was prepared from cefixime trihydrate IR batch C8 and ofloxacin SR batch F8 as given in Table 3.

Evaluation of Bilayer Tablets

Prepared bilayer tablets were evaluated for post compression parameters, results of C8F8 batch showed hardness between 5-6 kg/cm^2, friability as 0.136%, thickness about 7.8 mm, drug content of cefixime trihydate layer was found to be 99.54±0.45 and ofloxacin layer 98.25±1.65 and weight variation 4.2%.

All the tablets passed remaining post compression parameters within specified range.

In-vitro Drug Dissolution Test of Bilayer Tablet

The *in-vitro* drug dissolution study of bilayer tablets were performed using USP type I apparatus (Basket). Bilayered tablets prepared with optimized formulation of immediate release layer (C8) have shown disintegration time (30 ± 0.9 sec.).It was observed from Drug dissolution study of Cefixime trihydrate that it gets

99.53±0.49, almost completely dissolved within 30 minutes.

Dissolution Test

Cumulative percent drug release *vs.* time was plotted for cefixime trihydrate and ofloxacin compared with their marketed products represented in Figs. (**9** and **10**) respectively. The dissolution study suggested that the cefixime trihydrate IR layer had released more than 85% of drug within 10 min. which was desired. The cefixime trihydrate was released completely within 30 min in phosphate buffer 7.2. While ofloxacin released in very less amount (15.69%) within 2 h in acid buffer. After replacing media with acetate buffer (pH 4.5) and phosphate buffer (pH 7.4), it was found that ofloxacin dissolution was found to be increased and complete drug was released in 24 hours.

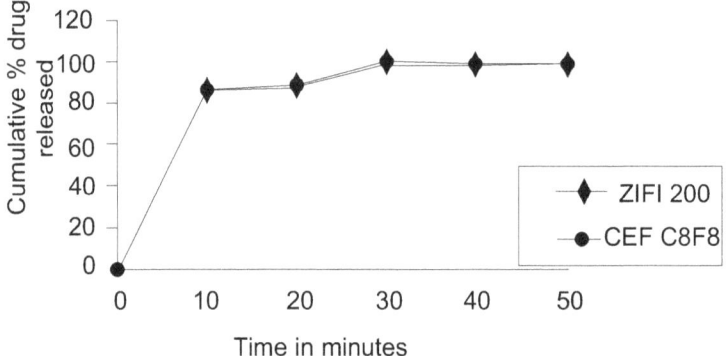

Fig. (9). Comparative dissolution profiles of cefixime trihydrate from bilayer tablets of C8F8 and marketed product ZIFI 200 (n = 3, mean ± S.D.).

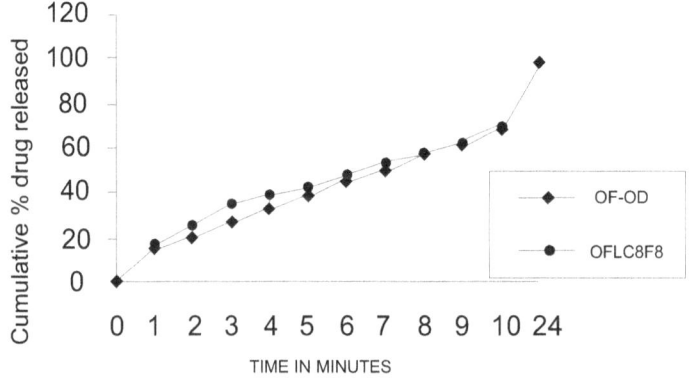

Fig. (10). Comparative dissolution profiles of ofloxacin from bilayer tablets of C8F8 and marketed product OF-OD (n = 3, mean ± S.D.).

Stability Study

Stability testing on batches of bilayer tablets was carried out. After checking the physical parameters, there observed no significant change in all the batches after stability study.

SUMMARY AND CONCLUSION

There are various difficulties associated with the currently available treatment of sexually transmitted disease (STDs) like increasing resistance against individual antibiotic, very less alternative medicines available to be used in pregnancy, unavailability of single medication having a wide spectrum of activity against multiple pathogens, high dose of drug required for treatment with multiple dosing.

In this study, selected drug combination was Cefixime trihydrate and ofloxacin which acts against STDs like gonnorhoea and trachomatus. This combination shows dual mode of action, as Ofloxacin-prevents nucleic acid synthesis and Cefixime-inhibits cell wall synthesis. Also these drugs are compatible with each other and acts synergistically.

The present research study was aimed to develop and evaluate the bilayer tablet containing Cefixime trihydrate and Ofloxacin. Bilayer tablets were prepared by using optimized best batches of immediate and sustained release layer.

Initially, IR tablets of Cefixime trihydrate was developed by using varying concentration of superdisintegrant *i.e.* sodium starch glycolate, crosscarmellose sodium, crospovidone and MCC PH-102 as a diluent. Superdisintegrants were used with aim to reduce the disintegration time and ultimately to increases dissolution of drug. The disintegration time of optimized batch (C8) was found to be less as compared to other, and also, *in-vitro* study showed 95-100% drug release within 30 min.

Subsequently sustained release tablets for prolonged drug release of Ofloxacin were formulated and evaluated. The optimized batch F8 was found more effective with 10% w/w concentration of HPMC-k100M polymer and ratio 30: 70 of MCC PH-101 and Lactose monohydrate. The release profile of optimized ofloxacin SR tablets was found similar to the marketed product OF-OD, with f2 value (Similarity factor) of 72.

Finally, bilayer tablets were formulated by using optimized immediate (C8) of cefixime trihydrate and sustained release layer (F8) of ofloxacin. Bilayer tablets quickly releases the immediate release layer where more than 85% of cefixime get released within 10 min., subsequently from sustained release layer the drug released in sustained manner, which would be required to maintain plasma drug concentration for effective treatment for longer duration of time.

In-vitro drug release study was performed separately for two drugs and samples analyzed by HPTLC method showed that immediate release layer of cefixime trihydrate is completely released within 30 minutes, followed by sustained release of ofloxacin which prolongs for 24 hours.

Stability study also showed no changes in the physical parameters as well in *in vitro* drug release.

CONSENT FOR PUBLICATION

Not Applicable.

CONFLICT OF INTEREST

The authors declare no conflict of interest, financial or otherwise.

ACKNOWLEDGEMENTS

Declared none.

REFERENCES

[1] The ACOG Committee on Adolescent Health Care. The American College of Obstetricians and Gynaecologist. 2nd ed., Sexually Transmitted Diseases, Tool Kit for Teen Care 2009.

[2] Kingston M, Carlin E. Treatment of sexually transmitted infections with single-dose therapy: a double-edged sword. Drugs 2002; 62(6): 871-8.
[http://dx.doi.org/10.2165/00003495-200262060-00001] [PMID: 11929335]

[3] Centers for Disease Control and Prevention (CDC). Update to CDC's Sexually transmitted diseases treatment guidelines, 2010: oral cephalosporins no longer a recommended treatment for gonococcal infections. MMWR Morb Mortal Wkly Rep 2012; 61(31): 590-4.
[PMID: 22874837]

[4] Tripathi KD. Essentials of medical pharmacology. Section -12, Antimicrobial Drug 6th ed.. 2008; 676-.

[5] Shiyani B, Gattani S, Surana S. Formulation and evaluation of bi-layer tablet of metoclopramide hydrochloride and ibuprofen. AAPS PharmSciTech 2008; 9(3): 818-27.
[http://dx.doi.org/10.1208/s12249-008-9116-y] [PMID: 18612830]

[6] Deshpande RD, Gowda DV, Mahammed N, Deepak N. Maramwar. Bi-layer tablets- An emerging trend: a review. IJPSR 2011; 2(10): 2534-44.

[7] Panchal HA, Tiwari AK. Novel approach of bilayer tablet technology: An review. J Pharm Sci Technol 2012; 4(4): 892-904.

[8] Divya A, Kavitha K, Kumar MR, Dakshayani S, Jagadeesh SSD. Bilayer tablet technology: An overview. J Anim Plant Sci 2011; 1(8): 43-7.

[9] Patel M, Ganesh NS. Kavitha, Tamizh M. Challenges in the formulation of bilayered tablets: A

review. IJPRD 2010; 2(10): 30-42.

[10] Reddy KR, Mutalik S, Reddy S. Once-daily sustained-release matrix tablets of nicorandil: formulation and *in vitro* evaluation. AAPS PharmSciTech 2003; 4(4): E61.
[http://dx.doi.org/10.1208/pt040461] [PMID: 15198556]

[11] Costa P, Sousa Lobo JM. Modeling and comparison of dissolution profiles. Eur J Pharm Sci 2001; 13(2): 123-33.
[http://dx.doi.org/10.1016/S0928-0987(01)00095-1] [PMID: 11297896]

[12] Pharmacopoeia of India. New Delhi: Ministry of Health and Family Welfare, Government of India, Controller of Publications 2007.

[13] Padmavathy J, Saravanan D, Rajesh D. Formulation and evaluation of ofloxacin floating tablets using HPMC. Int J Pharm Pharm Sci 2001; 3(1): 170-3.

[14] Ashraful ISM, Banu H, Sahariar MR. Bilayer tablets of paracetamol and aceclofenac: formulation and evaluation. International Journal Of Pharmacy &Technology 2011; 3(4): 3668-81.

[15] Khandagle KS, Gandhi SV, Deshpande PB, Kale AN, Deshmukh PR. High Performance Thin Layer Chromatographic determination of Cefixime and Ofloxacin in combined tablet dosage form. J Chem Pharm Res 2010; 2(5): 92-6.

[16] Kulkarni A, Bhatia M. Development and evaluation of regioselective bilayer Floating tablets of Atenolol and Lovastatin for Biphasic release profile. Iran J Pharm Res 2009; 8(1): 15-25.

[17] Remya K, Beena P, Bijesh P, Sheeba A. Formulation development, evaluation and comparative study of effects of super disintegrants in cefixime oral disintegrating tablets. J Young Pharm 2010; 2(3): 234-9.
[http://dx.doi.org/10.4103/0975-1483.66794] [PMID: 21042477]

[18] Higuchi T. Mechanism of sustained action medication. Therotical analysis of rate of release of solid drugs dispersed in solid matrices. J Pharm Sci 1963; 52: 1145-9.
[http://dx.doi.org/10.1002/jps.2600521210] [PMID: 14088963]

[19] Lachman L, Lieberman H, Kanig J. The Theory and Practice of Industrial Pharmacy. 3rd ed.., Bombay: Varghese pubilishing house 1990.

[20] Chien Y. Novel Drug Delivery Systems. 2nd ed. New York: Marcel Dekker. Inc 1992; pp. 1-139.

SUBJECT INDEX

A

Abortive infection system 137
Acid (s) 9, 16, 21, 56, 94, 95, 96, 97, 98, 141, 143, 147, 183
   acetic 94, 98, 141
   acetylsalicylic 96, 97
   ascorbic 183
   boric 94, 95
   formic 141
   Fusidic 16
   glycolic 9
   Hyaluronic 21
   lactic 141
   nucleic 56, 94, 143, 147
   oleic 20
   organic 141
   penicillanic amino 79
   phenolic 96
   poly-lactic (PLA) 9
   salicylic 77, 95, 96, 97
   saponified lipid 94
Acinetobacter baumannii 133, 145
Activity 9, 12, 13, 16, 17, 19, 21, 23, 24, 77, 84, 88, 89, 91, 96, 103, 122, 124, 126, 133, 135, 138, 139, 141, 142, 143, 144, 147, 170, 172, 176, 180
   anthropogenic 84
   anti-bacterial 13, 16, 19, 23
   antibiofilm 133
   anti-fungal 12, 17, 21, 24
   anti-infective 126
   antiparasitic 144
   anti-viral 9, 12
   bactericidal 12, 142
   bacteriostatic 77, 96, 141
   fungicidal 23
   metabolic 88, 122
   methyltransferase 170
   phagocytic 89
   potassium permanganate's antiseptic 103
   proteolytic 88, 176
   reduced migratory 89
Additional transcription unit (ATU) 62
Adeno-associated virus 65
Agents 6, 8, 13, 15, 16, 17, 172, 178, 181
   anti-fungal 6, 13, 15, 16, 17
   anti-viral 178
   chemotherapeutic 178
   host-targeted 172
   immunomodulatory 181
   immunosuppressive 8
Allergy and infectious diseases 51
Allogeneic bone marrow transplantation 7
Amino acids 81, 82, 138, 167
   hydrophobic 138
Amino acid's addition 80
Aminoglycosides 80, 91, 122, 123
Anti-bacterial activity test 19
Antibiotic resistance mechanism 124
Antibodies 47, 48, 58, 60, 63, 64, 65, 66, 129, 138, 139
   polyclonal 139
Antibody dependent enhancement (ADE) 67
Anti-CoV drug progression 172
Asthma 141, 183
Atherosclerosis 88, 92
Autoimmune diseases 7, 181

B

Bacillus subtilis 140
Bacitracin 10, 97, 135
Bacteria 91, 121
   antibiotic-resistant 121
   planktonic 91
Bacterial 82, 120, 134
   diseases 120
   helicase 82
   proteases 134
Bacterial infections 85, 90, 121, 136, 137
   antibiotic-resistant 85
Bacteriocins 133, 141, 142
Bacteriotoxic foam dressing 94

Subject Index

Baculovirus system 59
Behçet's disease 7
Biofilm-encased bacteria (BEB) 77, 91, 92, 96
Broad-spectrum antiviral agents (BSAAs) 171, 172

C

Cancer 7, 83, 140, 141, 144
   cervical 141
   therapy 144
Candida albicans 95, 139, 144
Central nervous system (CNS) 47
Chemical 95, 177
   features display 95
   structures of protease inhibitors 177
Chemotherapy, photodynamic antimicrobial 127
Clostridium tetani 138
Collagenase 92
Conjunctivitis 4
Contagious respiratory disease 43
Coronavirus 42, 140, 164, 165, 176
   disease 42, 164
   infecting pneumonia 165
   protease 176
   respiratory syndrome 140, 165
COVID-19 42, 180, 183
   disease 180, 183
   vaccine 42
Cryptococcosis 139
Cryptococcus neoformans 139

D

Diarrhea 48, 141
Disease(s) 4, 6, 7, 8, 42, 47, 48, 49, 66, 67, 78, 83, 88, 93, 120, 132, 140, 141, 143, 144, 145, 149, 180, 181, 183, 197
   allergic 141
   cardiovascular 141
   chronic 78, 83, 88, 93, 140
   inflammatory 181

modifying antirheumatic drugs (DMARDs) 181
   microbial 149
   neurologic 66
   parasitic 180
   respiratory 42
   virus-associated 132
Disorders 2, 24, 81, 120, 147, 183
   chronic obstructive pulmonary 183
   systemic 24
   urinary tract 81
DNA replication process 121
Double-membrane vesicles (DMVs) 166, 170
Drug-repositioning technique 171
Dry eye disease 2, 9

E

Ebola virus infections 173
Emerging diseases 140
Endocytosis 46, 143, 182
Endopeptidases 137
Endothelial progenitor cells (EPCs) 87, 89
Enterococcus faecium 124, 140
Enzyme-linked immunosorbent assay 145
Enzyme protease 169
Escherichia coli 94, 124, 135, 136, 144
Extended-spectrum beta-lactamases (ESBLs) 124

F

FDA-approved anti-HIV protease inhibitors 177
Fluconazole liposome 21
Fluorescence-linked immunosorbent assay 145
Food processing 137
Fourier transformed infrared spectroscopy 204
Fullerene-polyglycerol sulfates (FPS) 148

H

Hemolytic anemia 81

Hemostasis 87
Heparan sulfate proteoglycans 148
Hepatitis 139, 145, 174, 175, 176
Herpes simplex virus 133
HETCAM test 12
HIV 140, 176, 177
   protease 176, 177
   therapy in adults and RSV infection 140
HMG-CoA reductase enzyme 181
Homeostasis 141
Homotypic interactions 167
Horizontal 82, 84
   genetic transfer 84
   gene transfer 82
Host cell 131, 167, 169
   infected 131
   reactions 167
   receptor 169
Host innate immunity defense systems 128
Human 61, 65, 121, 129, 140, 176
   ACE-2 receptor protein 65
   embryonic kidney 61
   immunodeficiency virus (HIV) 121, 129, 140, 176
Hybridoma technology 138

I

Idiopathic diseases 7
Immunological assays 67
Immunomodulators 129, 131, 175
   proteins 129
   virus-encoded 131
Immunosuppressive diseases 4
Infection 2, 5, 6, 7, 8, 12, 24, 43, 45, 46, 47, 48, 65, 66, 76, 78, 85, 93, 121, 124, 125, 132, 137, 138, 140, 142, 144, 146, 167, 168, 171, 180, 181, 197
   antibiotic-resistant nosocomial 125
   antimicrobial-resistant 76
   dental 146
   dermal 78
   external eye 12
   genito-urinary tract 197

lower respiratory tract 121
lung 47, 167
nonmycobacterial 138
nosocomial 140
parasitic 5, 144
pulmonary 137
relieve eye 5
surgical site 142
systemic 93
upper respiratory tract 43
urinary tract 48
viral respiratory 85, 181
Infectious 5, 6, 42, 51, 78, 120, 121, 122, 124, 128, 143, 144
   diseases 42, 51, 78, 120, 121, 122, 124, 128, 143, 144
   endophthalmitis 5, 6
Influenza 175, 183
   A virus (IAV) 175
   virus infection 183
Infrared spectroscopy 200, 204
Inhibition of viral proteases 176
Injury, ischemia-derived 88
Innate defense regulatory (IDR) 133
International committee on taxonomy of viruses (ICTV) 165
Irritable bowel disease 141

J

Janus Kinase (JAK) 182

K

Keratitis 4, 5
   exposure 5
Keratitis formation 4
Ketoconazole 17, 21
Klebsiella pneumonia 124

L

Lactobacillus acidophilus 141
Lactococcus lactis 135

Lateral 48, 181
   flow assays 48
   myocardial infarction 181
Leuconostoc mesenteroides 140
Lipid nanoparticle (LNP) 63
Listeria monocytogenes 135

M

Mechanisms, efflux pump 123
Metalloproteases 88
Methicillin-resistant *Staphylococcus aureus* 76, 136
Methods 23, 96, 147
   electrospinning 23
   photocatalytic 147
   wound treatment 96
Methylene blue dyes 94
Microbial infections 120, 143
Micrococcus luteus 135
Minimum inhibitory concentration (MIC) 10, 85
Monoclonal antibodies 138, 139, 140
Multidisciplinary disease 5, 6
Multi 121, 122, 123, 135, 138, 167
   drug resistance (MDR) 121, 122, 123, 135, 138
   organ dysfunction 167
Mycobacterial Infections 138
Mycobacterium tuberculosis 6, 12, 123, 127

N

Nausea 48, 61, 167, 201
Neisseria meningitides 138
Niosomes 2, 17, 18, 20, 21, 22
   clotrimazole 17
   conventional 17, 18
   natamycin-loaded 17
Non-infectious 5, 6
   endophthalmitis 6
   keratitis 5
Non-oxidative mechanisms 147
Nucleocapsid 44, 47, 48, 60, 61, 166, 167
   phosphoprotein 61
   phosphoprotein residue 60
Nucleoside 172
   antiviral 172

O

Ocular 1, 2, 4, 6, 7, 8, 9, 13, 20, 24
   delivery systems 9
   hypertension 20
   immunity 8
   infections 1, 2, 6, 7, 8, 20, 24
   permeability 13
   surgery 4
   tolerability 9
Oils 11, 14, 21, 86
   castor 11, 21
   olive 14, 21
   soybean 11
Ointment, commercial acyclovir ophthalmic 12
Onchocerciasis 6
Osteomyelitis-caused Injury 108
Oxidative stress 95, 99, 126, 147

P

Pan drug resistance (PDR) 123
Paramyxoviruses 173
Pathogenesis 43, 45, 128
Pathogenicity 164, 178
Pathogenic 128, 142
   microorganisms 128
   inhibition 142
Pathogens 6, 7, 8, 66, 87, 121, 122, 128, 129, 131, 136, 137, 139, 140, 141, 142, 143, 144, 145, 146
   anaerobic 136
   antibiotic-resistant 122, 146
   broad-spectrum 144
   diapedesis engulfing 87
   drug-resistant 139
   emerging virulent 66
   viral 140

waterborne 145, 146
Pathways 82, 83, 95, 129, 130, 171
   death sensors 130
   inflammatory 130
   metabolic 82
   oxidative 95
Penicillinases 83
Penicillin-binding proteins (PBPs) 79, 82
Pfizer-BioNTech's vaccine 63
Phagocytosis 87, 127, 129, 130
   macrophage 87
Pneumocystis pneumonia, treating 180
Pneumonitis 66
Poly-lactic acid (PLA) 9
Polymorphonuclear leukocytes 87, 126, 127
Polyvinyl alcohol (PVA) 21
Pressure 67, 82, 88, 122
   consistent osmotic 82
   reducing 100
Price comparison 110
Processes 58, 76, 90, 91, 92, 93, 99, 121, 122, 127, 167, 170, 171, 173
   abnormal healing 92
   chemical 58
   healing 76
Production, prostaglandin 127
Products, prophylactic 2
Properties 78, 82, 86, 93, 95, 122, 131, 132, 144, 167, 170, 172, 199, 202
   antigenic 167
   anti-inflammatory 131
   antimicrobial 86, 93, 132
   antioxidant 144
   antiviral 172
Proteases 63, 87, 129, 130, 131, 166, 169, 176, 178
   suppressing serine 178
   tissue-cleaning 87
   toxins 129
   transmembrane serine 178
Protein(s) 23, 24, 50, 51, 59, 60, 62, 63, 64, 80, 82, 94, 123, 131, 134, 137, 166, 167, 169
   adjuvant 59
   biosynthesis 134
   synthesis 80, 82
   toxin 137
   transcription 82
Proteinase 44
Proteosome 130
Proteus 145, 146
   mirabilis 145
   vulgaris 146
Pseudomonas aeruginosa 12, 133, 135, 136, 137, 138, 145, 146
   multidrug-resistant 136
   infections 137
Pulmonary arterial hypertension (PAH) 181

Q

Quinolone's structure 80

R

Reactive oxygen 87, 89, 99, 126, 127, 128, 147, 148
   intermediates (ROI) 126, 127, 128
   Species (ROS) 87, 89, 99, 127, 147, 148
Real time reverse transcriptase-polymerase chain reaction 48
Receptor binding motif (RBM) 44
Respiratory syncytial virus (RSV) 175, 181
Rheumatic problems 183
Rhinoconjunctivitis 141
RNA 46, 48, 54, 55, 56, 65, 131, 137, 148, 166, 169, 174, 175
   genomic 169
   antitoxin 137
   binding protein 169
   chain terminator 176
   editing 131
   genome 166
   mutagenesis 175
   polymerase inhibitor 174
   toxin-antitoxin 137
   vaccines 65
RNA-dependent 169, 175
   RNA polymerase activity 169

viral replication 175
RNA replication 173, 174
  blocking 173
RNA synthesis 167, 172, 173
  blocking 172
  targeting viral 172
RNA viruses 175
  negative-sense 175
ROS 147, 148
  associated protein 148
  induced oxidative stress 147

S

Salmonella enterica 145
Sarcoidosis 7
SARS and human ACE-2 receptor protein 65
SARS 44, 51, 175
  coronaviruses 44, 175
  recombinant spike protein 51
SARS-CoV-2, 48, 52, 63, 65, 170, 172
  infection 170, 172
  protein of 63, 65
  vaccines 48, 52
SARS-CoV 43, 45, 47, 48, 66, 140, 179
  infections 43, 45, 47, 48, 66, 179
    influenza virus 140
Scleritis 5, 7, 8
  autoimmune 7
  infected 7
  infectious 8
  viral 7
Seborrheic dermatitis 97
Self-nano emulsifying system 18
Silver bionanocomposites 145
Sinovac vaccine 58
Skin 134, 135, 142
  glands 134
  healing 142
  infections 135
  microbiota 142
  problems 142
Solid lipid 2, 11, 12
  microparticles (SLMs) 11

nanoparticles (SLNs) 2, 11, 12
Spectrophotometric analysis of drug 204
Spike 42, 44, 46, 47, 48, 50, 51, 56, 57, 61, 68, 169, 178
  glycoprotein 61, 168
  protein 42, 44, 46, 47, 48, 50, 51, 56, 57, 169, 178
Steroids 5
Streptococcal lysine 137
Streptococcus mutans 129, 135, 138, 140, 146
  pneumonia 138
  pyogenes 129, 135
  thermophilus 140
Streptomyces griseus 122
Streptomycetes 83
Sulfonamides' structure 81
Surgery 5, 7, 104, 124
  conjunctival tumor 7
  hernia 104
  hip replacement 124
Synthesis 82, 96, 126, 171, 217
  chemical 171
  folic acid 82
  nucleic acid 217
Synthetic 57, 143
  attenuated virus engineering 57
  nanomaterials 143
Systemic 7, 199
  adverse effects of high potency drugs 199
  disease 7
Systems 14, 128, 141
  host defense 128, 141
  self-emulsifying 14

T

Target receptor protein 148
Technology 136, 198
  therapeutic delivery 136
  two-layer tablet 198
Therapeutic 49, 134, 136, 142
  agents 134, 136
  benefits 142
  drugs 49

Therapy 48, 84, 93, 96, 99, 120, 127, 128, 136, 137, 138, 142
   antimicrobial photodynamic 127
   convalescent plasma 48
   conventional antibiotic 120
   hyperbaric oxygen 93, 99
Tissue(s) 2, 6, 23, 24, 89, 90, 92, 95, 99, 104, 105, 108, 126, 142
   damaged 90
   destruction 89
   immunity-related 142
Tixothrophic solution (TS) 111, 112
Toxicity 13, 16, 67, 81, 139, 182, 198, 201
   reverse digoxin 139
Toxoplasma gondii 127, 139
Transcriptional programs 131
Transfected cells 64
Transmembrane protease serine 169
Trauma 5, 7
Trichomoniasis 197

U

Ulcer area 101, 102, 108
   progression 102
   reduction 101
Ulcerative colitis 141
Ultradeformable bilosomes (UBs) 18

V

Vaccine 42, 67
   associated enhanced respiratory disease (VAERD) 67
   production methods 42
Vasculogénesis 89
Venezuelan equine encephalitis virus (VEEV) 175
Vibrio cholerae 142
Viral 65, 131, 132, 144, 148, 168, 169, 170, 171, 179, 180, 182, 183
   attachment ligands 148
   diseases 132, 171, 179, 183
   immunomodulator proteins 131
   infections 65, 144, 148, 168, 169, 170, 171, 180, 182
Viral replication 46, 65, 170
   transcription complexes 170
Viral vector vaccines 61
Virions 46, 166, 167, 170
Virus 51, 56, 60, 167, 172
   like particle (VLP) 51, 56, 60, 167
   replication process 172
Visceral leishmaniasis 144

W

Waals forces 147
Wastewater, treating 145
Weight variation test 212, 214
Whole-virus preparations 58
World health organization (WHO) 49, 51, 121, 123, 165
Wound(s) 77, 86, 87, 89, 90, 91, 92, 93, 94, 95, 96, 98, 99, 100, 101, 103, 104, 105, 107, 108, 111, 112, 142, 146
   area 100, 101
   burned 94
   dressings 146
   healing 77, 87, 89, 93, 96, 111, 142, 146
   progress 98
   treatment in aerosol (WTA) 111, 112

Y

Yellow fever 174, 176

Z

Zika virus infection 180
Zinc oxide 93, 97

www.ingramcontent.com/pod-product-compliance
Lightning Source LLC
Chambersburg PA
CBHW051144220526
45473CB00003B/653